IMMUNOASSAY AUTOMATION

IMMUNOASSAY AUTOMATION
A Practical Guide

Edited by

DANIEL W. CHAN

Department of Laboratory Medicine
Clinical Chemistry Division
The Johns Hopkins Hospital and University
Baltimore, Maryland

ACADEMIC PRESS, INC.
Harcourt Brace Jovanovich, Publishers
San Diego New York Boston London Sydney Tokyo Toronto

Academic Press, Inc.
1250 Sixth Avenue, San Diego, California 92101-4311

United Kingdom Edition published by
Academic Press Limited
24–28 Oval Road, London NW1 7DX

Library of Congress Cataloging-in-Publication Data

Immunoassay automation : a practical guide / [edited by] Daniel W. Chan.
p. cm.
Includes index.
ISBN 0-12-167632-3
1. Immunoassay--Automation--Handbooks, Manuals, etc.
2. Immunoassay--Instruments--Handbooks, manuals, etc. I. Chan, Daniel W. (Daniel Wan-Yui)
[DNLM: 1. Automation. 2. Immunoassay--instrumentation.
3. Immunoassay--methods. QW 570 I328]
QP519.9I42I43 1992
616.07'56--dc20
DNLM/DLC
for Library of Congress 91-47040
CIP

PRINTED IN THE UNITED STATES OF AMERICA
92 93 94 95 96 KP 9 8 7 6 5 4 3 2 1

Dedicated to Jackie and Maria
for their love and support

Contents

Preface

Automation is essential for the operation of clinical laboratories. The automation of immunoassay procedures has lagged behind routine clinical chemistry and hematology systems. The homogenous immunoassay procedure, which requires no physical separation of unbound from bound antigen, could be adapted to existing routine chemistry analyzers. The heterogenous immunoassay procedure would require development of dedicated analyzers. Most of the fully automated systems have their particular combination of reagent and instrument in a closed or "black box" format, i.e., specific reagents are used on their particular instrumentation. With the shortage of skilled technologists and economic pressure to improve efficiency, automation of immunoassay is highly desirable.

The focus of this book is the automation of immunoassay from the practical viewpoint of the clinical laboratory. Part One starts with a general introduction (Chapter 1). The important issues of automated immunoassay systems are discussed in Chapter 2. This includes homogenous versus heterogenous, competitive versus immunometric, reagent stability, data management, sample management, processing center, signal detection, semi- versus fully automated systems, and disadvantages of automation. Part Two deals with the selection (Chapter 3) and the evaluation of automated immunoassay systems from four different aspects—technical (Chapter 4), clinical (Chapter 5), operational (Chapter 6), and economical (Chapter 7). Part Three consists of 16 chapters. Each chapter discusses one automated immunoassay system including an introduction, a description of the instrumentation, the reagent, and the performance. The last chapter deals with testing devices designed for decentralized locations, e.g., physician's office, outpatient clinic, and home testing. These chapters are not intended to include every available system. The systems are selected for their popularity, interesting technical advances, and/or operational efficiency. In the fast-changing world of high technology systems, it is inevitable that some of the systems may have changed to a new design or have been totally replaced by a new model. However, the editor hopes that by demonstrating certain principles in the design and application of immunoassay, they will have long lasting value in the evolution of automated immunoassay systems.

Daniel W. Chan

PART ONE

Introduction

CHAPTER 1

General Introduction

Daniel W. Chan
Department of Laboratory Medicine,
Clinical Chemistry Division,
The Johns Hopkins Hospital,
The Johns Hopkins University, Baltimore, Maryland

I. WHY AUTOMATION?

Automation is highly desirable for a clinical laboratory since it improves the outcome of the testing procedure and the efficiency of the laboratory. For the research laboratory, automation is useful, particularly for repetitive experimental steps. As we enter into the 1990s, the chronic shortage of qualified technologists and technicians for laboratory will increase the need for automation to reduce labor intensive procedures. Furthermore, smaller clinical laboratories could justify performing a larger menu of tests "in house" rather than sending them to outside commercial laboratories. This not only reduces the "purchase service" budget and increases the revenue, but also improves the service aspect of the laboratory by reducing the turnaround time of testing. With the availability of automated devices, certain laboratory tests may be relocated to "near patient," that is, point of care, whether at the bedside or the outpatient location.

II. HISTORY OF AUTOMATION

During the last 20 years, major advances have been achieved in automating routine and general clinical chemistry procedures. First, the autoanalyzer and its multichannel approach of the SMA analyzers (Technicon, Inc.)

Immunoassay Automation: A Practical Guide

were introduced, for example, SMA6, 12, and SMAC analyzers. Next came the centrifugal analyzer for measuring enzyme activities. Since most chemistry tests used enzyme reaction, this allowed the testing of enzyme levels as well as concentration of substrates using enzyme as reagent. The most successful system with prepackaged reagent was first introduced by DuPont, Inc., as the ACA analyzer. Most tests were designed for routine chemistries. Recently, homogeneous immunoassays were adapted to the ACA analyzer for drugs and thyroid hormone testing. Finally, discrete and random access analyzers provided a wide spectrum of chemistry tests around the clock to meet the demands of emergency testing. Recently, more attention has been focused on automating the sample handling and processing steps, especially with the concern of infectious specimens from patients with hepatitis and AIDS (acquired immunodeficiency syndrome).

Automating specialized procedures such as immunoassay has lagged behind, especially for heterogeneous immunoassay, that is, assay that requires a physical separation of the bound and unbound antigens. The homogeneous immunoassay, which requires no physical separation of bound and unbound antigens, can be adapted to a general chemistry analyzer; however, the heterogeneous immunoassay requires a dedicated analyzer. Such dedicated instrumentation is more demanding in both design and maintenance, as well as in cost for the manufacturing process. The first attempt was to automate radioimmunoassay (RIA). Several systems were introduced in the late 1970s. These systems included the Centria (Union Carbide), Concept 4 (Micromedic), ARIA II (BD), and Gammaflow (Squibb). They were disappointing from both the manufacturers' and users' points of view. These systems, with limited throughput and testing menu, were not as reliable and cost-effective as the users wanted. Only laboratories with sufficiently large testing volume ever considered acquiring a system. The total number of systems sold was disappointingly below the manufacturers' expectations. These automated systems still used radioactivity. Automation of immunoassay would not be successful until nonisotopic systems became available.

III. THE CONCEPT OF AUTOMATION

The total clinical laboratory testing process starts with the ordering of a test by a physician, then blood collection and processing, the actual testing procedures, the data reduction, and result reporting. An automated system should include as many steps as possible in the total testing process. However, most current systems only automate the actual testing procedure. This procedure usually starts with the application of a patient sample to the system and ends with the generation of test results. Most systems are different only in the in-between steps. Variations include homogeneous immunoassay versus heterogeneous immunoassay, automated versus semiautomated system with manual incubation or pipetting step, and differences in the delivery format, the label or signal, and the detection device.

The traditional idea of automation is to adapt the reagent on an automated instrument for central clinical laboratory. Such instrumentation mechanized all the necessary steps in an immunoassay procedure, such as pipetting, incubation, washing, and detecting the signal. In a broader sense, the concept of automation could include disposable devices designed for quick, mostly qualitative tests, like the ICON (Hybritech, Inc.) and the test pack (Abbott Labs) for pregnancy testing. These devices use membrane technology with monoclonal antibodies immobilized on them. Often, this requires a rather sophisticated design. Each device can be used for only one sample and perform only one test. After adding the sample, the analyte binds to the antibody on the membrane. The addition of enzyme-labeled antibody conjugate forms a sandwich with the analyte-antibody complex on the membrane. After washing the unbound substances and after the addition of substrate, a qualitative result will be obtained in a few minutes by the presence of color development. Quantitative results could be obtained by reading on a photometer. These devices are self-contained "automation in a box" without instrumentation. Most of these devices are intended for using in "point of care testing," that is, in a decentralized environment, such as a doctor's office or home testing.

The next level of automation involves multiple tests on a system, usually with limited throughput. These systems are designed for small laboratories or decentralized locations. For example, the Vision by Abbott Labs will accept whole blood specimens. Each test pack consists of multiple tracks to allow automation of sample processing and analysis. The whole blood sample is centrifuged to yield serum before chemical analysis. Therefore, the first step in deciding on the format of automation is whether to create a small disposable box consisting of a single test to be used for point of care testing, a larger box with limited tests and throughput for a decentralized lab, or a fully automated system with a broad menu and high throughput for a central laboratory. Such a decision should be based on the application of testing for the unique clinical setting.

IV. APPLICATION

Where do we need automated immunoassay devices and systems? How do we use these devices to benefit laboratory and its clients—physician and patient? I believe that these are important questions, which should be addressed jointly by the clinical laboratory personnel and manufacturer. We must first decide where the application for automated systems are; then we can design systems to fulfill these needs.

The three types of automation discussed earlier may have different applications. The top level of automation consists of instrumentation with high throughput and a large menu of tests. It is intended for the central clinical laboratory. An experienced technologist may be able to perform as many as several hundred patient samples during a working shift using a manual procedure; however, this includes only one or two different assays. Therefore, the most effective automation should be able to perform a large variety of test mixes at the same time, even if the total tests per hour (throughput) may not be significantly higher than the manual procedure. The second level of automation uses a smaller unit designed for low throughput and a somewhat limited menu of tests. These systems are mainly intended for outpatient clinics and physician offices. The third level of automation with disposable devices consists of a single test without instrumentation. The main target users are the physician office and home testing.

In reality, all three levels of automation may be applicable in all clinical laboratories, whether large or small. A large clinical laboratory may perform all tests in the day shift. During the evening shift, its testing may resemble a medium-size clinical laboratory. While on the night shift, it may be more like a small clinical laboratory. Therefore, a large clinical laboratory may want to acquire systems intended for large, medium, or small laboratories. For example, a laboratory may want to use a fully automated system during the day shift for routine pregnancy testing; however, it may want to use disposable devices for emergency pregnancy testing at other hours.

V. FUTURE TRENDS

An often-asked question is where the testing of patients will be done in the future—the central clinical laboratory, decentralized locations, the physician's office, or the patient's home. The decision of where the tests will be done may be driven by several divergent forces. These include the quality expectation of the laboratory service by the physician and patient, the economic issues of cost effectiveness, and the reimbursement policy by the third-party payer. It will also be influenced by the technical feasibility and the production cost of such devices by the manufacturer. Finally, it will be the consumer, whether it is the laboratory technologist, director, or patient, who will decide the acceptability of any automated devices to be used for testing.

The convenience of home testing will be hard to replace by other means unless a "house call" laboratory service can be provided. It is possible that a trained technologist could perform laboratory tests in the patient's home using a portable testing device. Alternatively, a sample can be collected by the patient and transported to a testing center. Reports could be telephoned or transmitted by computer.

The next level of testing could be performed by a testing center in a convenient location away from the patient's home. This could be located at a local shopping center, a supermarket, a doctor's office, or a hospital outpatient location, such as a clinic or emergency room. In such locations, all tests could be performed on site or sent to a central testing facility. It depends on the need of turnaround time, the complexity of the test, and the cost. I believe that the turnaround time issue will be less critical in the future as more attention is paid to expediting the preanalytical variables such as order entry, sample collection, transporation, processing, and result reporting. Examples are pneumatic tubes, robotic devices for sample handling, and computer interfaces. At the present time, such preanalytical variables often cause significant delay in the total testing process.

For testing of hospitalized patients and in commercial laboratories, two types of automation may be needed. The first one is a flexible system with a large menu, preferably random access, for both emergency and routine testings. The total throughput is less critical than the menu of tests. The other type of automation should have higher throughput as first priority since it is mainly for routine or batch analysis. The random access feature is less critical. This system will be applicable only to large laboratories. Since the economy of large-scale testing is indisputable, I believe more centralization of laboratory testing will occur to improve efficiency. Therefore, such a high-throughput instrument will be in demand.

A quality improvement program should be established as part of the automation. The program should consist of parameters to monitor the outcome of the testing. A laboratory could monitor the performance of testing even if it is performed at a different site, by computer. Therefore, the actual location of testing will become less important.

Finally, automated immunoassay systems should be designed to meet the clinical need and expectation of the user. They should include as many steps as possible in the total testing process. A system composed of individual modules may be the best approach. In one extreme, such modules may be a disposable unit to perform a single test. On the other hand, the module may be able to perform a group of tests suitable for a unique clinical setting, such as an emergency room, critical care unit, or outpatient clinic for a specific medical discipline. Clinical settings would be the determining factor of the test menu on a particular system, rather than the traditional laboratory disciplines of chemistry, microbiology, and hematology. Such modular systems would be most suitable for the changing needs of clinical laboratory testing in the 1990s and beyond.

CHAPTER 2

Automation of Immunoassay

Daniel W. Chan
Department of Laboratory Medicine,
Clinical Chemistry Division,
The Johns Hopkins Hospital,
The Johns Hopkins University, Baltimore, Maryland

I. INTRODUCTION

To design an automated immunoassay system, one should first examine the total laboratory testing process and decide what steps are to be automated. Next, one could divide the immunoassay procedure into components and design a system to automate these components.

The total laboratory testing process (Table 1) starts with the ordering of laboratory tests, preferably by computer. A complete test menu should be provided, with information for proper utilization of each test. Instructions should be given for a particular blood collection device with bar-code label for positive identification. The sample should be centrifuged in a closed system and transferred onto the automated system for direct sampling. The actual testing procedure may include a separation step of the bound from unbound antigen if it is a heterogeneous immunoassay. No physical separation step is needed if it is a homogeneous immunoassay. The detection system could be multiapproach, such as spectrophotometry and fluorimetry. Finally, electronic data processing and quality control should facilitate result verification and reporting. A computer terminal located at the user's site will shorten the turnaround time of testing.

Table 1 Total Laboratory Testing Process

1. Laboratory testing menu and test request information
2. Preanalytical variables—specimen collection and transportation
3. Laboratory testing procedure—instrument, reagent, and quality control
4. Result reporting and turnaround time
5. Result interpretation and followup testing.
6. User communication

A standard operating procedure will provide quality control of the preanalytical variables. Together with an automated analyzer and a data management system, it will ensure good quality assurance of the total testing process. Therefore, one can achieve the ultimate goal of automation—good quality and efficiency of the laboratory testing.

II. COMPONENTS OF AUTOMATION

An automated system consists of three major components: instrument, reagent, and computer. A system will not be successful unless all three components are functioning well. Experience has shown that the chemist can produce good reagent and the engineer can often design and build reliable instruments. The computer, particularly the software, seems to be the weak link. The problem may not be the programmer's inability to write a working computer program, but rather that it is "user unfriendly." Most programmers have neither work nor training in a clinical laboratory environment. This problem could be overcome by testing the software program in a clinical laboratory before finalization.

These three components are interdependent. The format of the reagent will determine the design of the instrument. The limit of the instrument design may require modification of the reagent and the immunoassay procedure. The computer program could optimize the reaction condition, the sequence of reagent addition, and the order of sample testing. It will expedite data processing and management, as well as result reporting. Therefore, we should consider the issues of automation as an integrated system.

III. ISSUES OF AUTOMATION

Immunoassay is an analytical procedure involving an antigen and antibody binding reaction. After the binding takes place, separation of bound antigen and antibody complex from unbound antigen is needed before the unknown antigen can be quantitated. Heterogeneous immunoassay requires a physical separation, while homogeneous immunoassay needs no physical separation. The decision on homogeneous versus heterogeneous assay will be critical for the design of an automated immunoassay analyzer. Next, one should consider the competitive immunoassay approach versus the immunometric assay approach. Other issues to be considered include reagent stability, data management, sample management, processing center, signal detection, semi- versus fully automated system, and the disadvantages of automated system.

A. Homogeneous or Heterogeneous Immunoassay?

Homogeneous immunoassay requires no physical separation of bound and unbound antigen. The major advantage is the ability of adapting homogeneous immunoassay to the existing clinical chemistry analyzer. A clinical laboratory could achieve greater efficiency by not having to purchase an additional dedicated immunoassay analyzer. For example, the EMIT assay (enzyme multiplied immunoassay technique) by Syva Co. for therapeutic (TDM) and abuse drugs has been adapted to automated instruments including centrifugal analyzers, such as the Cobas-Fara (Roche Diagnostics) and Monarch (Instrumentation Lab), and to random access chemistry analyzers, such as the Hitachi 700 series (BMD), Olympus AU-5000 series (Olympus), and DAX (Technicon). The other popular homogeneous immunoassay for TDM and toxicology is the fluorescence polarization immunoassay (FPIA) by Abbott Labs and Roche Diagnostics. The Abbott systems include TDx and ADx analyzers. The Roche system uses FPIA on the Cobas-Fara and MIRA Analyzers.

These automated homogeneous immunoassay systems use small sample size and low reagent volume and provide fast turnaround time. The calibration curve is stable for at least several weeks for the TDx and ADX analyzers. This allows a laboratory to perform tests at all hours without having to recalibrate the system. The efficiency is enhanced by saving technical time, quality control, and reagent expenses.

Homogeneous immunoassay is generally only useful for measuring small analytes. Most homogeneous immunoassay takes advantage of the size difference between unbound antigen (small) and antigen-bound antibody complex (large). The differences in the sizes may limit the spectroscopic changes. This will in turn limit the dynamic ranges of the assay and, to a certain extent, the sensitivity as well. Since there is no separation of the patient sample from the final signal detection, the sensitivity may be further compromised. Interferences in the patient's sample may cause high background signal or compete with the binding site. Some tests require sample pretreatment to eliminate interferences. For example, digoxin assay requires an acid precipitation (TDx) or a column treatment step before analysis (EMIT). In general, small analytes such as drug, thyroid, and steroid hormone, which are present in relatively high concentration, will work well using homogeneous immunoassay system.

Heterogeneous immunoassay is more versatile. It can measure both small and large analytes. With a physical separation step, it eliminates most interfering substances present in the patient's sample before quantitation. The separation step together with the potential of using a larger sample size will improve the sensitivity. The immunometric assay tends to have a broader dynamic range of the standard curve. The peptide hormone and tumor marker are ideally measured by immunometric assay. For example, human chorionic gonadotropin (hCG) can be measured by immunometric assay using two antibodies, one against the alpha and the other against the beta subunit. The disadvantages of heterogeneous immunoassay are that it is more labor-intensive and time-consuming, and requires a dedicated immunoassay analyzer. Such automated systems require more complicated design to include washing and separation steps.

B. Competitive or Immunometric Assay

Traditional radioimmunoassay (RIA) is based on the principle of competitive protein binding. The radioactive-labeled antigen competes with the unlabeled antigen for a *limited* amount of binding sites on the antibody. This approach with labeled antigen is also called "labeled analyte" technique. Although most RIAs use simultaneous incubation of antigen and antibody, sequential addition of unlabeled antigen with antibody before the addition of labeled antigen may improve the sensitivity of the assay. "Sensitivity" as defined by the minimum detectable amount of a RIA is determined by (1) the affinity constant of the antibody, (2) the nonspecific binding, (3) the specific activity of the labeled antigen, and (4) the experimental error in the measurement of bound and unbound antigen. RIA procedure could be optimized by changing (1) the antibody concentration, (2) the amount of labeled antigen, (3) the reaction volume, time, temperature, and pH, (4) the separation step, and (5) the counting time. In the development of an immunoassay, the competitive approach conserves the use of antibody in the assay, since the antibody concentration is limited.

Immunometric assay could be optimized for better sensitivity than the competitive immunoassay. The maximal sensitivity can be achieved with:

1. Large concentration of labeled antibody with high specific activity.
2. Low amount of nonspecific binding by the labeled antibody.
3. High affinity constant of the labeled antibody and antigen reaction.
4. Small experimental errors in measuring the bound labeled antibody.

The decision on whether to use competitive or immunometric assay will depend on the size of the analyte. For small analytes (e.g., drug, thyroid, and steroid hormone), competitive immunoassay is the choice. For large analytes (e.g., peptide hormones), immunometric assay is the choice. Immunometric assay provides both sensitivity and specificity needed for peptide hormones [e.g., parathyroid hormone (PTH) and adrenocorticotropin (ACTH)]. The sensitivity requirement for the hormones could be achieved by using the immunometric assay as discussed previously. The specificity requirement of measuring the intact molecule of PTH would exclude the PTH c-terminal fragments, which could accumulate in renal disease. Therefore, the specificity of PTH assay is better using the immunometric format than the competitive immunoassay.

C. Reagent Stability

Reagent should be designed to have long stability. Table 2 lists the desirable length of reagent stability. Most reagents have adequate shelf life before opened. A long shelf life is desirable so that a single lot of reagent can be used for a long period of time, that is, >1 year. This will minimize the reagent lot check-in process, which could be time-consuming and expensive. The stability of the opened reagent stored at 4°C will allow the same calibration curve to be used. Most reagents are capable of achieving this step. A desirable characteristic of reagent stability on the instrument of 1 month is more difficult to achieve. Most people do not appreciate the importance of this feature. The ideal automation is random access with testing on the first-in-first-out basis. If the system is to be used on a 24-h basis, the reagent will be expected to be stable and available for testing at all times. Calibration curve stability is important in the efficient operation

Table 2 Desirable Length of Reagent Stability

Reagent condition	Length
Shelf life of unopened reagent	2 years
Opened reagent at 4°C	3 months
Opened reagent on the instrument	1 month
Calibration-curve stability	1 month
Quality-control frequency	1 day

of the system. A 1-month stability will allow the laboratory to perform less frequent tests without recalibration. Quality control performed on a daily basis will ensure the readiness and the adequacy of testing.

D. Data Management

The data management system is the commanding center. To say that it is crucial is an understatement. A data management system should be designed to be "user friendly." Priorities should be set to achieve the important goals of automation. Table 3 lists the desirable characteristics of a data management system.

The technologist will become the data manager in the future. In order

Table 3 Desirable Characteristics for a Data Management System

Be a control center for the automation
Manage as many steps as possible in the total testing process
Be user friendly
Easy access to the routine daily function
Diagnostics of instrument functions for troubleshooting purpose
On-line quality control
Sample identification—bar-code label
Patient identification—report
Data reduction—selection of models
Lab management functions—work-load recording, turnaround time, quality assurance, and productivity

to manage the automation effectively, the data management system should control as many steps as possible in the total testing process as defined in Table 1. The system should be designed for the clinical laboratory, that is, be user friendly. The number one priority for such a system is to provide physicians the test results as quickly as possible while maintaining high quality. A user-friendly system should allow a technologist to perform the crucial daily functions efficiently, that is, turn out patient results with a quality checking system. If a system requires a technologist to get through pages of computer screen to reach the operating step, it is not designed for the routine clinical laboratory. For a "stat" or emergency lab request, minutes or even seconds of waiting to reach a particular step will affect turnaround time.

Diagnostics of instrument function or malfunction are important for troubleshooting purposes. Troubleshooting can be performed by the operator or with remote diagnostics through modem or satellite connection to the manufacturer. Modern instruments should contain built-in sensors for the proper operation of the system. One example is "detector of short sample" by the pipettor. In the event of an instrument malfunction, an error message should be sent to the operator. Some instruments are capable of performing not only diagnostics, but also self-correction or adjustment for certain important parameters, such as self-calibration of the instrument. Continuous monitoring and self-adjusting may be necessary for a truly "walk-away" automation.

A real-time, on-line quality control (QC) system allows the technologist to make a quick decision on the acceptability of the laboratory result. In this verification step, an "exception" list of results could be generated for further investigation. Results not in the exception list will be allowed to pass through to the reporting step. The rules for the exception list should be user defined. Table 4 contains indicators for the exception list. Problems associated with each individual test result could be flagged by the computer. For example, the result may exceed the highest standard or the linearity of the assay. Quality control rules could be set up, like the traditional rules of one QC value greater than 3 SD (standard deviation)

Table 4 Indicators for the QC Exception List

Outside the linearity of the assay
Lost of linearity
Failed QC rules
Failed delta checks
Interferences in the sample
Exceeds critical action or absurd values

rule or two QC values exceeding 2 SD. If the QC results are not acceptable, those patient samples could be held for retesting. A delta-check system could be established to compare each patient result with its previous result. If the difference exceeds the delta-check limit, the result can be identified for further action. The same situation can be applied to the critical action value or the absurd values. The critical action value is defined as the value where immediate action should be taken to notify the physician. The patient is in great danger of severe illness when the lab value exceeds these limits. The absurd value is defined as the value that is physiologically impossible. At such values, the laboratory result is most likely to be an error due to transcription error, such as a decimal point in the wrong place. There are certain interferences present in the patient sample that could affect the test result, such as hemolysis, lipemia, and icteric conditions. Such conditions could be detected by the instrument using a spectrophotometric check and calculating a certain interference index.

Sample identification should be done by a bar-code device with a unique identifying label generated as early as possible in the history of the sample. For example, each blood collection tube should have a bar-code label. This label will provide positive identification throughout the entire testing process. It should contain all the testing information and provide a link to the patient identification. The ability to store the test result is probably more important than result reporting. Most clinical laboratories are computerized. An automated system should be able to communicate with the host computer with a bidirectional interface. A buffer to store laboratory data will be important in the event that the host computer is "down." In short, a data management system should be able to perform all the testing functions even without a functioning host computer.

Other management functions will be useful for a laboratory to evaluate the testing data, work-load recording, turnaround time, productivity, quality assurance, and to show administrators the efficiency of the operation and perhaps justification for a second automated system. However, these management functions are less critical and should not interfere with the daily operating routines.

E. Sample Management

The sample management system is becoming increasingly important as the concern about infectious specimens rises. In fact, an automation would not be complete without the sample management step.

The sample management system should allow a sample to be pipetted into multiple reaction-mixture cups. A random access device is preferred since test requests vary with each individual patient. Furthermore, random access will allow a laboratory to perform testing continuously, that is, first-in-first-out. Therefore, it eliminates the batching and the scheduling of tests.

A sample preparation step may be necessary for certain tests, such as pretreatment of a sample to remove interfering protein or dilution of a sample with high concentration of the analyte. Since most samples are being tested for the first time, the system should be able to reanalyze the same sample with on-board dilution capability if the result exceeds the linearity of the assay.

A sample management system could include sample collection, processing, preparation, and introduction to the instrument. The sample collection has always been performed by a technologist. With the popularity of home testing, certain devices have been introduced to obtain a fingerstick blood sample. Positive identification (e.g., barcode label) should be applied at the blood-collecting step. The primary blood-drawing tube should be centrifuged and transferred to the testing step. The use of a gel tube will facilitate this process. Centrifugation along the axis of the tube will allow direct sampling through the top of the tube. Another approach is the use of automated cap removal devices. Either approach will allow the sample management system to be fully automated.

The sample introduction system should be designed to minimize carryover. Carryover is not a major problem for routine chemistries since the physiological ranges of most analytes are rather limited. However, carryover could be a significant problem for specialized chemistries, such as hormones and tumor markers. It is not uncommon to have a 10^5-fold difference in the values of tumor markers. For example, the alpha-fetoprotein (AFP) value is less than 10 ng/ml in healthy individuals. In patients with hepatocellular carcinoma, the AFP level may exceed 10^6 ng/ml. An ideal target for carryover is less than 1 ppm (10^6). For most analytes, 10 ppm may be acceptable. To minimize carryover, the design of the sampler, such as the shape, size, and materials, is important. Adding a washing step in between each sampling may help reduce carryover.

F. Processing Center

The processing center performs the following tasks: dispensing multiple reagents, mixing the reagent with sample, incubation, and separation of bound from unbound antigen by washing, decanting, or aspiration. For heterogeneous assay, all these steps are necessary. The format of the delivery system is determined by the reagent. One may argue that the reagent is actually dependent on the instrument. For example, a reagent

Table 5 Delivery Systems

System	Advantages	Disadvantages
Coated tube	Easy to use Simple to design	Nonuniformity of coating Difference in reaction kinetics
Coated bead	Easy to use	Limited capacity
Microtiter plate	Standard format	Nonuniformity of reaction kinetics and coating Limited capacity
Magnetic particle	Fast reaction Uniform coating Easy separation	Requires a magnet

using ferrous particle coated with antibodies will require an instrument with a magnet for the separation of the bound from unbound antigen. The advantages and disadvantages of the delivery system are outlined in Table 5.

The processing center will depend on a well-designed and reliable robotic system with great precision. Most tasks in the processing center involve moving steps and traveling certain distances to pick up and deliver reagent. These mechanical moving parts are under a great deal of wear and tear. A system should be designed to have as few moving parts as possible, to minimize the need for servicing.

G. Signal Detection

The type of signal detection system is determined by the signal or the label of the reagent. The choice should be based on the technical performance and economic considerations. Technically, a system should be able to achieve the sensitivity of most clinically important analytes and with acceptable precision. For example, the sensitivity of TSH assay should be down to 0.05 μIU/ml and preferably 0.01 μIU/ml. Economically, a system should be easy to build and relatively inexpensive. It should be common and easy to troubleshoot. Three types of detection systems that fit these criteria have been used in most automated systems:

1. Spectrophotometry with the use of enzyme immunoassay (EIA).
2. Fluorimetry with the use of fluorescent immunoassay (FIA).
3. Luminometry with the use of luminescent immunoassay (LIA).

Spectrophotometry is probably the most popular detector. EIA can be homogeneous, such as the EMIT assay, or heterogeneous. In the heterogeneous assay, two most frequently used enzymes are alkaline phosphatase and peroxidase. The Abbott EIA uses horseradish peroxidase conjugated to the antibody. The substrate, hydrogen peroxide and *o*-phenylenediamine.2HCl, is converted to a colorimetric product and measured at 492 nm with a Quantum spectrophotometer. Using the same approach as Hybritech and in some assays, the same antibodies, TOSOH Medics developed a fully automated system: AIA 1200 and 600.

Fluorimetry is widely used for both homogeneous and heterogeneous immunoassay. Some systems use enzymes to convert a substrate to a fluorescent product, while others use both spectrophotometry and fluorimetry in the same system. For example, the Affinity system by Becton Dickinson uses both EIA and FIA. In theory, fluorimetry is capable of detecting as little as 10^{-14} mol of a compound, while spectrophotometry can only detect 10^{-8} mol. In practice, the sensitivity is much reduced due to the background noise from the endogenous fluorophores, such as bilirubin, protein, and lipids. Time-resolved fluorescence and particle concentration technique may reduce this problem somewhat. The DELFIA system by LKB and the Cyberfluor system use the time-resolved approach. The Pandex system by Baxter and the modified approach of the Abbott IMX system use particle concentration FIA. The IMX system allows measurement of both small and large molecules. This system complements the Abbott TDX homogeneous FPIA system, which only measures small molecules and with limited sensitivity.

Luminometry is gaining popularity rather quickly. Luminescence has the potential of achieving the highest sensitivity. Most LIAs are heterogeneous assay and semiautomated, like the Amerlite system and the MagicLite enhanced system. Taking advantage of the inherent sensitivity, London Diagnostics developed an ultrasensitive thyrotropin (TSH) assay that is capable of measuring TSH down to 0.005 μ IU/ml. Recently, Ciba Corning developed a fully automated system—ACS 180—using this approach.

H. Semiautomated or Fully Automated Systems

An automated instrument could be built on multiple blocks. These building blocks may be linked by computer program or mechanically attached together. In most semiautomated systems, these blocks function separately. Technologists need to perform tasks in between blocks, for example, remove test tubes from the pipettor and place in the incubator or detector. Examples of such systems are the Photon-Era by Hybritech, Inc., or the Commander parallel processor by Abbott Labs. These systems are useful for high-volume testing since they handle the most labor-intensive steps. A fully automated system has robotics devices to handle the transfer of test tubes and all the steps in a immunoassay procedure. A technologist becomes a data manger and an instrument supervisor. Therefore, very little hands-on time is required.

A fully automated system is more complicated and requires a rather long development time. One approach is to develop a semiautomated system and market it to gain real experience in the field. In the meantime, continue to develop a fully automated system based on the semiautomated system. Most fully automated heterogeneous immunoassay systems are relatively slow. Most systems have throughput between 30-120 tests/h. Therefore, the high-volume testing laboratory may benefit from using a semiautomated system that takes care of the most labor-intensive steps, leaving the less time-consuming steps for the technologist.

I. Disadvantages of Automation

Automation has its negative side. The disadvantages of automation are outlined in Table 6. The most obvious disadvantage is the need for capital equipment acquisition. Most laboratories are experiencing difficulty in obtaining funds to purchase capital equipment. Although leasing and reagent rental agreements can alleviate the pain in purchasing equipment, this adds onto the cost of the operating budget. Similar reagents usually cost more for an automated system than for the manual assay. The difference in pricing may not be as great if automation results in testing being performed in singlet rather than in duplicate. Most fully automated systems use dedicated reagents. This means a closed system without any substitution of other reagents. The usual argument for the closed system is to ensure good quality control of the entire system. Economically, it is clearly important for the manufacturer to be able to make a profit for a

Table 6 Disadvantages of Automation

Capital equipment cost
Higher cost of reagent
Closed system with dedicated reagent
Long-term commitment
Total dependence in the automation
Throughput not necessarily greater
Requires maintenance, service, and training
Negative human factor

longer period of time and to recoup the cost of research and development on the system. The closed system "locks in" the laboratory to use all the reagents from the same manufacturer, even though they may not have the same quality. The choice of tests is also limited by that particular system. The commitment for an automated system is usually 3–5 years. While the quality of reagent may change, the instrument will also be obsolete.

The throughput of most automated systems using heterogeneous assay is between 60 and 120 tests/h. An experienced technologist performing manual tests may be able to keep up with the speed of an automated system. The limited throughput as well as the reliability issue cause many labs to acquire more than one system. The total dependency of an automated system means that the entire immunoassay system may be shut down. In the manual assay lab, one or perhaps two assays may be "down." It is unusual for all the assays to be "down." All instruments require maintenance and service. Most technologists performing immunoassays are very good in manual techniques; however, they are not as familiar with instrumentation. Since instruments require proper training and schedule maintenance, it is important that this be done faithfully. Finally, one should not overlook the human factor. Most instruments are advertised as "walk-away." However, as technologists walk away from the instrument, they are leary of the outcome of the testing—what if the instrument malfunctions and none of the results are acceptable? Do we have to stay late to troubleshoot the problem . . . perhaps restart the testing after hours?

PART TWO

Evaluation

CHAPTER 3

Selection of Automated Immunoassay Systems

Daniel W. Chan
Department of Laboratory Medicine,
Clinical Chemistry Division,
The Johns Hopkins Hospital,
The Johns Hopkins University, Baltimore, Maryland

I. INTRODUCTION

The need for automation, as well as the advantages and disadvantages, has been discussed in Chapter 2. In this chapter, I will focus on the selection of automated immunoassay systems as an introduction to the more detailed discussion of the evalution process.

Before you acquire an automated immunoassay system, you should decide whether automation is what you need. If so, what type of automation is most useful for your laboratory? For example, do you need a fully automated or a semiautomated system? What type of throughput do you need?

To establish criteria for the selection of an automated system, you should define the goals of automation. What do you expect the automation to do—improve turnaround time, consolidate work stations, reduce the number of FTE (full-time equivalents), improve assay performance, etc.? We will consider five major issues: clinical, technical, operational, economical, and human factors.

Immunoassay Automation: A Practical Guide

II. CRITERIA FOR THE SELECTION OF AUTOMATED IMMUNOASSAY SYSTEMS

A. Define the Goals

The first step in the selection of an automated immunoassay system is to define the goal and objectives of such automated systems (Table 1). One of the most important benefits of automation is the consolidation of work stations. Traditionally, immunoassays were performed manually. Each assay was performed by a technologist in a work station. An experienced technologist may be able to set up one assay. During the incubation period, a second assay could be started. By carefully scheduling "batch" runs, one could perform two assays in an 8-h shift. For shorter assays, it may be possible to perform three assays in a shift. However, with the difficulty of hiring medical technologists, especially experienced ones, automation may be the only solution to consolidate work stations and thereby reduce the labor requirements.

The reduction of labor requirements includes both the number and the skill level of the technologist. Instead of an experienced radioimmunoassay (RIA) technologist, a medical laboratory technician (MLT) may be able to operate such an automated system. Furthermore, the technologist can be cross-trained to perform routine, special chemistries and other areas of the laboratory. This makes scheduling of technologists much easier, particularly on weekend shifts.

Most automated systems are able to achieve calibration stability of 2–4 weeks. This allows more frequent testing without the increased cost of daily calibration. The total assay time of most automated systems are shorter than the manual assays. The turnaround time of the test as defined from the sample collection to the result reporting will be improved.

Automation generally improves the technical performance of the assay, such as its precision and sensitivity. Most assays could be performed in a single tube rather than the traditional duplicate tubes. This

Table 1 Goals and Objectives of Automation

Consolidate work stations
Reduce labor requirements
Increase test frequency
Improve turnaround time
Improve assay performance
Reduce total cost
Random access—eliminate "batch" concept
Improve overall efficiency

reduces not only the total assay time but also the cost of reagent. The total cost of the testing should be reduced, as the savings in labor and the reagent could offset the cost of instrumentation.

The random access feature of the automation should eliminate the "batch" concept. Tests could be performed as the patient samples arrive in the laboratory. There will be no scheduling of tests. It is simply first-in-first-out. This feature will enhance the turnaround time.

The overall goal of automation should be to improve the efficiency of testing. All the issues discussed earlier should contribute to the efficiency of the automation.

B. Clinical Issues

To meet the clinical requirements of testing, one needs to provide an accurate and meaningful test result to the requesting physician in a timely fashion. Accuracy could be achieved by the technical improvement of automation, which will be discussed under technical issues. To provide a test result in a timely fashion would depend on the test frequency and the time required to perform the testing. It is the turnaround time of testing that is most important.

Most manual immunoassays are performed on a scheduled "batch" mode. The frequency of testing a given analyte is dependent on the clinical requirement of turnaround time, the batch size, the frequency of calibration, and the cost factor. Even if it is clinically acceptable to have a turnaround time of more than 1 week, a test should be performed at least weekly. A weekly testing will allow the technologist to maintain the necessary technical expertise for good performance. If the batch size is too small to perform on a weekly basis due to economical issues, the test should be sent to an outside laboratory.

An automated immunoassay system with random access capability should eliminate the "batch" process. Patient samples could be analyzed according to the order of receipt or priority. Tests can be performed at any time of the day and on any day of the week. This would be cost-effective if the calibration curve is stable for at least 2–4 weeks. Therefore, random access and long-term calibration stability will improve the turnaround time.

C. Technical Issues

The major technical issues are accuracy and precision. The analytical evaluation of such issues will be discussed in the next few chapters. Here I will address the selection of automated system to achieve good accuracy and precision.

Automation should improve precision. Manual immunoassay included pipetting, washing, decanting, and counting steps. All these steps contributed to imprecision. Automation mechanized these steps to be performed precisely the same for each tube. Modern instrumentation uses robots, which should improve the overall precision. Each sample should be able to be tested in a single tube rather than in the traditional duplicate analysis of manual immunoassay. This not only improves the test technically but also its operation and economic issues.

Systems should be selected to have not only good precision but also accuracy. Accuracy could be affected by carryover from other samples, reagent used on the system, and mechanical devices on the instrument. It is also important to have built-in quality checks. Sensors for malfunction of system components should be used. For example, a quality check should examine the pipetting accuracy, adequate sample size, the mechanical moving parts, the appropriate reagent addition, the proper timing for incubation, and washing or reading the enzyme reaction.

D. Operational Issues

Operational issues include both the operation of the system and the impact of automation on the laboratory operation. The system should be easy to operate and require minimum maintenance and services. System malfunction should be apparent with error messages clearly indicated for troubleshooting. Self-diagnostics will be useful, possibly with a communication link to the manufacturer.

A telephone "hot-line" for troubleshooting should be available on a 24-h basis. If on-site services are needed, responses from the manufacturer should be quick. The response time will depend on the type of tests performed; in general, on-site response time of greater than 24 h is not acceptable. The software should be user friendly. Some of these issues were discussed in Chapter 2.

The impact of automation on the laboratory operation is mainly on the work-station consolidation. Automation of the test procedure may allow the technologist to perform other tasks such as quality assurance. The degree of consolidation of work stations will depend on the type of automation and the variety of test menu. This will reduce the labor requirement in both the skill level and the number of technologists needed. Work-station consolidation is probably the single most important benefit of the automation system.

E. Economical Issues

An automated immunoassay system should be cost-effective. In the analysis of the cost-effectiveness of a system, the total cost should be evaluated. The total cost includes instrument, reagent, disposables, labor, service contract, maintenance, and overhead expenses. The cost savings due to the impact on patient care may also be included, such as the reduction of the length of stay, the communication and reporting of results, etc. This component of cost saving is difficult to realize, especially from the laboratory point of view, since it mainly affects the other parts of the hospital. Most automated systems have higher cost for instrument and reagent. In order to reduce the total cost, there should be significant savings in the other components, particularly labor. The reduction in labor could be achieved by consolidating work stations and reducing the skill of technician.

F. Human Issues

Finally, one should not forget about human issues in automation. It is a person who operates the system. Therefore, issues related to the interaction between human and instrument should be considered. The first issue is safety. A system should be designed to ensure safety of the operator. Safety issues are related to injury due to mechanical moving parts, infections from biological hazards (e.g., AIDS, hepatitis virus), and potential fire hazards.

Computer programs for the operation of the system should be "user friendly." Psychological factors should be considered for a walk-away instrument. For example, error messages should be indicated as soon as a problem occurs. An audible alarm should be used to alert the operator of such an occurrence.

III. CONCLUSION

In this chapter, I have outlined the criteria in the selection of an automated immunoassay system. One should start by defining the goal and objectives of the automation to meet the particular needs of the laboratory, such as cost reduction, work-station consolidation, etc. Five major factors in the selection process are clinical, technical, operational, economical, and human issues. After the importance of each issue is considered, one should start an evaluation process based on the actual testing of the automated system. This will be discussed in detail in Chapters 4–7.

CHAPTER 4

Technical Evaluation

Daniel W. Chan
*Department of Laboratory Medicine,
Clinical Chemistry Division,
The Johns Hopkins Hospital,
The Johns Hopkins University, Baltimore, Maryland*

I. INTRODUCTION

Technical evaluation is the first step in the assessment of the performance of an automated immunoassay system. First, the system should be installed and function properly. After the operator has been trained and familiarized with the system, one could begin the technical evaluation. The system should be tested in the order of precision, sensitivity, accuracy, comparison with another method using patient samples, and lot-to-lot variation. Accuracy could be assessed by linearity, parallelism, recovery, interference, carryover, and calibration stability.

II. PRECISION

Precision, or more appropriately imprecision, is probably the most important technical aspect of the system. Automation should improve precision to the point that single testing is acceptable. Duplicate testing defeats the purpose of automation. When evaluating precision, the coefficient of variation (%CV) of the single determination on an automated system should be comparable to or better than the manual assay performed in duplicate.

A. Within-Run Precision

Both within-run and between-run precision should be evaluated. For within-run precision, three levels of quality control (QC) samples should be used to cover the useful range of the assay. Clinically, these levels should be selected within, below, and above the reference ranges for healthy individuals. For example, one level would be within the reference range of thyroxine (T_4) for healthy individuals (euthyroid range). The other two levels should be in the hypothyroid range (<5 μg/dl) and the hyperthyroid range (>12 μg/dl).

Ideally, these QC samples should be analyzed in replicates of 20. The within-run precision can be calculated from the mean ($\bar{x}$) and standard deviation (SD), that is, coefficient of variation (CV%) = $100 \times SD/\bar{x}$. A precision profile can be constructed. Most competitive assays show better precision in the mid-range of the calibration curve. The precision profile resembles a U-shaped curve. Immunometric assays tend to have a flat precision curve. At the extreme low concentration, approaching the detection limit, the sensitivity affects the precision. At the other end of the calibration curve where the absorbance is high for the enzyme immunoassay, the precision also suffers.

B. Between-Run Precision

Between-run precision is a more realistic performance indicator since patient samples are analyzed from day to day. Between-run precision is usually calculated from the daily QC results over a period of time, preferably over 20 days. For shorter-term evaluations, one may be able to run QC several times a day and obtain similar between-run precision data. In general, the between-run precision tends to have a higher %CV than the within-run precision, since variables are introduced from run to run or from day to day. The acceptable level of precision will vary from analyte to analyte and from laboratory to laboratory. The performance standard should be about 5%CV in the useful concentration ranges.

Another aspect of between-run precision is the variation of QC values from one lot of reagent to another lot. Whenever possible, this should be evaluated. One should obtain more than one lot of reagent to determine the mean and SD of each lot. In addition to the QC data, one should compare patient results on different lots. Usually, 5–20 patient samples will be sufficient for the experiment. QC samples may not always indicate the same variation as patient sample, due to matrix effect of lyophilization of QC material. It is the patient results that are most important. From my experience, I have seen significant differences in patient results between lots while the QC results are the same, or vice versa. The lot-to-lot variation will be discussed in more detail elsewhere in this chapter.

For a random access system, the precision should be determined in the random access versus batch mode to see if there are any differences. Some systems show better precision in the batch mode as compared to the random access mode.

C. Sources of Imprecision

Since precision is the most important aspect of the technical performance, identifying and controlling the source of imprecision is quite important. Table 1 lists a number of sources of imprecision. For the clinical laboratory user, the design of the system and the selection of reagent components are out of their control. The more automated the system, the less influence that the user will have in controlling the imprecision. It is therefore imporant to evaluate the imprecision before acquiring a system.

The selection of reagent components of a system has predetermined the extent of imprecision. Both the affinity constant and the concentration of the antibodies used in the reagent will affect the precision. For an assay using antibody coated to the solid phase, the amount of antibody coating will affect the extent of antigen binding. The coating process will affect the competitive assay more than the immunometric assay, since only a limited amount of antibodies is coated. Uncoated tubes will result in falsely low values. On the other hand, the antibody conjugate will determine the amount of signal generated. This will in turn affect the sensitivity and the precision of the assay. The substrate set will also determine the enzyme reaction and the final color production. The stability and the consistency of the substrate should be examined. The accurate assignment of the calibra-

Table 1 Sources of Imprecision

Reagent: antibody capture, antibody conjugate, calibrator, diluent, wash solution, substrate set, quality control
Antigen antibody reaction: timing, temperature, separation, washing
Enzyme substrate reaction: timing, temperature, and quenching
Detection: radioactive counter, spectrophotometer, or fluorometer
Data reduction: curve fit
Pipetting: calibration, setting, and reproducibility
Interference: nonspecific, specific, carryover, and high-dose hook

tor value and the stability of the calibrator is another factor. Other components that affect the precision are diluent, wash solution, quench solution, and quality control samples. The matrices, pH, ionic strength, and the lyophilization process will also influence the overall precision.

The binding of antigen and antibody is influenced by the incubation time, temperature, pH, the separation step, and the washing of unbound antigen (competitive assay) or the antibody (immunometric assay). If the incubation time is not sufficient for equilibrium to be achieved, the timing for the separation step becomes rather critical since the binding is still increasing. Any deviation from the preset time will result in poor precision. This may be more a problem for the semiautomated than the fully automated system. If the separation step involves a membrane device, the nonspecific binding to this membrane may be an area of concern. Adequate washing of the membrane is important.

The enzyme-substrate reaction is affected by similar conditions as the antigen-antibody reaction. However, the effect of temperature and time may be more crucial. For example, the Q10 value of the alkaline phosphatase is 1.7. The value of alkaline phosphatase will increase by 70% with a 10°C increase. This is much greater than the effect on most antigen–antibody reactions. Furthermore, the stabilities of both the enzyme and the substrate are less than the antibody. The color development is also subject to spectroscopic interference.

Imprecision could be introduced at the detection step. Error associated with the counting of radioactivity varies with the counts per minute (cpm) of each sample. The error in the measurement of absorbance could result from spectroscopic interference and the use of a secondary wavelength. Similar problems could be encountered for fluorescent immunoassay (FIA) using a fluorescent signal.

The selection of curve-fitting models for data reduction could affect the imprecision. The use of a logit-log model to linearize the standard curve could post imprecision at both ends of the curve. At such extreme concentrations, the standards fall off the curve. An example is the radioassay for folate determination. In the event that logit-log transformation does not linearize the standard curve, the use of a four-parameter logistic method may provide a better fit.

Pipetting is one step in the automation that affects the precision directly. The accuracy of the pipette should be checked against a known amount of solution. If problems exist, the pipette should be calibrated. The precision of the pipette should be evaluated by pipetting repeatedly a known amount of radioactivity or color solution. The precision of the pipette should be less than 2%CV. Periodic preventive maintenance is essential in maintaining good precision of the pipetting station.

Interferences could cause imprecision. Nonspecific interferences such as hemolysis, lipemia, and icterus as well as specific interferences like heterophilic antibodies will affect both the accuracy and precision. Samples with extremely high concentrations of analyte will affect precision in two ways. First, the high concentration of this sample could carry over into the next sample. Second, it may cause a high-dose hook effect. The apparent low value will be rather imprecise. This will be discussed in more detail in the accuracy section.

III. SENSITIVITY

Sensitivity is usually defined as the detection limit of an assay. Several approaches to the determination of sensitivity do not yield the same result. The following are three approaches.

A. Minimum Detectable Dose

The minimum detectable dose (MDD) is calculated from the mean + 2SD of 20 replicates of the zero calibrator performed within a run. It is usually calculated based on the response (absorbance or radioactivity) and read off the calibration curve to obtain the MDD. This approach usually gives the best (lowest) MDD possible mainly due to the better precision within the same run. This is the accepted industry standard and is usually the published MDD value. However, the MDD calculated in this manner is unrealistic and usually not reproducible from day to day.

B. Sensitivity between Days

This approach is similar to the MDD except the zero calibrator is determined as an unknown between days for a period of time. The mean + 2SD of the actual value is calculated from the zero calibrator as an unknown. This approach is more realistic since the claimed sensitivity should be achievable from day to day. This value is usually higher than the within-run MDD by 50–100%. For example, sensitivity of a highly sensitive thyrotropin (TSH) assay on the IMx system is 0.05 μIU/ml as determined by MDD. The sensitivity from day to day is found to be 0.1 μIU/ml based on 100 runs of TSH assay in our laboratory.

Another approach is to use patient samples with zero analyte concentration in determining sensitivity, since calibrator does not always resemble patient material. Biases have been incorporated into the calibrator. It is possible to adjust the zero calibrator to read on the negative side, thereby resulting in artificially lower responses and hence low MDD. Furthermore, it is more important to be able to differentiate patient diagnostic groups. For example, after a successful radical prostatectomy, a prostatic cancer patient with organ-confined cancer should have undetectable prostate-specific antigen (PSA). QC at this low level of PSA is important. We routinely use a female patient sample as QC since women, having no prostatic tissue, should not have any detectable PSA values. Using this patient sample approach, we found the working sensitivity of PSA IRMA assay (Tandem-R; Hybritech, Inc.) to be 0.2 ng/ml instead of an MDD of 0.08 ng/ml. This gives us confidence in reporting PSA values greater than 0.2 ng/ml.

C. Sensitivity by Dilution

Another approach to the evaluation of sensitivity is by diluting a patient's serum with the assay diluent to below the detection limit of the assay. For example, a highly sensitive TSH assay using this approach will be more realistic. The sensitivity is determined at the dilution where the percent recovery found is no longer close to 100% of the expected value. The percent recovery is calculated from the found/expected concentration. Similarly, one can also evaluate the expected changes in TSH values following dilution. Sensitivity is determined at the point where no significant changes in TSH values occur.

Another approach is the use of patient diagnostic groups. A highly-sensitive TSH assay should clearly differentiate hyperthyroid from euthyroid patients without any overlapping TSH values. Statistically, the mean + 3SD limit of the hyperthyroid patient's TSH values should not overlap with the mean −3SD limit of the euthyroid patient's TSH values. Additional criteria for assessing sensitive TSH assays were proposed by Klee and Hay (1987).

IV. ACCURACY

The analytical accuracy is the ability of a system to determine the true value of the analyte. If a definitive method exists to obtain the true value of the analyte, the accuracy of the test method can be determined by comparing the result to the definitive method determined. In most instances, only indirect assessment of the accuracy is possible. Several indirect measurements of the accuracy are commonly employed. These include recovery, linearity, parallelism, interference, carryover, and calibration stability.

A. Recovery

Recovery is an indirect assessment of accuracy. It tests the system's ability to measure a known amount of analyte. The experiment is done by adding a known amount of analyte (A) to a base (B) and measuring the concentration (C). The percentage of recovery can be calculated by $100\% \times (C-B)/A$. The recovery is affected by the precision of the system. If the base concentration (B) is very low, that is, near the detection limit, the error in determining B will become a factor. A similar situation also applies to the added amount (A). It is recommended that the recovery be assessed at three different concentrations of A. For most hormones except T_4, pure substances are difficult to obtain. Therefore, it is not possible to weigh out certain amounts of analyte (A) for the recovery experiment. In those situations, relative recovery will be used instead of absolute recovery.

B. Dilution

The dilution experiment is an assessment of the relative recovery of the system. A sample with analyte concentration near the top of the calibration curve is used. The diluent is usually the assay buffer or the zero calibrator. In addition, saline or another patient sample could also be used to assess the matrix effect. The dilution factor is usually recommended as follows: 1, $\frac{3}{4}$, $\frac{1}{2}$, $\frac{1}{4}$, $\frac{1}{8}$, $\frac{1}{16}$, $\frac{1}{32}$, $\frac{1}{64}$, or until the expected concentration penetrates the detection limit of the assay. At such low concentration, the dilution experiment could be used to assess the sensitivity as discussed previously.

The majority of immunoassays show nonlinear dose-response curves. A calibration curve is needed to calculate the unknown concentration. The linearity is an indication that the responses are proportional, and the final concentrations calculated from the curve are linear. It is important to show the parallelism between the standard curve and a patient sample diluted throughout the assay range. Good parallelism indicates that the assay fulfills one of the fundamental principles of immunoassay, that the unknown antigen give the same response as the standard antigen. Good linearity is important in the event that a patient sample needs to be diluted because the concentration is greater than the highest calibrator. Accurate results will be assumed if an assay shows good linearity.

If the calculated concentration does not match the expected concentration, there are several possibilities. The most common cause is the matrix effect of the diluent. I would recommend repeating the dilution experiment with several different diluents including saline, buffer with protein base, zero calibrator, and a patient serum. If protein concentration is the problem, the dilution with saline will show poor recovery while the patient serum as diluent will show good recovery. If diluting with zero calibrator causes nonlinear responses, it may indicate that the matrix used in the calibrator is not compatible with patient serum sample. The matrix for the calibrator may have to be changed. The diluent found to give good linearity should be used to dilute patient sample with values greater than the highest calibrator.

C. Interference

It is also useful to test the dilution beyond the calibrator curve. This may indicate assay problems like "high-dose hook effect" in an immunometric assay or the presence of interference. At extreme high analyte concentrations, the antibody binding sites may be saturated with antigens making the antibodies unavailable to form a sandwich, that is, antibody-antigen complexes. Furthermore, the immunometric assay that usually works with excess antibody becomes a competitive assay with limited antibody. The end result is the severe underestimation of the analyte concentration. This is a particular problem with analytes that could be present in wide concentration ranges, for example, tumor markers like alpha-fetoprotein (AFP). In a patient with AFP concentration of 6×10^6 μg/l, the apparent concentration by an IEMA (Tandem-E, Hybritech, Inc.) was 29 μg/l (Chan *et al.*, 1986). Without knowing the patient's clinical condition, one would severely underestimate the true AFP concentration in this patient. Often, a clue to the high-dose hook sample is imprecision. At such a high concentration, the response of binding is extremely imprecise. If assays are performed in duplicate, the CV of the replicate is poor. For example, a pediatric patient with hepatoblastoma was presented with an AFP of 59 μg/l. The CV of the replicate was 30%. Repeat testing in a subsequent run resulted in an AFP of 126 μg/l, CV 25%. In another run, the AFP was 75 μg/l, CV 26%. Upon dilution, the high-dose hook phenomenon was discovered.

Heterophilic antibodies have been reported to cause false positive results in immunometric assay (Boscatto and Stuart, 1988). Since most monoclonal antibodies are developed from a hybridoma using the mouse system, the presence of anti-mouse antibodies in a patient's serum will lead to false positive results. To minimize this problem, mouse serum has been added to the reaction medium to absorb mouse antibodies. Some assays use other scavenger antibodies or Fab fragments rather than the whole immunoglobulin in the assay. Genetically engineered chimeric antibody with a combined mouse and human immunoglobulin molecule has also been used. In addition to the problem of endogenous antibodies, immunotherapy of cancer patients with toxin-labeled antibody in the blood circulation as well as human anti-mouse antibodies (HAMA) will cause interference (Kricka *et al.*, 1990). High titers of rheumatoid factors will also cause false positive results in immunometric assays.

Other nonspecific interferences, such as lipemia, hemolysis, and icterus, may affect the separation and detection using the spectrophotometric or fluorometric measurement. In the serum, substances may be present that cross-react with the antigen for the antibody. In the digoxin assay, digoxinlike immunoreactive substances (DLIS) have been identified to cause false positives in neonates, pregnant women, and patients with renal or liver diseases (Valdes, 1985; Soldin, 1986). Some assays use a column separation pretreatment step to remove such DLIS (Skogen, 1987). It is almost impossible to outline all the interferences. Readers should be aware of and cautious about discrepant results, which may require further investigation.

D. Carryover

Carryover is a unique problem for the automated immunoassay system because it is no longer a problem for general chemistry analyzers. Consider the physiological ranges of most general chemistry tests, which are so narrow that 0.1% carryover will be acceptable. For most analytes of immunoassay, the physiological ranges are quite broad. It is particularly troublesome for tumor markers. For example, the AFP values in a patient with hepatocellular carcinoma could exceed 10^6 ng/ml, with a reference range from 0 to 10 ng/ml for healthy individuals. One would require a carryover rate of less than 1 part per million (ppm). For most analytes, 10 ppm will be acceptable. To assess carryover, one should run three high samples, followed by three samples with zero concentration. The carryover rate is calculated from the value of the first zero sample. The second and third zero samples also serve as an indication of how far the carryover will penetrate.

E. Calibration Stability

The stability-of-calibration curve can be determined by the daily QC results over a period of weeks or months. Trend analysis and other statistical analysis may be helpful. Some assays require running one calibrator with each run. The absorbance of this calibrator is compared to the stored curve. The ratio is calculated. Most IMx assays have the acceptance limit from 15 to 30%. The variation of this factor may be a useful indicator of the extent of shift in the calibration curve. One could compare the QC data with and without the adjustment of the calibration curve. If there is no difference, the adjustment may be unnecessary.

When to recalibrate the system is a difficult question. Should a system be recalibrated if the QC rule is unacceptable, or are there other causes for the failed QC? Judgment needs to be exercised. If the QC values show a declining trend, calibration may be in order. After the system has been recalibrated, what is the acceptable criterion for the calibrator? Is the fact that all three QC values are within acceptable limits sufficient to accept the calibration? Would you demand that all the QC should be within one SD of the mean? How much shift would you introduce as the result of recalibration? This is a real problem for systems that have long-term calibration stability. The bias introduced during the calibration may be a significant component of the overall imprecision of the system.

V. METHOD COMPARISON

Method comparison may be overemphasized by most laboratorians. It is often assumed that if method A compares well with method B, then method A must be good. One declares that the new method A is better than the old method B because they correlate well. Despite the potential shortcomings of method comparison, it is still useful if one realizes the limitations and defines the goal for such comparison. The usefulness of method comparison is shown in Table 2. If the reference method is a definitive method, the result of the method comparison could be used to establish the analytical accuracy of the new method. When the clinically defined patient samples are used in the method comparison, the clinical accuracy of the new method can be established. The comparison to the reference method

Table 2 Usefulness of Method Comparison

Reference method	New method
Definitive method	Analytical accuracy
Diagnosis established method	Clinical accuracy
Reference method	Identify outliers
Current method	Establish reference values
Market leader	Provide competition

can be used to identify outliers if the reference method has good precision. These outliers can be investigated for possible interferences. When the current method is the reference method, one can decide whether the reference ranges need to be changed. With a good correlation coefficient but slope not equal to one, one can adjust the reference ranges by the slope factor. If the correlation coefficient is poor, that is, significantly less than 1.0, it will be difficult to assess the reference ranges. When the reference method is the market leader, the result of the method comparison can provide information to establish a marketing plan against the competitor.

To perform the method comparison, one should randomly select 100–200 patient samples with analyte values throughout the entire calibration curve. If most samples are clustered narrowly in one end of the concentration range with very few points at the other end of the concentration range, the linear regression will be biased with those few samples. If samples are distributed in two groups at both ends of the concentration range, the slope of the linear regression will be determined by the mean of those two groups. A falsely elevated coefficient may be obtained together with an incorrect slope of the linear regression.

VI. LOT-TO-LOT VARIATION

The consistency of the technical performance of an automated immunoassay system will depend on the proper maintenance of the system and the lot-to-lot variation of the reagent. The issue of maintenance will be discussed in Chapter 6. Here I will address the lot-to-lot variation.

Whenever possible, the technical performance of multiple lots of reagents should be evaluated. I recommend evaluating three lots of reagents. After acquiring the system for routine use, one could use the same protocol for new lot check in. A recommended protocol is shown in Table 3.

To check in a new lot of reagent, one should record the lot number of all components. In the event of inconsistent performance, the component information will facilitate troubleshooting of the causes. The most frequent lot change is the tracer in the radioimmunoassay (RIA) and the conjugate in the enzyme immunoassay (EIA). In most instances, such changes are trivial and should not affect the performance of the assay. However, this may produce rather dramatic changes in the absolute absorbance or the amount of radioactivity. When the calibrator lot changes, shifts in QC and patient results may happen. The calibrator is not a standard. The calibrator value is set according to a master lot. During the process of value assignment, imprecision and inaccuracy could be introduced. The degree of inaccuracy will depend on the QC tolerance limit set by the producer. The

Table 3 Protocol for Lot Check In

1. Record lot numbers of all components.
2. Evaluate the absolute absorbance of the calibrator.
3. Evaluate the differences in absorbance between calibrators.
4. Evaluate the characteristics of the calibration curve.
5. Evaluate the replicate CV.
6. Evaluate QC shifts.
7. Compare patient results between the old and new lots.
8. Check linearity, if necessary.
9. Compare patient results obtained during the primary and secondary wavelengths, if more than one wavelength is used.

tolerance limit varies from 2 to 10% or 1–2 SD of the difference between lots. Therefore, users should decide what is the acceptable limit for their own laboratories.

The absorbance of the calibrator is a good indicator of lot-to-lot variation of the conjugate. In an immunoenzymatric assay (IEMA), the amount of enzyme conjugate to the antibody has the most effect on the absolute absorbance. When only one calibrator is used in an assay, the absorbance of this calibrator becomes quite important. The slope of the calibration curve changes significantly according to its absorbance. This will affect the sensitivity, linearity, and precision of the assay. It also determines when the secondary wavelength will be used. We have observed that the absorbance of calibrators varies from 1.0 to 1.5 between lots of the TANDEM-E creatine kinase MB (CK-MB) assay.

In addition to the absolute absorbance, differences in the absorbance of the calibrator should be evaluated. The differences in absorbance will affect the dynamic ranges and the sensitivity of the assay. This applies to both quantitative and qualitative assays. For qualitative assay, this is especially important since no quantitative values are produced. A positive or negative result will greatly depend on the differences in the absorbance of the zero and the positive cutoff calibrator. Minimum acceptable absorbance value should be set for such assays, such as the EMIT assay for abuse drugs, to avoid false positive results.

The parameters generated from the data reduction of the calibration curve could be evaluated. These parameters include the slope, intercept, ED_{50}, coefficient of correlation, and standard error estimate. Such parameters could be recorded for quality control and troubleshooting purposes. For assays with longer-term calibration curve stability, such as the IMX system, a calibrator is included with each run to adjust the curve in the mode 1 operation. Evaluation of the variation in this calibrator may help troubleshooting.

For assays performed in duplicate, the CV of the replicates may indicate any changes in precision of the new lot of reagent. Routine quality control samples should be run and compared to the historic data to detect any possible QC shifts. If all the QC results are higher or lower than the mean value, it may indicate a bias in the new reagent. Ideally, one would like to have all QC values within 1 SD of the mean. Since most QC samples are artifical and consist of different matrices, patient samples should be analyzed and compared to results obtained with the old lot. A minimum of three patients with different concentrations should be analyzed. Any indication of differences should increase the number of patients to perhaps 10. Both the mean and individual values should be evaluated for any biases.

If there is any indication of nonlinearity—for example, the patient with high analyte value is much lower than the value obtained by the old lot of reagent—a linearity study should be performed. If both the primary and secondary wavelengths are used, one should compare patient results obtained by both wavelengths. For example, an EIA using alkaline phosphatase has a peak absorbance at 405 nm. To extend the working range of the assay, one could read the absorbance at 450 nm, which is on the shoulder of the absorbance peak. At a given concentration of the bound conjugate, the absorbance will be lower. Therefore, the ranges of concentration can be extended further before reaching the nonlinear portion of the spectrophotometric curve. In order to use results interchangeably between the two wavelengths, one should prove that these two values are identical. One approach is to dilute a sample with high analyte concentration. The diluted sample should give the same value read in the primary wavelength as compared to the undiluted sample read in the secondary wavelength. Linearity should be proven in either one of the wavelengths.

REFERENCES

Boscato, L. M., and Stuart, M. C. (1988). Heterophilic antibodies: A problem for all immunoassays. *Clin. Chem.* **34,** 27–33.

Chan, D. W., Kelsten, M. L., Rock, R. C., and Bruzek, D. (1986). Evaluation of a monoclonal immunoenzymetric assay for alpha-fetoprotein. *Clin. Chem.* **32,** 1318–1322.

Klee, G. G., and Hay, I. D. (1987). Assessment of sensitive thyrotropin assays for an expanded role in thyroid function testing: proposed criteria for analytic performance and clinical utility. *J. Clin. Endocrinol. Metab.* **64,** 461–471.

Kricka, L. J., Schmerfeld-Pruss, D., Senior, M., Goodman, D. B., and Kaladas, P. (1990). Interference by human anti-mouse antibody in two-site immunoassays. *Clin. Chem.* **36,** 892–894.

Skogen, W. F., Rea, M. R., and Valdes, R., Jr. (1987). Endogenous digoxin-like immunoreactive factors eliminated from serum samples by hydrophobic silica-gel extraction and enzyme immunoassay. *Clin. Chem.* **33,** 401–404.

Soldin, S. J. (1986). Digoxin-issues and controversies. *Clin. Chem.* **32,** 2–12.

Valdes, R., Jr. (1985). Endogenous digoxin-like immunoreactive factors: Impact on digoxin measurements and potential physiological implications. *Clin. Chem.* **31,** 1525–1532.

CHAPTER 5

Clinical Evaluation

Daniel W. Chan
Department of Laboratory Medicine,
Clinical Chemistry Division,
The Johns Hopkins Hospital,
The Johns Hopkins University, Baltimore, Maryland

I. INTRODUCTION

The goal of a clinical evaluation is to assess the ability of a system to provide accurate test results in a timely fashion for the clinical need. The need could be for disease screening, diagnosis, or management. The clinical performance of a system could not be assessed without a sound technical performance. In the clinical laboratory, you often have only one chance to get the correct result, while in the research laboratory it may be possible to analyze a sample multiple times over a period of time. Therefore, a system with poor technical performance, such as imprecision, should be eliminated from consideration. The clinical evaluation will not be necessary.

The clinical evaluation should begin with the establishment of a reference range for healthy subjects. For certain tests, it may be useful to determine the reference range for certain nondiseased individuals or benign conditions. A decision level using the predictive value model rather than the upper limit of normal may be more appropriate. For tests mainly used for the disease management, such as tumor markers, it is necessary to monitor patients during the treatment process. Finally, an accurate test result may not be useful unless it is reported in a timely fashion for the clinical need.

II. DIAGNOSTIC ACCURACY

A. Reference Values

Reference values should be established for a new system using the population from your area. This can be compared with the published values. The determination of reference values is rather time-consuming and requires a large healthy population, $n = 120$ or more. Traditionally, reference values are defined as the central 95% interval of the healthy population. The theoretical lower limit of the sample size to estimate the 2.5% to 97.5% is $1/0.025 = 40$. The precision of the estimate increases with the larger population. It is recommended that the practical limit should be at least three times the theoretical limit (Solberg, 1987).

Statistical analysis using the mean ±2 SD for a population with Gaussian (normal) distribution is the most frequently used method. For non-Gaussian distribution, percentile method is probably the simplest approach. One would rank the results from the lowest to the highest value. The values at the 2.5-th and the 97.5-th percentiles become the reference values. The ranks at these percentiles are calculated from $0.025(n + 1)$ and $0.975(n + 1)$. For example, if the total population is 120, the rank at the 2.5-th percentile is $0.025(120 + 1)=3$ and at the 97.5-th percentile is $0.975(120 + 1)=118$. Therefore, the reference values are the values at the ranks 3 and 118 (Solberg, 1987).

The reference values determined using healthy subjects in this fashion are applicable to analytes with physiologically well-defined normal concentrations. Examples are serum sodium and glucose concentrations. The euthyroid ranges for thyroxine (T_4) could be determined by this approach with values above and below indicating hyper- and hypothyroid ranges. For tests with relative specific applications, such as creatine kinase MB (CK-MB) in the diagnosis of acute myocardial infarction (AMI) or tumor markers in the diagnosis and management of cancer, a decision level is more appropriate than the upper limit of the normal population. The decision level for CK-MB should be established using the AMI "rule out" (Chan *et al.*, 1985). For tumor markers, in some cases using benign patients as the nondisease group is better than the healthy population. The decision level can be determined using a predictive value model.

B. Predictive Value of Diagnostic Test

The predictive value model includes sensitivity, specificity, and efficiency of a test. The definition is shown in Fig. 1. A perfect test should have 100% sensitivity, specificity, and efficiency. However, no tests show perfect

	Patients with positive test result	Patients with negative test result	Totals
Patients with disease	TP	FN	TP + FN
Patients without disease	FP	TN	FP + TN
Totals	TP + FP	FN + TN	TP + FP + TN + FN

TP = True positives — number of diseased patients correctly classified by the test

FP = False positives — number of nondiseased patients misclassified by the test

TN = True negatives — number of nondiseased patients correctly classified by the test

FN = False negatives — number of diseased patients misclassified by the test

Sensitivity = positivity in disease, expressed as a percent:

$$\frac{TP}{TP + FN} \times 100$$

Specificity = negativity in health or in the absence of a particular disease, expressed as a percent:

$$\frac{TN}{FP + TN} \times 100$$

Predictive value of a positive test = percent of patients with positive test results who are diseased:

$$\frac{TP}{TP + FP} \times 100$$

Predictive value of a negative test = percent of patients with negative test results who are nondiseased:

$$\frac{TN}{TN + FN} \times 100$$

Efficiency of a test = percent of patients correctly classified as diseased or nondiseased:

$$\frac{TP + TN}{TP + FP + FN + TN} \times 100$$

Figure 1 Predictive value model.

predictive values. By varying the decision level, sensitivity and specificity will change in the opposite directions. A higher decision level will reduce the sensitivity while increasing the specificity. An optimal decision level can be selected based on the highest possible efficiency. An example is the comparison of three CK-MB assays for the diagnosis of AMI. An optimal decision level was selected using this approach to be 9 μg/l for the TANDEM-E assay, 14 U/l for the Isomune assay, and 7 U/l for the electrophoretic assay (Chan *et al.*, 1985).

A useful approach to evaluate multiple tests for the same analyte is the receiver operating characteristic (ROC) curve. The ROC curve can be constructed by plotting sensitivity versus 1− specificity or true positive rate versus false positive rate. The advantage of ROC curve is the display of the performance over the entire decision levels. One can pinpoint the

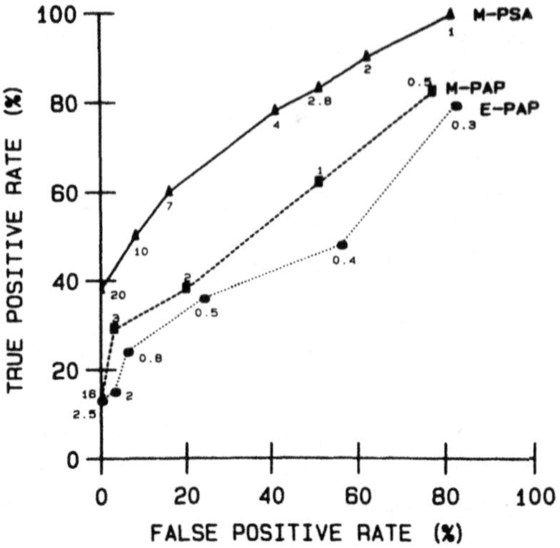

Figure 2 Receiver-operating characteristic (ROC) curves for PSA, M-PAP, and PAP. The data for all 128 patients with prostatic disease are plotted, with several quantitative decision levels (as indicated in the figure) for each assay. Units are μg/l for M-PAP and PSA, and U/l for E-PAP. Reprinted with permission from Rock *et al.* (1987).

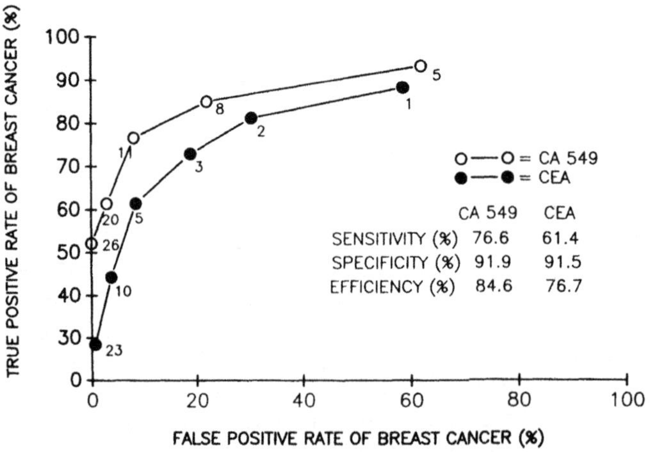

Figure 3 Receiver-operating characteristic (ROC) curves for CA 549, kilounits/l, and CEA, μg/l. The sensitivity, specificity, and efficiency are based on the decision level of CA 549, 11 kilounits/l, and CEA, 5 μg/l. The data includes patients with breast cancer and benign breast diseases, 331 for CA 549 and 322 for CEA. The decision values are indicated on the curve. Reprinted with permission from Chan *et al.* (1988).

decision level where the optimal sensitivity and specificity can be achieved. By superimposing the ROC curves of more than one test method, one can select the best methodology. A better test is one that displays a higher true positive rate and a lower false positive rate. Examples are shown in Figs. 2 and 3. Prostate-specific antigen (PSA) is better than prostatic acid phosphatase (PAP) for the diagnosis of prostatic cancer (Rock *et al.*, 1987), and CA 549 is better than carcinoembyronic antigen (CEA) for identifying active breast cancer (Chan *et al.*, 1988). The preparation of an ROC curve has been discussed in detail by Zweig and Robertson, 1987.

C. Distribution of Patient Values

The predictive value model is difficult to use for analytes that are not diagnostic for a single disease. Tumor markers are good examples. Most, if not all, tumor markers are elevated in more than one disease condition. CEA has been shown to be elevated in colorectal, lung, breast, and pancreatic carcinoma as well as in benign conditions. The reference values for CEA in the healthy population are higher for smokers than for nonsmokers. Using the predictive value model, it is necessary to select a population that includes disease and nondisease groups. What patients should be included in these two groups? The clinical question asked should be used to define the disease group. If the question is the diagnostic efficiency of CEA for active colorectal carcinoma, the disease group should include only the patients with active colorectal carcinoma. The nondisease group is more difficult to decide. Should one include both healthy and benign conditions? If so, how many benign groups should be included? Should the patients in remission be included as well, since they do not have active disease? The outcome of the sensitivity and specificity will greatly depend on the inclusion of the number and groups of patients. In this situation, the actual distribution of patient values may be more informative.

The distribution of tumor marker values is usually shown as the percentage of patients with elevated values using various "cutoff" values in groups of healthy, benign, and cancerous patients. These groups are selected from past experiences of other similar markers. An example is CA 549 (Table 1). The normal women group is used as the healthy population for comparison. The nonmalignant or benign groups are selected to include the most likely causes of marker elevation: benign liver, breast, and pregnancy. The non-breast metastatic cancer groups are selected to show the specificity of the CA 549 using endometrial, colon, lung, prostate, and ovarian carcinoma. Grouping breast cancer patients into one single category is not satisfactory since CA 549 is a marker for active breast cancer.

Table 1 Distribution of CA 549 Values[a]

		Number (and %) of patients with CA 549 values, kilo-units/liter					
Diagnosis	Number of Patients	0–8	>8	>11	>15	>20	>25
Normal women	100	85(85)	15(15)	5 (5)	0 (0)	0 (0)	0 (0)
Nonmalignant							
Benign liver	42	19(45)	23(55)	11(26)	3 (7)	0 (0)	0 (0)
Benign breast	69	63(91)	6 (9)	1 (1)	1 (1)	0 (0)	0 (0)
Pregnancy	30	26(87)	4(13)	0 (0)	0 (0)	0 (0)	0 (0)
Nonbreast metastatic cancer							
Endometrial	8	7(88)	1(12)	1(12)	1(12)	1(12)	0 (0)
Colon	41	25(61)	16(39)	7(17)	3 (7)	1 (2)	1 (2)
Lung	40	22(55)	18(45)	13(33)	11(28)	6(15)	6(15)
Prostate	30	13(43)	17(57)	12(40)	5(17)	5(17)	3(10)
Ovarian	60	22(37)	38(63)	30(50)	21(35)	15(25)	10(17)
Breast cancer							
Adjuvant	88	61(69)	27(31)	10(11)	6 (9)	4 (5)	0 (0)
Metastatic							
Complete remission	16	11(69)	5(31)	3(19)	1 (6)	1 (6)	1 (6)
Partial remission	52	12(23)	40(77)	33(63)	27(52)	22(42)	16(31)
No response (progressive)							
Local	12	5(42)	7(58)	5(42)	3(25)	2(17)	2(17)
Metastasis	94	7 (7)	87(93)	83(88)	79(84)	73(78)	69(73)

[a] Reprinted with permission from Chan *et al.* (1988).

The adjuvant group consists of patients after mastectomy and treated with adjuvant chemotherapy presented with no evidence of disease. The CA 549 values are not expected to be elevated. The metastatic group includes patients in complete remission, partial remission, and progressive breast cancer with local or distant metastasis. The progressive group should have the highest percentage of elevated CA 549 values. The partial remission should have a lower percentage of elevated CA 549 values. The complete remission should have the lowest percentage of elevated CA 549 values.

III. DISEASE MANAGEMENT

The evaluation of the performance of an automated immunoassay system in disease management is mainly for analytes like tumor markers that are used in the monitoring of treatment and progression of cancer. As discussed earlier, the selection of patient groups are important to illustrate the usefulness of the analyte in various clinical settings. A marker could be used to determine the success of surgery, to detect the recurrence of cancer, and to monitor the effectiveness of the treatment modality.

To determine the success of surgery, one would expect that an elevated marker prior to surgery should fall after a successful operation. The extent of the decrease in the marker value will depend on the pretreatment tumor involvement. An example is PSA. One would expect that an elevated PSA value in a patient with organ-confined prostatic cancer will fall to undetectable level after a successful radical prostatectomy. In a patient with prostate cancer extended outside the capsule like seminal vesical involvement or positive lymph nodes, PSA will not fall completely after radical prostatectomy. Followup of patients after surgery have confirmed such findings. Walsh *et al.* (1988) reported a long-term study of 297 men followed for 1–13 years after radical prostatectomy (Table 2). For the 180 patients with organ-confined cancer, only 11 (6%) had elevated PSA levels (>0.5 μg/l). Three of these patients had documented recurrence while the other eight had no evidence of cancer. The frequency of elevated PSA levels increased with advancing pathologic stage. Of the entire group, 12% had elevated PSA without evidence of recurrence. It was assumed that these patients had residual disease. All patients with recurrence had elevated PSA levels.

To detect the recurrence of cancer after a successful initial treatment, one would expect the marker value to be steady, possibly within the reference values of healthy individuals. When the marker value starts to show a trend upward, it may indicate the recurrence of cancer. An example is the monitoring of breast cancer patients after mastectomy and during

Table 2 PSA and Tumor Status in 297 Men Followed 1–13 Years after Radical Prostatectomy[a]

Pathologic stage	Postoperative PSA			
	<0.5 ng/ml	>0.5 ng/ml		
	NED[b]	NED	recurrence[c]	(percent)
Organ confined	169	8	3	6
Capsular penetration	51	3	10	20
Seminal vesicle involvement	9	10	9	68
Positive lymph nodes	4	15	6	84
Total	233	36	28	

[a] Reprinted with permission from Walsh *et al.* (1989).
[b] No evidence of disease.
[c] Local recurrence and/or metastatic disease.

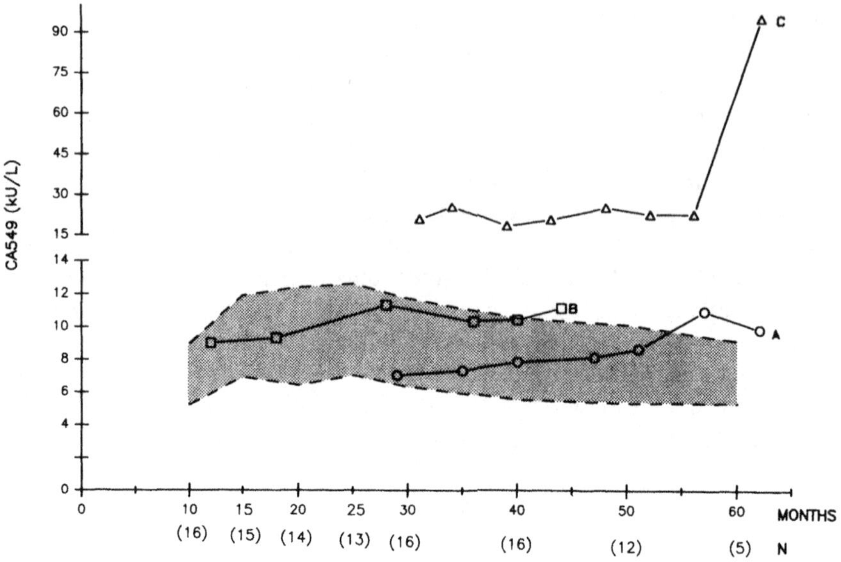

Figure 4 Monitoring the clinical sources of adjuvant breast cancer patients ($n = 19$). Mean (bottom line of the shaded area) and mean + 2 SD (top line) of CA 549 values for 16 patients: ○, patient A; □, patient B; △, patient C; N, number of specimens. Reprinted with permission from Chan *et al.* (1988).

adjuvant chemotherapy with the CA 549 assay (Chan *et al.*, 1988). An elevated CA 549 value may suggest the development of metastasis (Fig. 4).

To monitor the effectiveness of cancer therapy, one would expect that the marker value should increase with progression of cancer. With regression of cancer, the marker value should decrease. For stable patients, the marker value should not change. An example is alpha-fetoprotein (AFP) in the monitoring of hepatocellular carcinoma (HCC) (Kelsten *et al.*, 1988). In this study, the changes of AFP values were correlated with the intrahepatic tumor volume. One could evaluate individual patients in the treatment and progression of cancer. It is also possible to evaluate each event and correlate with the change in marker values. One can group all the events related to the progression of disease, stable disease, and regression of cancer, then evaluate whether the marker value changed in the right direction in all these situations (Chan *et al.*, 1986). Another example is the monitoring of metastatic breast cancer using CA 549 (Chan *et al.*, 1988). In this study, changes of greater than 25% of CA 549 and CEA values are defined as significant. They are correlated with the progression and regression of tumor, fatal progression, and the change from no evidence of disease to metastasis.

REFERENCES

Chan, D. W., Taylor, E., Frye, R., and Blitzer, R. (1985). Immunoenzymetric assay for creatine kinase MB with subunit-specific monoclonal antibodies compared with an immunochemical method and electrophoresis. *Clin. Chem.* **31,** 465–469.

Chan, D. W., Kelsten, M., Rock, R., and Bruzek, D. (1986). Evaluation of a monoclonal immunoenzymometric assay for alpha-fetoprotein. *Clin. Chem.* **32,** 1318–1322.

Chan, D. W., Beveridge, R. A., Bruzek, D. J., Damron, D. J., Bray, K. R., Gaur, P. K., Ettinger, D. S., and Rock, R. C. (1988). Monitoring breast cancer with CA 549. *Clin. Chem.* **34,** 2000–2004.

Kelsten, M. L., Chan, D. W., Bruzek, D. J., and Rock, R. C. (1988). Monitoring hepatocellular carcinoma by using a monocloncal immunoenzymometric assay for alpha-fetoprotein. *Clin. Chem.* **34,** 76–81.

Rock, R. C., Chan, D. W., Bruzek, D. J., Waldron C., Oesterling, J., and Walsh, P. (1987). Evaluation of a monoclonal immunoradiometric assay for prostate-specific antigen. *Clin. Chem.* **33,** 2257–2261.

Solberg, H. E. (1986). Establishment and use of reference values. In "Textbook of Clinical Chemistry" (N. Tietz, ed.), pp. 371–378. W. B. Saunders, Philadelphia.

Walsh, P. C., Oesterling, J. E., Epstein, J. I., Bruzek, D. J., Rock, R. C., and Chan, D. W. (1989). The value of prostate-specific antigen in the management of localized prostate cancer. In "Therapeutic Progress in Urological Cancer" (G. Murphy and S. Khoury, eds.), pp. 27–33. Alan Liss, New York.

Zweig, M. H., and Robertson, E. A. (1987). Clinical validation of immunoassay: A well-designed approach to a clinical study. In "Immunoassay: A Practical Guide" (D. W. Chan, ed.), pp. 97–128. Academic Press, San Diego.

CHAPTER 6

Operational Evaluation

Daniel W. Chan
Department of Laboratory Medicine,
Clinical Chemistry Division,
The Johns Hopkins Hospital,
The Johns Hopkins University, Baltimore, Maryland

I. INTRODUCTION

One of the important benefits of automation is to enhance the efficiency of the laboratory operation. Two major issues of automation are the improvement of system operation and the impact of automation on laboratory operation. The first issue includes data management, servicing, and throughput of the automated system. The second issue relates to the impact on the laboratory as the result of the mechanization of the testing procedure, the consolidation of work stations, and the work flow. The operational enhancement will improve the turnaround time of the testing and the efficiency of the laboratory. To evaluate an automated immunoassay system, one should examine these operational issues.

II. SYSTEM OPERATION

A. Data Management

The data management system is the command center of an automated immunoassay system. In Chapter 2, Table 3 listed the desirable characteristics of a data management system. An automated system should have as many of these features as possible. As the medical technologist becomes a data manager, the data management system is critical for an efficient operation. The system should be user friendly with easy access to most daily routine functions. Results should be available to technologists on the computer screen in a logical fashion for quick verification and quality control checks. These functions should be user-defined.

This is particularly important for random access systems where multiple test results from a given patient will be reported. For example, thyroid function tests could be arranged in the order of diagnostic sequence: thyroxine (T_4), thyroid hormone uptake (TU), free thyroxine index (FTI), thyrotropin (TSH), and triiodothyronine (T_3). The calculation of FTI from T_4 and TU results will be useful in evaluating TSH and T_3 results. On the other hand, if the physician wants to begin the diagnostic sequence using highly sensitive TSH and free T_4 assays, the test menu could be set up differently to accommodate the particular need. An on-line quality control system will facilitate result reporting. The quality control issue has been discussed in Chapter 2. Other useful programs include work-load recording, quality assurance, productivity, turnaround time, and management functions.

B. Service

An automated system should require minimum servicing, both scheduled and unscheduled. Reliability of an automated system is one of the critical factors. Automation usually means consolidation of procedures into a system. The cost of acquiring such a fully automated system with high throughput is high. Most laboratories may not be able to afford more than one system. Therefore, malfunction of the system could shut down the entire immunoassay laboratory.

A detailed maintenance schedule should be set up to include daily, weekly, monthly, quarterly, and yearly services of the system. Modern instruments should contain sensors to detect error. When an error is detected, an error message should be apparent to the operator. Self-diagnosis of malfunction will facilitate troubleshooting, especially if a communication link exists between the manufacturer and the system. A 24-h hot line should be available for troubleshooting and technical information. One should ask the manufacturer for a commitment to service unscheduled problems. What response time can you expect by telephone and in person? Where is the service center located for the service technician? Where are the parts located and how will the parts be shipped to your laboratory?

Training of the operator is essential for the operation of an automated immunoassay system. This will reduce the number of service calls to the manufacturer. A well-organized training program should include the theory and principle of the system, system operation, data management, maintenance, and troubleshooting. Both lectures and hands-on practice are useful for the training. Training for in-house biomedical engineers may be helpful for more complicated systems. The availability of a box of parts may allow certain repairs to be performed by the user on site.

The turnaround time of most tests performed in a clinical laboratory is the most visible performance indicator. A late result may be useless no matter how accurate and precise it is. Therefore, one should stay away from a company with a poor reputation of service.

C. Throughout

It is difficult to compare throughout of various systems. Most companies listed the maximal throughput which is often unrealistic. Most available systems are between 30 and 180 tests/h. One should evaluate not only the throughput in terms of test/hour but also patient samples per hour and samples per working day. This is particularly important if the test is being done in duplicate. If the system is a batch analyzer, one should evaluate how many batches can be performed in a shift. It is more realistic to evaluate the throughput based on your own workload and the physician's ordering pattern. For example, if the batch size is 90 tests and the time for a batch 3 h, you may be able to perform only two batches in a shift. This is much less than the 240 tests you would expect if you use the throughput of 30 test/h. The throughput based on patient samples will depend on the calibration and quality-control frequencies as well as the batch size. The less frequent the calibration and quality control of a system, the closer the real throughput of patient samples will be to the theoretical throughput. This also applies to a random access analyzer. However, the true throughput of a random access analyzer is closer to the theoretical throughput, since the nonproductive time will be less than with a batch analyzer.

III. IMPACT OF AUTOMATION

The impact of automation on the laboratory operation is mainly on the mechanization of the testing procedure and the consolidation of work stations. Random access features of automation will facilitate the work flow and improve the turnaround time. Finally, automation may alter the testing location and the personnel of testing.

A. Mechanization

To evaluate an automated system, one should examine the steps of testing that are mechanized. The total laboratory testing process was defined in Table 1 of Chapter 2. Most systems only perform step 3, the testing procedure. However, step 2, the preanalytical variables, is most problematic for laboratories. Sample collection is time-consuming. Typically, a phlebotomist would collect the specimen from the patient. Transportation of the sample of the laboratory could be accomplished by sending the sample through a pneumatic tube or by a messenger. The tube would be centrifuged and the serum separated from the red cells. Then the serum sample would be aliquoted into separate tubes or cups for analysis by different work stations. Each work station performs one specific radioimmunoassay (RIA) test.

Automated systems should include the sample processing step, such as centrifugation and dilution. Whole-blood analyzers will eliminate the centrifugation step. Systems designed for decentralized testing may include a sample collection device. A totally automated system including the six steps of the total testing process is possible by combining computer technology for order entry and result reporting with a robotic device for sample application and analysis.

Automation will change the job function of a technologist from a technician to a data manager and quality control officer. It will eliminate manual pipetting and thus the "carpal tunnel" syndrome suffered by some technologists. Through work-station consolidation, it will reduce the labor requirements, in terms of both skill level and number. This will be discussed later in more detail in the economic considerations.

B. Work-Station Consolidation

Most automated systems are operated at about the same speed as an experienced technologist when only one assay is being performed. The ability to perform multiple assays is the advantage of an automated system. Therefore, the major benefit of automation is in the consolidation of work stations. One should evaluate how many work stations could be consolidated. The reduction in bench space and personnel should be evaluated. The disadvantage of consolidation is total dependency on the system. In the event of malfunction, the entire immunoassay testing will be shut down. One should consider backup options and redundant systems to ensure continued testing.

Automated systems, either batch or random access, should result in the consolidation of work stations. The extent of such consolidation will depend on the degree of random accessibility. An automated batch analyzer may allow partial consolidation, as with the TDx analyzer by Abbott (Chapter 23). The batch completion time is about 30 min. In an 8-h shift, one could perform 10–12 batches of 20 routine samples. Multiple TDx work stations are needed in order to perform both "stat" and "routine" requests. Efficiency is poor for small laboratories that may only perform one or two samples per batch. For larger laboratories, multiple instruments are needed to achieve satisfactory throughput and turnaround time.

A hybrid batch–random access system capable of analyzing multiple tests in a batch format will achieve intermediate consolidation, as with the ES-300 analyzer by BMD (Chapter 16). This type of automation will perform the day's work load with patient samples collected by the beginning of the day. Subsequent samples arriving later in the day will be analyzed in the next batch run in the afternoon or evening, depending on the length of the batch completion time.

A truly random access system with a broad menu and high throughput should allow maximum consolidation into one work station for immunoassay testing, such as the AIA-1200 analyzer by Tosoh Medics (Chapter 10). This type of system should eliminate scheduling of analytical runs. Tests will be performed as the sample arrives in the laboratory. The turnaround time should be improved. The advantage of a single work station is no sample aliquoting, no transferring to different work stations, and no hunting for a missing specimen. The personnel savings in such consolidation could be significant.

C. Random Access—A Case Study

To assess the impact of a random access automated system on the laboratory operation, we conducted a study in the clinical chemistry laboratory at the 1100-bed Johns Hopkins Hospital using the AIA-1200 analyzer manufactured by Tosoh Medics, Inc. We analyzed 847 routine patient samples during a 1-week period. Emergency or "stat" samples are excluded. The following nine assays were tested: T_4, T_3, thyrotropin (TSH), human chorionic gonadotropin (hCG), carcinoembryonic antigen (CEA), alpha-fetoprotein (AFP), prostate-specific antigen (PSA), prolactin, and ferritin.

The distribution of patient samples during the week is shown in Fig. 1.

1. Turnaround Time

In this study, the turnaround time is calculated from the time that the sample is received to the time that the result is available for reporting. The

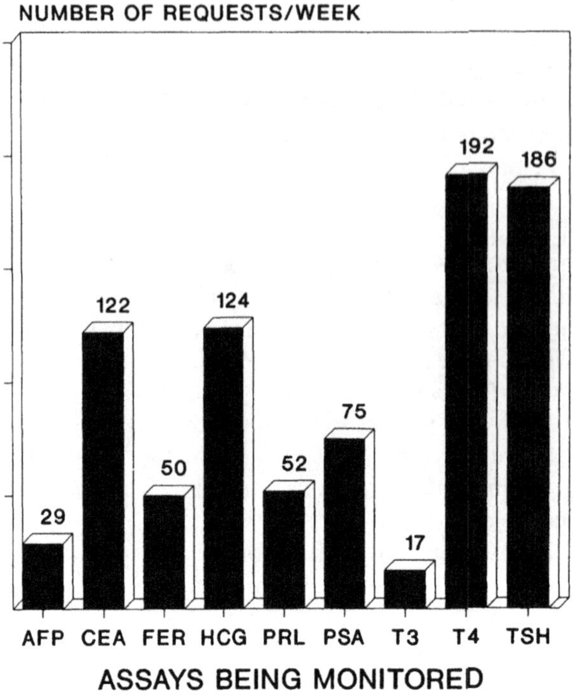

Figure 1 Test distribution for 1 week. Total = 847 of the selected assays.

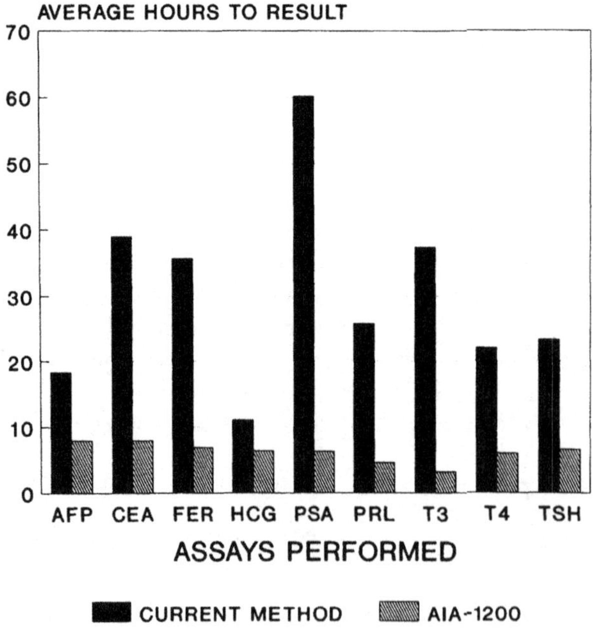

Figure 2 Turnaround time for batch vs. AIA-1200. Data excludes weekend samples since AIA-1200 was not run on weekends.

Table 1 Current Method

Test	Reagent	Manufacturer	Instrument
AFP	IEMA	Hybritech	Photon-Era
CEA	IEMA	Hybritech	Photon-Era
HCG	IEMA	Hybritech	Photon-Era
PRL	IEMA	Hybritech	Photon-Era
PSA	IRMA	Hybritech	γ-Counter
T_4	FPIA	Abbott	TDx
T_3	FPIA	Abbott	TDx
TSH	MEIA	Abbott	IMx
FER	MEIA	Abbott	IMx

average turnaround time is shown in Fig. 2. Significant improvement of turnaround is achieved using the random access analyzer AIA-1200 as compared to the current batch operation. The current methods are listed in Table 1. The improvement in turnaround time is mainly due to several factors. The first is the frequency of batch runs in a batch program. The fewer the batches, the longer the turnaround time. For example, PSA exhibits the longest turnaround time, 60 h, because PSA is performed twice a week. The hCG has the shortest turnaround time, 11 h, because there are 14 runs per week. The current test frequency is shown in Table 2. The second factor is the requirement of dilution. For samples with values greater than the linearity of the assay, the test will be repeated in the next run. This will prolong the turnaround time. Therefore, it is an advantage to have a greater linearity. When dilution is needed, it will be much easier on a random access analyzer since there will be no need to wait for the next run.

2. Batch Time

Batch time is the time needed to complete a run. The batch time is relatively constant, about 1.5–2 h. When compared to the AIA-1200 analyzer, the batch time is actually shorter on the Abbott TDX and IMx analyzers and longer on the Hybritech Photon-Era analyzer (Fig. 3). This shows that the random access analyzer will lose its advantage when oper-

Table 2 Test Frequency

Test	Runs/week	Test	Runs/week
AFP	3	T_4	5
CEA	5	T_3	3
PRL	3	TSH	5
hCG	14	FER	2
PSA	2		

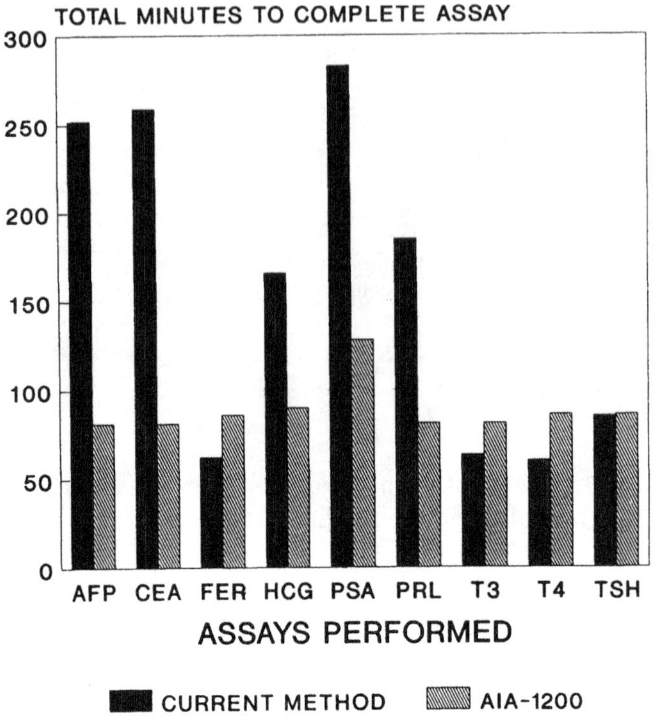

Figure 3 Batch completion time. Result data entry time excluded.

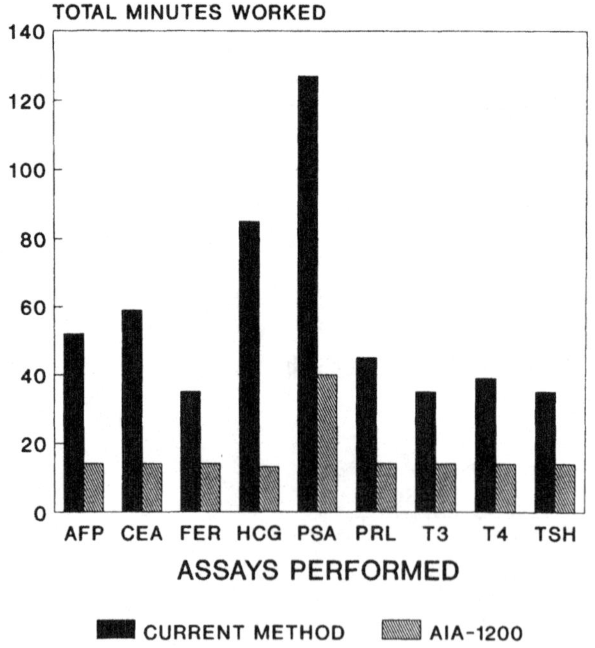

Figure 4 Batch technologist time. Result data entry time excluded.

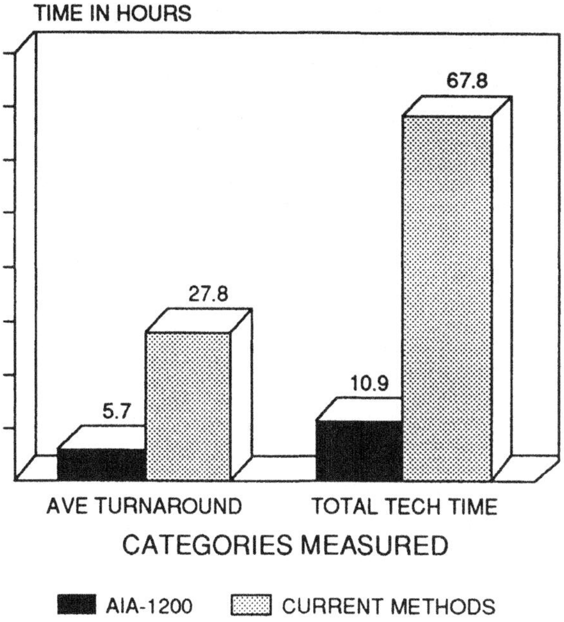

Figure 5 Summary of the comparison. Total of 798 specimens. Weekend runs not included.

ating in a batch mode and should be operated continuously in random access mode.

3. Technologist Time

The technologist time is measured as actual hands-on time per batch of testing. The technologist time on the random access analyzer is much less than the current manual method. This may represent the degree of automation. The least amount of technologist time on the batch analyzer is found with the Abbott TDX and IMx. The semiautomated Photon-Era analyzer comes in second. The manual PSA IRMA assay is the most time-consuming assay (Fig. 4). Furthermore, the current systems are not interfaced with the computer. The set up time should be reduced with computer interface. The batch time is longer for PSA on the TOSOH system because the batch size is larger than other assays, since PSA is performed only twice a week.

In summary, the advantages of a random access system are evident as shown in Fig. 5. The average turnaround time of the random access system is 5.7 h, versus 27.8 h on a batch analyzer. The average technologist time needed for a random access analyzer is 10.9 h, versus 67.8 h for the current method in performing the 798 specimens during the week of study.

CHAPTER 7

Economical Evaluation

Daniel W. Chan
Department of Laboratory Medicine,
Clinical Chemistry Division,
The Johns Hopkins Hospital,
The Johns Hopkins University, Baltimore, Maryland

I. INTRODUCTION

As the health care expenditure of the nation increases, there are increasing pressures to reduce cost at the level of the health care provider. The laboratory, in turn, is under considerable pressure to reduce costs. With the diagnostic related groups (DRGs) program, the laboratory becomes a cost center rather than a revenue generator. The health care provider is no longer reimbursed on cost plus, but on a given admission of patients to the hospital. Some hospitals have shifted their patient activities and laboratory testing from inpatient to outpatient services. At this moment, the reimbursement of outpatient testing is more favorable since there are no DRGs for outpatient activities. However, this situation will probably change in the near future. DRGs for outpatient service are definitely a possibility. Therefore, the key to economic success is to establish a cost-improvement program.

The cost-improvement program should include (1) increased productivity, (2) reduced labor requirement, (3) reduced system cost, and (4) reduced total cost. The total cost should include the cost of quality assurance and the impact of automation on the laboratory services, which, in turn, affects other areas of the hospital. Poor quality is expensive! In the laboratory, poor quality means repeat testing and a bad reputation. Outside the laboratory, it could jeopardize patient care, turnaround time, and

Immunoassay Automation: A Practical Guide

patient's length of stay in the hospital, and could mean possible litigation.

We will examine these four aspects of cost improvement in the economical evaluation of an automated immunoassay system.

II. PRODUCTIVITY

Productivity is defined as the output of product per full-time equivalent (FTE) of laboratory personnel. The product could be measured by the number of tests or work units. The higher the work unit per FTE, the higher the productivity. The work unit per FTE is a better indicator than the number of tests per FTE, since tests vary in their complexity. The more complicated the test, the larger the amount of time required to perform the test. For example, a highly sensitive thyrotropin (TSH) immunometric assay may require longer total system time than a single-step T_4 (thyroxine) assay.

First, let us examine the output of product. Most laboratory product is the testing of patient samples. The measurement of productivity should be based on the patient result. In the process of arriving at the final productivity, one should examine other testing support activities. These include calibration, quality control, duplicate testing, dilution of sample with values in excess of the highest calibrator, and repeat testing due to the malfunction of the system. A system that requires frequent calibration, quality control, and repeat testing will result in lower productivity of patient results. Automated systems should have a calibration curve stability of at least 2 weeks. Some systems are capable of achieving a calibration stability of several months. The calibration stability may vary with different analytes. For example, the Abbott TDx system can achieve a calibration stability of several months for the carbamazepine; however, the quinidine assay is stable for about 2 weeks. Individual users should evaluate each assay and establish criteria for quality control (QC) acceptance for a particular system.

The other factor that will affect productivity quite significantly is whether the testing should be performed in singlet or in duplicate. The argument for duplicate testing is to improve the precision and the reliability of the test result. In the general chemistry area, testing for electrolytes and glucose has been done in singlet for a long period of time, mainly due to automation. Now that fully automated immunoassay systems have become available, we should be able to perform these tests in singlet, just as we do the tests in general chemistry. However, the clinical impact of singlet testing should be considered. The impact of a single abnormal result far exceeds its general chemistry counterpart. Diagnosis is often made or confirmed with a single laboratory value. Examples are pregnancy testing, tumor marker, and other hormones in the diagnosis of endocrine disorders. As a clinical chemist, would you tell the doctor and the patient that she is pregnant or he has cancer if the decision is based on a crucial lab value? This is not only an economic decision, but also a moral and legal decision. A fully automated system is more reliable than the manual assay, but it is not foolproof! An automated system often improves precision; however, occasional outliers have been observed. For example, a system with antibody-coated tubes has been found to have one or two tubes without antibody coating. Unless the system is capable of detecting uncoated tubes, a negative result may be erroneously reported. You have to decide what price you are willing to pay for such occasional problems.

Quantitative measurement of productivity can be expressed in terms of work units per FTE. A commonly used work unit is the College of American Pathologists (CAP) work-load unit. In simple terms, one work-load unit is 1 min of personnel time. By adding up all the work-load units of a given system, one can calculate its productivity. In certain states, laboratory work is reimbursed at *X* cents per work-load unit. The revenues generated can be estimated. The cost of operating a laboratory can be analyzed by the cost per work-load unit as well. Using the work-load unit, automated systems could be compared in the total amount the work-load unit each generated. One can divide these units by the number of FTE needed to operate the system to arrive at the productivity figure.

III. LABOR REQUIREMENT

The labor component represents the greatest potential in cost improvement. Both the skill level and the number of FTE needed to operate the system will be affected by automation. The labor component represents the denominator of the productivity equation. With a given level of product output, the smaller the labor denominator, the higher the productivity.

The shortage of qualified technologists in the 1990s in both numbers and skill level underscores the importance of automation. Radioimmunoassay (RIA) is demanding for skilled technologists. Traditionally, performing RIA is not only a science, but also an art. Laboratories often designate special RIA technologists. Automation should improve this situation. However, a misconception exists that automation will not require skilled technologists. Automation requires and demands different levels of skill. Instead of needing a skilled pipettor in the RIA era, it demands a skilled instrument operator capable of performing maintenance and troubleshooting. It also demands the ability to manage larger amounts of data in a short period of time. Expertise in computer and data management is needed. Furthermore, quality control becomes even more important.

Automation demands different skills and training, but not necessarily less skill. The good news is that the number of technologists should be reduced due to the consolidation of work stations. Therefore, automation may help reduce the shortage of technologists. In the future, automation of the total testing process may lead to robotization of the clinical lab.

Any reduction in the labor requirement is not beneficial unless this saving can be turned into additional productivity. If the savings in technologist time is fragmented and difficult to convert to a significant block of time, the anticipated increase in productivity will be hard to realize. For a batch analyzer, the reduction in technologist time from 8 h to 6 h per day may not allow another batch to be run. There will be no increase in the output of product even though the productivity figure may have increased.

Automation of immunoassay will change the work habits of the technologists. RIA is often an individual task. Each technologist is responsible for a single test procedure from the beginning to the end. To fully utilize the automated system, one may wish to have one technologist feed the system continuously while another is verifying results, checking QC, and reporting patient results. Operating an automated system will become more a team effort.

IV. THE SYSTEM COST

The cost of acquiring and operating a system includes instrument, reagent, disposables, maintenance, service contract, and quality control.

Most manufacturers, as well as laboratorians, often negotiate the price for the instrument and reagent while other operating costs are not appreciated. Examples include the service contract, maintenance, disposables, and quality control. The annual service contract is often priced at about 10% of the instrument cost. For a $200,000 instrument, it represents an annual service contract of $20,000. Most service contracts only cover from 9 a.m. to 5 p.m., Monday thru Friday. Additional expenses are needed to cover other hours. If you are planning to use the system at all hours, you have to be prepared to pay more. One should also examine other aspects of the service contract. For example, are all parts covered? Does it include preventive maintenance? How many times per year? Maintenance is critical for the readiness of a system. How much time will it take to perform daily, weekly, monthly, and quarterly maintenance? If you are planning to operate the system on a 24-h basis, would you have time to do the daily maintenance? Do you have to shut down the system for a period of time and can you afford to do that? Do you need more than one system when considering both scheduled maintenance and unscheduled downtime? If so, it will cost you more.

Unscheduled downtime can be costly for both the laboratory and the hospital. The laboratory already has the technologist scheduled to work but cannot produce any useful products. The laboratory result is not available for the requesting physician. Not only does the turnaround time suffer, but also the patient's stay in the hospital may be lengthened. Troubleshooting starts with a well-designed system. Many features of a well-designed system were discussed in the earlier chapters. A good training program provided by the manufacturers is important for the operators to be able to troubleshoot problems. A 24-h hotline and helpful staff will expedite problem correction.

Disposable items can be costly on a daily basis if a system uses disposable curvettes, pipettes, tips, etc. For those systems with prepackaged reagents, the cost of reagent may include, but not always, one or more of the disposables. Some systems require a reaction cell for the separation step, which may not be included in this reagent cost. It is important to examine every aspect of the testing to include the cost of all disposables.

Quality control (QC) is essential but does not generate revenue. The cost of QC is determined by the frequency of QC and the QC material. The need for running QC with every batch of patient sample could be costly. Some systems require running one calibrator with each batch of patient sample to readjust the calibration curve. The cost of QC may be higher if the system requires unique QC materials from the manufacturer of the system to be used. The unique QC material could be expensive if it is the only material workable on the system due to matrix effect or interferences.

Manufacturers make most profit from the reagent and disposables but not as much from the instrument. The cost of reagent should be analyzed not only per test, but per patient. A number of factors will affect reagent usage and hence reagent cost (Table 1). Examples are single versus duplicate testing, frequency of calibration, QC, retesting of samples with values greater than the assay dynamic range, and malfunction of the system. The other factor is waste. Every system has waste due to the design of the system, the stability of reagent after it is opened (i.e., the shelf life), and the particular work load in your laboratory. A system with

Table 1 Factors That Affect Reagent Usage

Replicate testing
Calibration frequency
Quality control frequency
Repeat testing due to system malfunction
Dilution for over the range
Waste factor

lower reagent cost per test may in fact be more expensive if it has a higher waste factor. The waste factor is usually between 5 and 20%. Many companies will discount the reagent, but not the calibrator. Some will charge you extra for the substrate in the enzyme immunoassay system. It is advisable to ask the cost for all the necessary materials to operate the system.

Finally, the instrument cost is becoming unpredictable. In most closed systems, the instrument cost is not as important to the manufacturer since you have to purchase the reagent and disposable from them. The pricing of automated immunoassay systems is more an art than a science. It is often determined by the market forces at a given time. In general, purchasing of the system is probably the most economical approach since the manufacturer will most likely give you a better reagent price. In other situations, it may be more advantageous to rent or lease. For example, during the phase of rapid changing technology, it may be wiser to rent so that your system will not be obsolete before the end of the useful life.

V. THE TOTAL COST

In addition to the cost items discussed earlier, some other hidden costs are usually not appreciated. One should examine the total cost to include quality assurance (QA) and impact on the health care provider. Quality assurance has become increasingly important. The Joint Commission of American Health Care Organization (JCAHO) has emphasized the outcome measurement of a quality improvement program. The cost for such a program has been estimated to cost hospitals about 2–5% of the operating budget. In a clinical laboratory, the cost of QA including QC could be as high as 20–30%.

The impact of turnaround time and of the level of laboratory service on the hospital is difficult to measure. One indicator is the length of stay of patients in the hospital. Any avenue to reduce the length of stay will save hospital money. In the DRG environment, the shorter the stay the more economical it will be. An automated system could provide more frequent testing and better turnaround time. This may lead to faster diagnosis and workup of the patient. It will expedite the discharge of the patient. For example, a rapid creatine kinase MB (CK-MB) assay may be helpful in removing patients from the coronary care unit (CCU). Good automation means quality. Poor quality is expensive for the hospital. Litigation is expensive. It may be difficult to measure the cost savings as the result of quality improvement.

VI. SYSTEM ACQUISITION

After considering the productivity and the cost issues, the challenge is how to acquire the system. In these days of cost containment, it may need some creative financing to acquire capital equipment. In addition to outright purchase, other options include leasing and reagent rental with the use of the system. The decision as to which option is most beneficial will depend on your unique situation. Let us consider these options.

A. Purchase Option

Purchasing the system is usually, but not always, the lowest cost option. If you only purchase the instrument but not the reagent from the same manufacturer, you would have to pay top money to acquire the system. On the other hand, if you purchase the entire system including instrument and reagent, you would probably be able to negotiate the best price. Most of the fully automated systems are closed systems—that is, they use dedicated reagent. Therefore, the decision on whether to purchase the entire system or not may not be an issue.

To secure funding for acquiring the system may be difficult and time-consuming. You would have to request a specific equipment purchase from your institution. This may require planning for more than 1 year in advance. You have to justify the request to a capital equipment committee. The members of this committee seldom know any technical details of the equipment.

Taking ownership of the system will provide greater flexibility in the choice of reagent. One can use suppliers of the reagent other than the manufacturer of the instrument. This may have both quality and economical advantages. The laboratory may choose to make its own reagent from bulk chemicals. This approach is more economical for large laboratories, especially multiple branches of commercial laboratories. Other savings could come in the area of service contracts. By using an in-house biomedical engineer rather than purchasing a service contract from the vendor, savings could be substantial.

There are several disadvantages to owning the system. In an era of rapid changing technology, the system may be obsolete before the end of its useful life. It also ties up a large amount of cash that the laboratory could use for other purposes. If the system does not perform as expected, it will be more difficult to return it. The service contract could be expensive since it usually costs at least 10% of the system's price.

B. Leasing Option

Leasing is preferable if cash is not available for outright purchase of the system. This option allows better cash flow since it spreads the payment over a longer period of time. The usual leasing period is 3–5 years. If owning the system is desirable, one should negotiate a lease with purchase option at the end of the leasing agreement. Most systems will be fully depreciated by the end of the term. Therefore, purchasing of the system will be quite inexpensive. This is particularly attractive if the system is well built and the expected useful life is longer than the leasing term. Some companies will include a service contract at a deep discount as part of the leasing agreement.

The company is as interested as you in maintaining the system properly to ensure the useful life of the system.

Leasing could be expensive if the interest rate used in the calculation is much higher than the prevailing rate. It is not uncommon to charge 50–100% above the prime lending rate. The penalty of such a high rate is worsened with nonprofit hospitals. Such hospitals may be able to sell tax-free bonds at lower than the prime rate to finance the purchase of capital equipment.

C. Reagent Rental Option

Reagent rental is probably more expensive than the two options mentioned above. In addition to the added charges of using the equipment, the reagent cost may be inflated. However, this option allows a great deal of flexibility for the user. Even though reagent rental has a period of agreement similar to leasing of 3–5 years, it usually has a cancellation clause of 60–90 days. In the rapid changing technology of clinical chemistry or computers, it may be an advantage to stay flexible. Perhaps some new technology may be so much more efficient that the savings in labor may be greater than the interest charge of renting the system.

The concern of using "lock-in" reagent from the manufacturer of the instrument may not be as real nowadays. Most automated immunoassay systems have dedicated reagents. These reagents are formulated and formatted with such a unique concept that other automated systems will not be compatible. In addition, better quality control can be assured if both instrument and reagent are produced by the same manufacturer. The competition is so strong among manufacturers that the technological advantages and quality improvements are comparable between systems. The laboratory should not be as concerned about choosing the best assay from different companies.

The "system use" option is another term for the reagent rental option. This option was particularly popular with the introduction of the Abbott TDx analyzer. For the first time, a small laboratory was able to perform immunoassay for TDM drugs and hormones that had otherwise been sent to an outside laboratory. In the 1980s, many hospital laboratories ventured into the commercial laboratory business with outpatient services. The "old" commercial labs became competition for the hospital labs. There were greater incentives to set up testing even for very low-volume tests. The long-term calibration curve stability also enhances the capability of these small laboratories in providing low-volume tests.

The other advantage is that one need not purchase the service contract. If the system fails, the manufacturer will either repair or replace it. For these small hospital labs, if the venture proves to be unprofitable, they may cancel the reagent contract and return the entire system. The benefits outweigh the risks.

D. Creative Options

What if all three of the above options fail? If you determine that an automated immunoassay system is what you really need, you have to be creative. Examples follow.

1. Cost Improvement

Try to justify a plan to your administrator even if no funds are available. You should evaluate the total cost and formulate a cost-improvement plan. You should be able to save labor so it can be used to expand services by generating new revenue. You might be able to replace an expensive service contract and save costly repair expenses. You may be able to shorten the length of patient's stay in the hospital. You may be able to improve quality assurance and save the hospital expensive litigation. Try to focus on the total cost discussed earlier.

2. Used System

If the price of a new system is out of your reach, try a used system. Companies are more willing to discount for a used system. A "used" system could be defined as a demonstrator unit used by a sales person. This could be a system evaluated by others during a beta site evaluation. It may even be newly built for a customer but the order was canceled. Acquiring a used system requires careful screening. Some instruments are not reliable after use. One should avoid instruments with a lot of moving parts, such as a centrifuge or a centrifugal analyzer.

3. Loaner System

If you have limited funds and need a bigger discount than the manufacturer is willing to give, consider working with the company as an external evaluation. You could provide a demonstration site for potential customers to come and see the system in operation. You will, of course, be expected to purchase reagents. If you do not have funds available right away, ask for a loaner.

4. Partnership

Consider a partnership agreement with the manufacturer. This could be a joint venture of the lab services. It will be attractive for new services. This could be a value-added package to include other lab supplies purchased from the same vendor. The agreement may involve other services or benefits that the vendor may value, such as consultation provided by the clinical lab to the vendor, test site for new products, product integration, and training of personnel from the company.

5. Joint Purchase

An individual lab has limited test volume and hence less "clout" with the manufacturer in negotiating a discount. Consider joining forces with other hospitals in the area to form a single purchasing group. The higher volume of the combined lab will result in a lower price per test. Hospital groups across the country may also benefit from such an arrangement. For example, the volunteering hospital association (VHA) of nonprofit hospitals has negotiated VHA pricing for its member hospitals.

PART THREE

Automated Immunoassay Systems

CHAPTER 8

Introduction of Automated Immunoassay Systems

Daniel W. Chan
Department of Laboratory Medicine,
Clinical Chemistry Division,
The Johns Hopkins Hospital,
The Johns Hopkins University, Baltimore, Maryland

I. INTRODUCTION

Part III of this volume consists of chapters describing individual immunoassay systems. The chapters are arranged alphabetically according to the name of the system. It is impossible to include every available automated immunoassay system. The systems covered in this book do represent a rather wide spectrum of instrumentation intended for various laboratory settings. Some systems are suitable for large laboratories, for example, the AIA-1200 analyzer (Chapter 10), while others may be used in small laboratories in locations ranging from hospital or clinic to physician's office, such as the Eclipse ICA (Chapter 15). Although these systems are different in many respects, they are dedicated analyzers for immunodiagnostics. Most general chemistry analyzers could be adapted to perform homogeneous immunoassays for small molecules, mainly drug assays. With the exception of the Cobas-Fara II (Chapter 12), these systems are not included in this book, among them the BMD-Hitachi 717 and 747 analyzers.

Both semiautomated and fully automated immunoassay systems are included in this book. Large laboratories, particularly commercial laboratories may find semiautomated systems such as the Magic-Lite system

Immunoassay Automation: A Practical Guide

Table 1 Automated Immunoassay Systems[a]

Descriptor	System															
	Affinity	AIA-1200	Amer-lite	Cobas-Fara	Cyber-Fluor	DELFIA	Eclipse	ES-300	IMX	Magic/ ACS180	Opus	Photon-Era	SR-1	Stratus	TDx	Vista
Manufacturer	BD	Tosoh	Amer-S	Roche	CyberF	LKB	Biotope	BMD	Abbott	Ciba	PB	Hybritech	Serono	Dade	Abbott	Syva
Chapter	9	10	11	12	13	14	15	16	17	18	19	20	21	22	23	24
Automation																
Total	Y	Y	N	Y	N	N	Y	Y	Y	N/Y	Y	N	Y	Y	Y	Y
Semiautomated	N	N	Y	N	Y	Y	N	N	N	Y/N	N	Y	N	N	N	N
Analyte																
Number	9	15	15	14	11	25	4	17	36	16	10	12	17	30	60	6
Type	H,D(l)	H,T	H,D(l)	D	H	All,D(l)	H,D(l)	H,D(l),T	H,T,I	H,T	H,D	H,T(a)	H	H,D,T	D,H	H
Assay																
Homogeneous	N	N	N	Y	N	N	N	N	N	N	N	N	N	N	Y	N
Heterogeneous	Y	Y	Y	N	Y	Y	Y	Y	Y	Y	Y	Y	Y	Y	N	Y
Competitive	Y	Y	Y	Y	Y	Y	Y	Y	Y	Y	Y	N	Y	Y	Y	Y
Immunometric	Y	Y	Y	N	Y	Y	Y	Y	Y	Y	Y	Y	Y	Y	N	Y
Label	E	E	E	F	F	F	E	E	E	A	E	E	E	E	F	E
Signal	S	F	L	F	F	F	F	S	F	L	F	S	S/F	F	F	F
Separation	C	M	C	N	C	C	P	C	PF	M	CF/MF	B	M	CF	NA	M
Prepackaged	Y	Y	N	N	N	N	Y	N	N	N	Y	N	Y	N	N	N

Sample																
Tray capacity	32	100	96	30	96	96	16	160	24	60	20	60	30	30	20	50
Primary tube	N	N	N	N	N	N	N	N	N	N/Y	N	N	N	N	N	N
Multiple tests	N	Y	Y	N	Y	Y	N	Y	N	N/Y	Y	N	Y	Y	N	Y
Random access	Y	Y	N	N	N	N	Y	N	N	N/Y	Y	N	Y	Y	Y	N
Selective	Y	Y	N	Y	N	N	Y	Y	N	N/Y	Y	N	Y	Y	Y	Y
Batch	Y	Y	Y	Y	Y	Y	Y	Y	Y	Y/Y	Y	Y	Y	Y	Y	Y
Stat add	Y	Y	N	Y	N	N	N	N	N	N/Y	Y	N	Y	Y	N	N
Replicate	1	1	2	1	2	2	1	1	1	2/1	1	2	1	1	1	1
Throughput																
Incubation time	30–60 min	40 min	15–60 min	5–15 min	0.5–2 h	1–4 h	17 min	50–210 min	30–45 min	30 min/ 15 min	6–21 min	1–3 h	NA	8 min	20–45 min	NA
Time to first result	30–60 min	50 min	30–90 min	5 min	0.7–2.4 h	1.2–4.5 h	17 min	1–4 h	40–60 min	NA/15 min	10–25 min	2–4 h	35–102 min	10 min	25–50 min	NA
Time between results	2 min	0.5 min	NA	0.5 min	NA	NA	NA	NA	NA	NA/20 s	30 s	NA	NA	NA	NA	18 s
Maximum	30	120	192	120	192	96	60	100	36	180	20–75	60	55	60	60	120
Calibration																
Full curve	2w	4w	0	2–4w	0	0	L	2w	2w	0/1w	2–8w	0	4w	2w	3w	4w
Single calibration	N	N	NA	N	NA	NA	NA	0	0	N	N	N	0	N	N	N

[a] Key. Analyte type: H, hormone; D, Drug; T, tumor marker; I, infectious disease; (l), limited; (a), FDA-approved. Label: E, enzyme; F, fluorescence; A, acridinium ester. Signal: S, spectrophotometric; F, fluorometric; L, luminescence. Separation: C, coated tube; M, magnetic; P, particle; PF, particle filter; MF, multilayer film; B, coated bead; CF, coated filter paper; N, no. Throughput: maximum, number of tests per hour; NA, not available or applicable. Calibration: full curve, W, week; O, every run; L, lot specific; single calibration, O, every run; N, no.

(Chapter 18) to be more cost-effective for high-volume testing than a totally automated system like the Affinity system (Chapter 9). Most hospital laboratories require both routine and emergency testing. Patient samples arrive in the laboratory around the clock. A truly random access analyzer like the Affinity system, rather than a batch analyzer such as the Photon-Era analyzer (Chapter 20), may be most convenient to the laboratory. The turnaround time should be improved with continuous testing.

All systems described should be available when this book is published. Some systems have been used for several years, for example, the TDx system (Chapter 23), the Stratus system (Chapter 22), and the Photon-Era analyzer. Other systems are relatively new, for example, the Vista system (Chapter 24), the SR-1 system (Chapter 21), and the Eclipse ICA system.

II. SUMMARY OF THE AUTOMATED IMMUNOASSAY SYSTEMS

A summary of the automated immunoassay systems included in this book is outlined in Table 1. The table is organized according to the chapters. You will find a summary of key features of these systems for quick comparison, starting with the system name, manufacturer, and chapter number. The degree of automation may be total or semiautomated. The number of analytes and their types are given, as hormone, drug, tumor marker, and infectious agents. The assay formats include homogeneous, heterogeneous, competitive binding, immunometric (sandwich), label (enzyme, fluorescent compound, etc.), and the signal (spectrophotometric, fluorometric, luminescent, etc.). The separation of bound from unbound antigen may be achieved by various techniques including magnetic particle, multilayer film, particle, bead, filter paper, etc. Some systems use prepackaged reagents.

The sampling aspect includes the tray capacity for samples, the ability to sample from the primary blood drawing tube and perform multiple tests on one sample, the ability of the system to perform random access, selective, or batch testing, and the capability to add a "stat" sample. Testing could be performed in either singlet or duplicate. The throughput of the system should be examined in terms of the incubation time, the time required for the first result and subsequent results, and the maximum throughput. Finally, the calibration-curve stability will be compared with the frequency of calibration using either the entire curve or a single calibrator. Some systems recommend a full calibration once a month; however, on a daily basis, one calibrator test is performed to adjust the calibration curve.

Chapter 18 includes both the Magic Lite enhanced system and the automated ACS-180 system. Different characteristics of both systems are indicated by Magic/ACS-180.

III. FUTURE SYSTEMS

The future immunoassay system will be more automated than the current systems in the total testing process as discussed in earlier chapters. These will include both the pre- and postanalytical steps. The preanalytical step is mainly sample handling and order entry. The postanalytical step will focus on the information processing, for example, result reporting and interpretation. Random access will be the standard feature of the automated system.

Technical advances in the signal amplification and detection will improve the sensitivity of the assay. Chemiluminescent detection like the Amerlite system (Chapter 11) and Magic Lite system (Chapter 18) have inherent advantages in sensitivity. Perhaps newer labels in the future will enhance the detection limit. Time-resolved fluorescence units like the CyberFluor immunoanalyzer (Chapter 13) with new labels incorporating more light-emitting capability will further improve sensitivity. A modular approach in system design will allow the same technology to be used in low- or high-throughput instruments using the same reagent. These systems could be placed in commercial or hospital laboratories, clinics, emergency rooms, intensive care units, and physicians' offices, as well as remote testing centers and patients' homes.

CHAPTER 9

Affinity Immunoassay System

Daniel W. Chan and Cynthia Kelley
Department of Laboratory Medicine,
Clinical Chemistry Division,
The Johns Hopkins Hospital,
The Johns Hopkins University, Baltimore, Maryland

I. INTRODUCTION

The Affinity is a fully automated, random access system for the performance of immunoassay using prepackaged reagents. Each test is performed with an individual test unit, an ImmUnit. The ImmUnit contains six wells: one well for the sample, four wells for reagents, and one well for the mixing, incubation, and detection steps. Antibodies are coated on the surface of a tube within the ImmUnit. The detector can measure either absorbance or fluorescence.

The Affinity system is a desk-top instrument, relatively compact in size, 28(W) × 25 (D) × 15½ (H) in. A test may be run in either routine or stat mode. The calibration curve is stable for at least 2 weeks. On-line quality control is available. The system is designed to handle low- to medium-volume testing with random test selection capability. The system is suitable for a 24-h laboratory operation.

This chapter describes the Affinity system, both instrumentation and reagent. The performance of the system is evaluated with data generated from our laboratory. We will discuss mainly the technical, clinical, and operational performance.

Immunoassay Automation: A Practical Guide

II. SYSTEM DESCRIPTION

A. Instrumentation

The Affinity system consists of two major components: computer, and instrument for testing. Figure 1 displays the major areas of the instrument.

1. Computer

The Affinity computer consists of hardware and software. The membrane keypad is equipped with audio feedback. It provides the input information and commands to the instrument. Options include editing, result availability, and instrument status. It loads either routine or stat samples and unloads a single tray or an entire carousel. The liquid-crystal display (LCD) provides a two-line, 40-character-per-line display. It shows the current operational status of the instrument, including a time clock. It prompts the operator to load and unload samples, indicates any warnings or errors, and lists selections for any OPTIONS functions. The thermal printer is dot-matrix with 40 characters per line. It sits on top of the instrument.

The Affinity software is stored in a $3\frac{1}{2}$-in diskette with 720K memory. The single disk drive is located at the lower right-hand corner of the instrument. The software controls the Affinity's mechanical actions, such

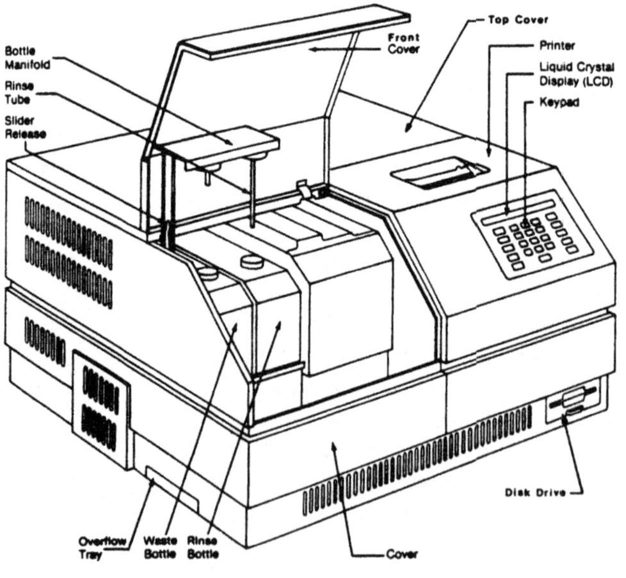

Figure 1 Major areas of the Affinity system.

as transferring samples from the sample tray and carousel, reading the bar code, and executing the appropriate actions. It also controls other tasks such as ensuring that calibrator and control sets are complete, efficient scheduling, processing, and testing of samples, recognizing stat samples, and automatically report test results.

2. Instrument Testing Components

The instrument testing components consist of sample tray, work station, carousel, and detector assembly.

The molded, plastic sample tray contains 16 positions for the placement of ImmUnits. The ImmUnits fit into the sample tray in only one direction.

The work station is located between the sample tray and the carousel. It consists of the following assemblies: a bar-code reader, a shuttle mechanism, a punch apparatus, a transfer pipette, and a rinse/waste pipette. When a tray containing ImmUnits advances to the work station, a bar-code reader above the tray reads the ImmUnit label. The label contains the lot number, the individual identification number, the test request, and the testing parameters. The shuttle moves ImmUnits between the tray, the work station, and the carousel. All the appropriate steps including pipetting, mixing, and rinsing are performed in this area.

The carousel is a rotating, circular rack with 32 slot positions. It is enclosed within a housing at 37±0.8°C with hot air. All incubations occur in the carousel. It also acts as a transport for ImmUnits between the work station and the detectors.

The detector assembly measures either fluorescence or absorbance. There are two detectors. A fluorescent detector is positioned at 90° to the light source, which is a tungsten–halogen lamp. Interference filters located on a rotating filter wheel to provide selection of desired wavelengths are used as monochromators. The fluorescent signal is quantified by photon counting. This provides a high signal-to-noise ratio and good sensitivity, particularly at low analyte concentration. A photodiode detector is used to measure absorbance.

B. Reagents

1. ImmUnit

The ImmUnit is a self-contained, ready-to-use, analyte-specific package that consists of six cups attached to a headpiece (Fig. 2). Each ImmUnit is designed to perform one test. The first cup is for the sample. On top of this cup is a label with a star-shaped perforation to aid in sample dispensing and help prevent sample evaporation. The next four cups con-

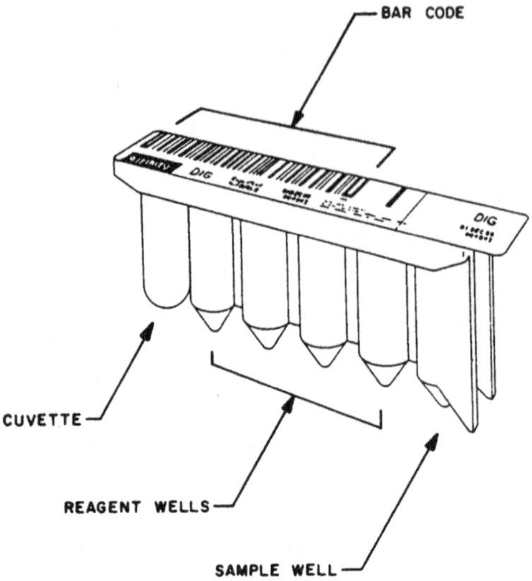

Figure 2 The Affinity ImmUnit.

tain reagents. An example is thyrotropin (TSH). Cup 2 contains reagent A: substrate-hydrogen peroxide. Cup 3 contains reagent B: chromogen-3,3′,5,5′-tetramethylbenzidine (TMB). Cup 4 contains stop solution–aqueous citric acid. Cup 5 contains enzyme conjugate: horseradish peroxidase (HRP) coupled to goat anti-hTSH antibody (IgG) in a Tris-buffered protein solution. The sixth cup is a clear plastic cup, which serves as a reaction or measurement cuvette.

A bar-code label displays a three-character test code (e.g., DIG for digoxin), a production lot number (the lot expiration date), and an ImmUnit identification number. This ID number could be used as a patient identification number. The information on the label is displayed alphanumerically as well as in bar-code format. One end of the bar-code label forms a tear-off adhesive tab with the same information. This tab may be placed on the test worksheet for test identification. The label also has two boxes, which could be filled in with a black pen. One is designated CAL for calibrator testing, and the other is designated CON for control testing.

2. Assay Principles

Two different methodologies are used in the Affinity system: a competitive binding assay for small analytes, and a sandwich immunoenzymetric assay (IEMA) for large analytes.

a. Competitive Immunoassay Analytes with low molecular weight, such as thyroxine (TT_4) and digoxin (DIG), are measured using this approach. A limited amount of antibodies is immobilized on the surface of a polystyrene tube. Horseradish-peroxidase–labeled antigen is added to compete with the unknown antigen for the binding site on the antibody. After incubation, the unbound antigen is washed away. The transfer pipette aspirates chromogen, 3,3′,5,5′-tetramethylbenzidine (TMB), from reagent cup 3 and substrate, hydrogen peroxide, from reagent cup 2 to the coated tube. After incubation, citric acid from reagent cup 4 is added to stop the enzyme reaction. The colored solution will turn from blue to yellow. The absorbance is measured at a primary wavelength of 450 nm and a secondary wavelength of 630 nm as a reference to eliminate the tube-to-tube differences. The absorbance is inversely proportional to the analyte concentration. The greater the analyte concentration, the lower the absorbance.

b. Immunoenzymetric Assay Analytes with high molecular weight, such as thyrotropin (TSH), prolactin (PRL), and luteinizing hormone (LH), are measured based on this approach. Two different antibodies in excess are used in the sandwich assay. Each antibody is directed against a different epitope on the antigen molecule. One antibody is bound to the surface of the antigen molecule. One antibody is bound to the surface of the polystyrene tube. The other antibody is conjugated with horseradish peroxidase. In the simultaneous IEMA, the sample is incubated in the antibody-coated tube with the conjugate antibody. In the sequential assay, the sample is incubated first in the antibody-coated tube without the conjugate. After a washing step, the conjugate is introduced for a second incubation. At the end of the incubation period, the tube is washed to remove any unbound conjugate. The transfer pipette aspirates chromogen (TMB) from cup 3 and substrate (hydrogen peroxide) from cup 2 into the coated tube. At the end of the enzyme incubation, citric acid is added from cup 4 to stop the enzyme reaction. The ImmUnit is read in the same way as described for the competitive immunoassay.

c. Data Reduction Four-parameter logistic analysis is used to calculate calibration curves. Data from the calibrator points are fitted to a hyperbolic equation using a least-squares technique that weights the data points according to a matched-response algorithm. The weighting factors reduce the effect of outliers on the curve, and the iterative process determines the best curve fit for the data.

Before the calibration curve is calculated, several checks will be performed. A minimum number of calibrator points should be present. The signal values are reasonable. The difference between the signal for the lowest and highest concentration calibrators exceeds a defined limit. If all these factors are within the limits, the curve is accepted.

III. SYSTEM PERFORMANCE

The performance of the Affinity immunoassay system was evaluated over 2 years in the clinical chemistry laboratory of the Johns Hopkins Hospital. Some assays have been revised more than once. Here we will summarize our most recent findings.

A. Technical Performance

1. Precision

The intraassay precision was calculated with a number of consecutive, single data points as indicated in Table 1. Three levels of quality control samples were used in the determination. The intraassay precision has improved over the evaluation period, with the data presented here representing the latest reagent. The interassay precision was determined by the quality control results over the number of days indicated in Table 2. Occasional outliers were observed. Overall, the precisions were acceptable. Most coefficients of variation (CVs) were 10% or less.

2. Sensitivity

The sensitivity was determined by the mean + 2SD of the zero calibrator (Table 3). Overall, the sensitivity was acceptable. The sensitivity of TSH was determined to be 0.05 mIU/ml. This level was also confirmed by diluting patient samples with low TSH values with assay diluent.

3. Linearity

The linearity of each test was determined by diluting patient samples with the assay diluent. We were able to verify the linearity up to certain values as shown in Table 4. In most cases, these were the highest values of the available samples tested. The linearity of TT4 varies from sample to

Table 1 Intraassay Precision

		Mean and CV%						
Analyte	Unit	Level I		Level II		Level III		*N*
TT4	μg/dl	2.6	8%	8.6	6%	12	4%	20
TUP	%	26	6%	34	5%	46	6%	10
TSH	μIU/ml	2.7	3%	8.1	3%	30	3%	20
hCG	mIU/ml	14.3	9%	99	2%	697	4%	20
PRL	ng/ml	7.8	12%	23	7%	136	4%	20
DIG	ng/ml	0.94	4%	1.8	7%	3.3	6%	10

Table 2 Interassay Precision

Analyte	Unit	Mean and CV%						N
		Level I		Level II		Level III		
TT4	μg/dl	2.5	6%	7.9	10%	11.7	9%	10
TUP	%	26	7%	35	8%	47	7%	33
TSH	μIU/ml	3.0	5%	8.4	5%	30.5	5%	20
hCG	mIU/ml	16.2	11%	97	2%	670	3%	10
PRL	ng/ml	8.0	11%	21	7%	42.9	7%	24
DIG	ng/ml	0.83	8%	1.7	7%	3.0	5%	26

sample. Therefore, no upper limit of linearity was indicated. The linearity claimed by the manufacturer was also shown for comparison.

4. Method Comparison

Comparison methods used in this study were the TDx and IMx analyzers from Abbott Labs (North Chicago, Illinois 60064); the Tandem assays from Hybritech Inc. (San Diego, CA 92121); and radioimmunoassay (RIA) from Ciba-Corning (Medfield, Massachusetts 02052) and Diagnostic Products (Los Angeles, California 90045). The linear regression analysis of the method comparison with the Affinity method on the *Y* axis and the comparison method on the *X* axis are shown in Table 5. The correlation was mostly acceptable with *r* between 0.917 to 0.999. The slope of the linear regression line varied from 0.77 to 1.26.

5. Calibration Curve Stability

We found the calibration curve to be stable for at least 2 weeks.

B. Clinical Performances

1. Reference Values

The reference values were determined for a specific group of healthy individuals or patients (Table 6). Euthyroid patients were used for TT4 and

Table 3 Sensitivity

TT4	0.1 μg/dl
TSH	0.05 μIU/ml
hCG	2.7 mIU/ml
PRL	0.74 ng/ml
DIG	0.3 ng/ml

Table 4 Linearity

	Linearity	
Analyte	Tested	Claimed
TT4	See text	25 μg/dl
TSH	32	50 μIU/ml
hCG	970	1000 mIU/ml
PRL	190	200 ng/ml
DIG	5.9	6 ng/ml

TSH. Hyperthyroid patients were useful to assess the sensitivity of TSH assay. Nonpregnant individuals were used to determine the normal human chorionic gonadotropin (hCG) values. Healthy males and females were used for prolactin study. Reference values should be established by each laboratory using their own populations.

2. Digoxinlike Immunoreactive Factor

Digoxinlike immunoreactive factor (DLIF) has been observed in specific patient populations without taking digoxin. These populations include neonates, renal and/or hepatic failure, and pregnant women. Apparent digoxin values have been reported in a number of immunoassays as discussed in Chapter 4, Technical Evaluation. We evaluated the Affinity digoxin assay using these patients. Similar results were observed as compared to the TDx digoxin II assay. All digoxin values were below the therapeutic level, less than 0.6 ng/ml, indicating the presence of low-level DLIF.

Table 5 Method Comparison

Affinity (Y)	Comparison (X)	Unit	Range	Slope	Intercept	r	N
TT4	IMx	μg/dl	0–20	1.26	0.19	0.917	47
FTI	Corning/DPC		0–30	1.12	1.22	0.941	133
TSH	IMx	μIU/ml	0–50	1.12	0.25	0.932	108
			0–5	1.21	0.03	0.984	88
hCG	Tandem-E	mIU/ml	0–1000	0.86	1.04	0.999	41
PRL	Tandem-E	ng/ml	0–200	0.77	0.017	0.966	34
DIG	TDx	ng/ml	0–5.6	1.00	0.12	0.985	120

Table 6 Reference Values

Analyte	Patient	Mean ± 2SD
TT4	Euthyroid	4.1–15.0 μg/dl
TUP	Normal	26–36%
TSH	Euthyroid	to 4.3 μIU/ml
TSH	Hyperthyroid	0–0.06 μIU/ml
hCH	Nonpregnant	0–7 mIU/ml
PRL	Normal male	0–18 ng/ml
PRL	Normal female	0–13 ng/ml

C. Operational Performances

1. System Operation

The Affinity is an easy instrument to operate. After the ImmUnits have been loaded, the instrument requires no "hands-on" by the operator. To prepare a tray to be loaded, the ImmUnits are placed in the slots within a tray. The ImmUnits can be placed in any order since the Affinity has both random access and batch running capabilities. Each ImmUnit has an identification tab over the sample cup that can be peeled off and attached to a work sheet. A required minimum volume of sample specific to each test is dispensed into the sample cup using a volumetric pipette. Only one test result can be determined per ImmUnit. All controls and calibrators need to be designated with a black marker by coloring in the appropriate portion of the bar-code label. Calibrators need to be loaded in order of increasing concentration. A full calibration is stable for a minimum of 2 weeks. Controls for each test must be run daily and are loaded as a complete set. Calibrators, controls, and samples can be run in duplicate or singlet. If they are run in duplicate, the corresponding ImmUnits cannot be split up and must be loaded side-by-side as a pair.

To load a tray, the operator can press either the "Routine" or "Stat" key. All routine samples are placed in the tray from right to left and are loaded by the instrument onto the carousel in that order. Stats are placed in the tray from left to right according to the number of spaces preprogrammed for stats. Both routines and stats can be loaded on the same tray as long as there is a space to separate the two loading sequences. After pressing a loading key option, lift the instrument cover and place the tray into the loading track. Once the cover is closed, the instrument will begin to load the ImmUnits through the shuttle area and onto the carousel. It is possible to interrupt a tray that is being loaded to add stats or load more routines by pressing the "unload/tray" key. The Affinity will immediately stop loading the tray, release it from the shuttle area, and return the tray to the home position. Open the cover and add the samples. After a complete tray has been loaded, the window will indicate that the instrument is "ready to load next tray." The carousel will hold up to 32 ImmUnits.

The throughput of Affinity varies according to the specific assay. The average throughput is less than 30 ImmUnits per hour. After an initial incubation time of 30–60 min, a test result will become available every 2 min. The throughput is faster in the batch mode than in random access mode.

When the sample testing is done, the used ImmUnits can be unloaded in one of two ways. While other samples are being loaded from a tray, the used ImmUnits are being unloaded simultaneously into the tray. Once the tray has been released, discard the old processed ImmUnits. To unload all of the tests, including those ImmUnits still processing, press the "unload/carousel" key. The Affinity will request an empty tray in the window area and begin unloading the carousel. Any tests in progress will be aborted. Results can be programmed to "print as loaded" or "store results as completed." All results, system alerts, and test alerts appear on the printout located at the top right-hand side of the Affinity.

2. Maintenance

The Affinity requires very little routine maintenance. Inspect the tray area, rinse solutions, and waste bottles for any spills or leaks. Clean up any spills with water or 10% bleach solution. Occasionally the waste container will need to be emptied and the rinse bottle replaced with a full one. Replace the printer paper as needed. Biweekly the resident val unit (RVU) should be replaced. The RVU is used by the instrument for spot primes and to check the filters. It holds a permanent position in the carousel and looks like a regular ImmUnit. The only time the RVU unloads from the carousel is when the "unload/carousel" key is pressed.

After continued use, the punch will eventually become dirty and could cause carryover problems. Turn the instrument off and remove the front cover. Also, remove the pump and valve cover. Using a screwdriver, loosen the punch screw. The punch screw is located above the shuttle area on the right-hand side. Once the screw is loosened, lift it completely out of the instrument. Clean with hot, soapy water and bleach. Place the punch back into position and screw it down tightly. This procedure need only be done as required, usually once a month. Any other problems with hardware or parts that may need to be replaced require a call to service.

3. Reliability

There are three types of alert messages that can appear on the Affinity LCD (liquid crystal display). They are load alerts, test alerts, and system alerts. Throughout our clinical trials, we have encountered some of these alert messages.

Load alerts appear when there are problems with loading test ImmUnits. A common error seen here is load alert 1: "CANNOT READ BARCODE IN TRAY SLOT XXX." This error indicates that the instrument could not read the bar-code label on an ImmUnit, possibly for several reasons. There could be a defect in the printed label, the tray could be out of alignment with the shuttle area, or the bar-code reader was dirty. The Affinity will try to reload an ImmUnit three times before it rejects that test unit. After rejecting the ImmUnit, it will remain in the tray. Load alert 1 causes a major problem if the instrument is running in duplicate. The paired ImmUnit will continue to be processed and cause the printed results to be offset by one test unit. Also, a recalculation of means will be required. Other load alerts that are common are load alert 2, "CALIBRATOR SET NOT COMPLETE," and load alert 3, "CONTROL SET NOT COMPLETE." These alerts occur when the calibrator or control sets are not loaded as defined in the protocol. Load alert 7, "CURVE MISSING FOR --- LOT," will be displayed on the LCD when an ImmUnit does not have a calibration curve in storage corresponding to the same lot number. This often happens when loading controls behind a calibration curve and the curve is not automatically accepted by the Affinity but appears pending. Until the curve is manually accepted or there is a previous curve in storage for that particular lot number, the control results will not print. A curve must be generated within 24 h or the test data will be erased.

Test alerts appear on the printouts and provide information about results. For example, test alert 1, "REFERENCE RANGE," indicates that the value is outside of the reference range defined in the protocol. When one or more control values are outside of a given range, test alert 5, "CONTROL OUT OF RANGE," will appear on the printout. Test alert 21, "CONFIDENCE FACTOR LOW," is sometimes seen after a calibration curve is generated. The confidence factor is an internal calculation used to determine if a calibration curve is acceptable.

The operator should review the data to determine if the curve is acceptable. Most test alerts do not require immediate corrective action—they are designed to keep the operator aware of a possible problem. If any of the test alerts persist, they should be investigated to rule out a possible ongoing problem.

System alerts are the most severe of the three types of alerts. In the case of a system alert, the instrument repair service should be contacted. These alerts are designed to inform the operator of a malfunction with the system's performance. Depending on the type of problem, the instrument will print a message, but at times it will abort tests in progress. Examples of some system alerts that we have encountered in our clinical trials are "SHUTTLE ERRORS," "CAROUSEL ERRORS," "TRANSFER PIPETTE ERRORS," and "SAMPLE PROCESSING INTERRUPTED."

IV. CONCLUSION

The Affinity is an automated, random access immunoassay system. The prepackaged reagents eliminate reagent preparation. The throughput is slow for high-volume laboratories. Most medium-sized laboratories will find it acceptable. Multiple systems could be used to increase throughput and provide backup capability. This relatively compact in size instrument will require only limited space. As more assays become available, the system will be quite attractive for a routine laboratory. In the future, sampling from primary blood collection tubes will further automate the entire immunoassay testing process.

CHAPTER 10

AIA-1200 Immunoassay System

Daniel W. Chan and Pamela L. Thornton
Department of Laboratory Medicine,
Clinical Chemistry Division,
The Johns Hopkins Hospital,
The Johns Hopkins University, Baltimore, Maryland

I. INTRODUCTION

Fully automated, random access chemistry analyzers have been used in the clinical laboratories since the early 1980s. However, this type of automation for immunoassay has just begun. Traditionally, immunoassay is performed in batch mode. The testing frequency is determined by the batch size and the turnaround time requirement. If the batch size is too small, it may not be economically justifiable. For manual radioimmunoassay (RIA), testing frequency less than once a week is not practical technically. The random access feature of the automation will change the way immunoassay is done. Testing can be performed around the clock. There will be no batch and no scheduling. Every test is available at any time. Emergency and routine testings are the same. Together with work-station consolidation, fully integrated automation can be accomplished.

The AIA-1200 immunoassay system is a fully automated, random access analyzer using prepackaged reagents (Fig. 1). Each reagent pack contains magnetized beads coated with specific antibodies and alkaline phosphatase conjugated to antibody (IEMA, immunoenzymetric assay) or antigen (competitive immunoassay (Fig. 2). The entire system is manufactured by Tosoh Medics, Inc., 800-A Gateway Blvd., South San Francisco, California 94080.

Immunoassay Automation: A Practical Guide

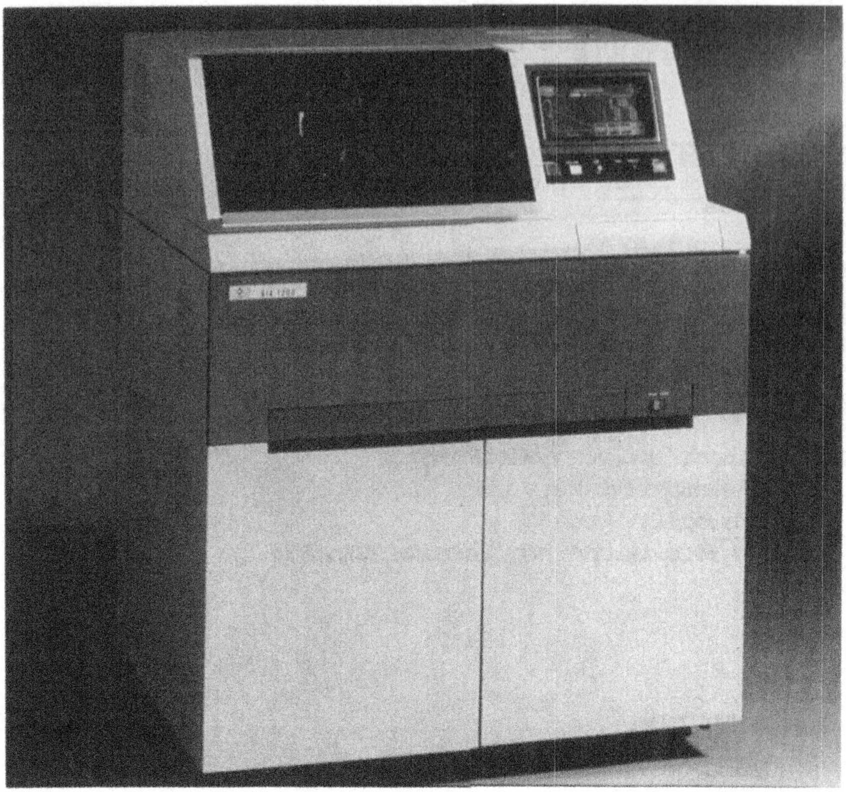

Figure 1 Photograph of the AIA-1200 analyzer.

This chapter describes the AIA-1200 immunoassay system, both instrumentation and reagent. The performance of the system is evaluated with data generated from my laboratory. We will discuss the technical, clinical, and operational performances.

II. SYSTEM DESCRIPTION

A. Instrumentation

The AIA-1200 system consists of five major modules: computer, test cup sorter, analyzer, pressurized fluid delivery, and power-source driver modules. An internal diagram shows various steps of the AIA-1200 system (Fig. 3).

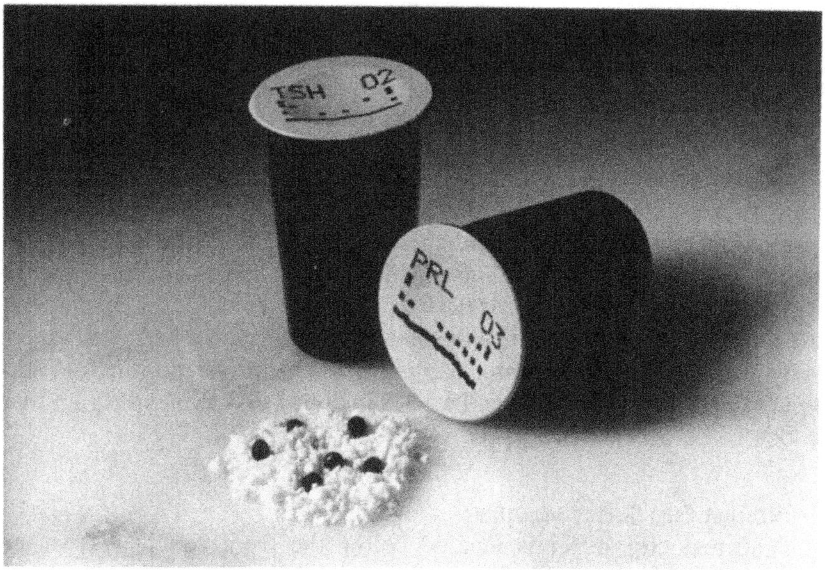

Figure 2 Reagent cups containing magnetized beads coated with specific antibodies.

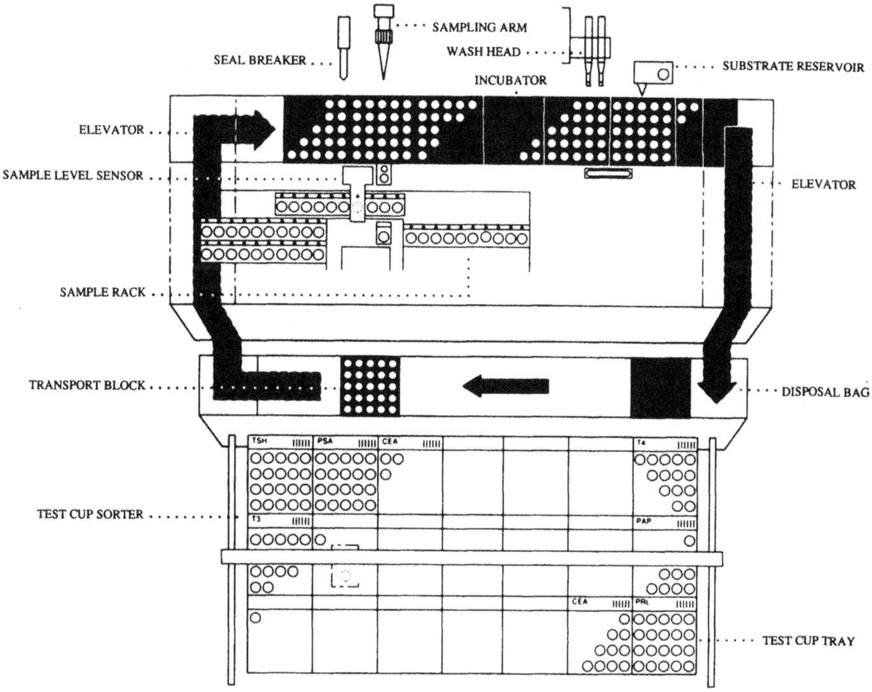

Figure 3 Internal diagram of the AIA-120 analyzer.

1. Computer Module

The AIA-1200 system has nine microprocessors that direct the operation of the system. It has a total of 1 megabyte (MB) of combined random access memory (RAM). There are two RS-232C ports on the system, which can be interfaced with the host computer. The operating software controls the timing and execution of all mechanical activity. In addition, it performs calculations and provides temporary storage of test results. The operator can program system configuration, protocol parameters, and test requests through the control station, which includes an electroluminescent (EL) display unit and a infrared (IR) touch panel. Below the EL display is a hard panel that contains control buttons for power, panel lock, and emergency stop. The thermal printer can perform a print screen function and output requested by the system. Two 3.5-in floppy disk drives with 1.6 MB are located below the hard panel.

2. Test Cup Sorter Module

The test cup sorter is located below the front panel. The sorter drawer holds 21 trays with 20 test cups per tray. The sorter arm/head contains several functional units: a bar-code scanner, an IR cup detector, and a vacuum pickup mechanism. The bar-code on the test cup contains the analyte identification and the lot number. The scanner manages the system inventory by reading the bar-code on the test cup trays and calculating the contents of the sorter drawer. The vacuum pickup mechanism is responsible for the transfer of test cups from the tray to the transport block.

3. Analyzer Module

The analyzer module performs the following steps: transporting the test cup, loading the sample racks, sample pipetting, incubation, wash and substrate pipetting, and fluorometric detection. The testing process starts with moving the test cups on the transport block to the seal-breaking station. The aluminum top seals of each reagent pack are broken for reagent reconstitution. The transport block moves to the sampling station. A sample rack can carry as many as 10 sample cups and disposable pipette tips. The sample level sensor measures the volume of each of the samples before they reach the pipetting station. If the sample volume is inadequate for the tests requested, an error message will be displayed. A cover is placed over the samples to minimize evaporation. A separate "stat" sample rack with one sample cup and one pipetting tip is located in front of the sampling arm. If more than one test is requested for a sample, the tip is rinsed and reused until all the tests are completed.

The incubator unit houses a magnetic stirring mechanism and electric heating pads. The temperature is maintained at 37 ± 0.1°C. The immune reaction is temperature dependent. The rate of reaction increases with higher temperature. The incubation time is chosen at 40 min, where only 40–60% of the reaction is completed. The equilibrium of the antigen–antibody reaction requires 3–4 h. Therefore, control of the timing and the temperature is important. The magnetic stirring mechanism keeps the antibody-coated beads in suspension with an agitation rate of 85 cycles/min. After incubation, the test cup is washed 11 times with a total of 7 ml wash solution. The substrate probe delivers 0.22 ml of preheated substrate.

The fluorometric detector consists of a source lamp, dichroic bichromatic mirrors, lenses, photodiodes, and preamplifiers. It measures the rate of fluorescence produced by the enzymatic conversion of the substrate 4-methylumbelliferyl phosphate to 4-methylumbelliferone. The detector measures five test cups simultaneously. Five detector channels are standardized to a sixth channel, a reference channel. The top–top rate fluorescence measurement is obtained by irradiation of light at 365 nm from the top of the cup and detection of emission light at 450–550 nm by the detector located over the top of the cup. This type of fluorescence measurement eliminates background correction, substrate contamination from other assays, and the reaction quenching step.

4. System Operation

The main menu of the system consists of nine functions: calibration, sample program, worksheet, sorter map, assay start, pause, result review, report, and special menu. The special menu includes disk data demand, work-load statistics, system close, mechanics check, operator date and time, recovery from emergency stop, disk utilities, maintenance, system specifications, system mode set, analyte registration, assay specifications, washer parameter set, and system engineer tools. A typical daily operational flowchart is shown in Fig. 4.

The first test result is available in approximately 1 h. Thereafter, five results are reported every 2.5 min. The maximal theoretical throughput is 120 tests per hour. Various report formats can be selected including master report, preliminary report, and final report. Statistical analysis of quality control results are also available. The detailed system operation will be discussed later, in the section on system performance.

B. Reagent

1. Test Cup

The black plastic test cups in the AIA-1200 reagent pack contain either antibody or antigen conjugated to alkaline phosphatase. Each test

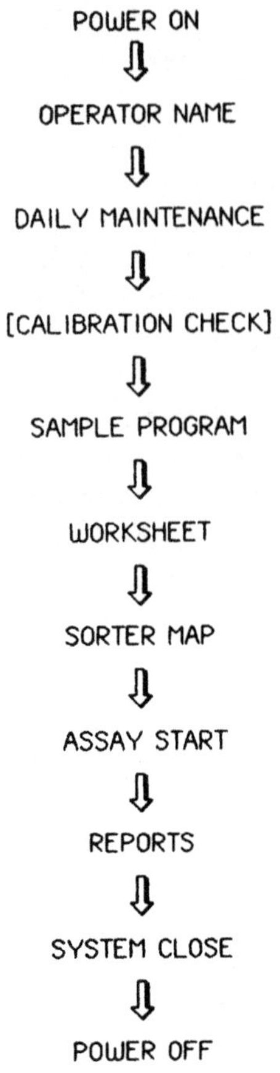

Figure 4 Daily operation flow chart.

cup contains an exact number of magnetized beads. These polymer beads are 1.5 mm in diameter and coated with ferrite. The polymers have functional groups with antibody chemically immobilized. The conjugate-bead mixture is lyophilized in individual cups (Fig. 5). Each cup is sealed with aluminum foil with analyte name, code, and lot number on it. Twenty test cups are placed in a plastic tray, which is packaged in a moisture-resistant aluminum pouch. The test cups should be stored at 2–8°C.

2. Assay Principle

Two different methodologies are used in the AIA-1200 system (Fig. 5): a one-step sandwich immunoenzymetric assay (IEMA) for large analytes, and a competitive binding assay for small analytes.

a. Immunoenzymetric Assay Analytes with high molecular weight, such as thyrotropin (TSH), carcinoembryonic antigen (CEA), and alpha-

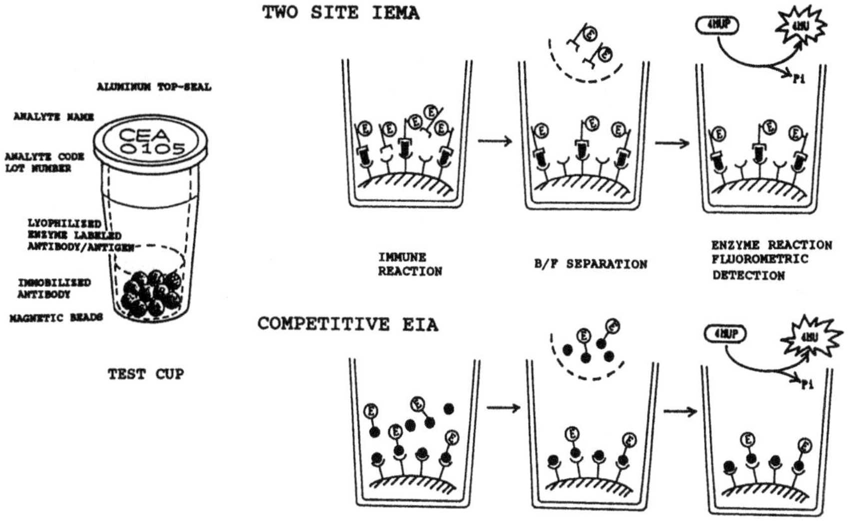

Figure 5 The Tosoh assay principles showing two types of immunoassay: the competitive EIA and the two-site IEMA. B/F, bound/free.

fetoprotein (AFP), are measured based on this approach. Two different antibodies in excess are used in the sandwich assay. Each antibody is directed against a different epitope on the antigen molecule. One antibody is bound to the magnetic bead. The other antibody is conjugated with alkaline phosphatase. During the 40-min incubation, the antigen forms a sandwich with both antibodies. Then the unbound antibody-conjugate is washed away. The amount of enzyme activity bound to the bead is directly proportional to the analyte concentration. The greater the analyte concentration, the higher the fluorescent signal.

b. Competitive Binding Assay Analytes with low molecular weight, such as thyroxine and digoxin, are measured using this approach. A limited amount of antibodies is immobilized on the magnetic beads. Alkaline phosphatase–labeled antigen is added to compete with the unknown antigen for the binding site on the antibody. After incubation, the unbound antigen is washed away. The amount of enzyme activity bound to the bead is inversely proportional to the analyte concentration. The greater the analyte concentration, the lower the fluorescent signal.

c. Enzyme Reaction Alkaline phosphatase converts 4-methylumbelliferyl phosphate (4MUP) to 4-methylumbelliferone (4MU), which is fluorescent. The fluorescent signal is measured every second, starting at 10 s after the addition of the substrate for up to 100 s. The reading may stop before 100 s if the fluorescent intensity reaches the upper limit of detection (12 μM of 4MU). The rate of the fluorescence increase is calculated to

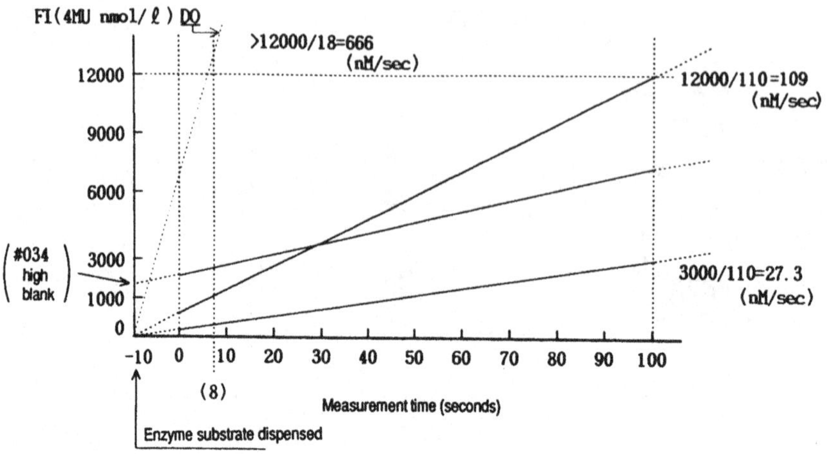

Figure 6 Measurement of enzyme reaction.

be the enzyme activity (Fig. 6). At least eight data points within the limits of the detector range are needed for the calculation. A "DO" flag is printed if the detection limit test failed. The substrate solution should be stored in a dark, cool place to avoid the increase of background fluorescence due to the conversion of 4MUP to 4MU. If the background fluorescence is greater than 1.5 μM 4MU, an error message number 034 will be printed.

d. Calibration A calibration protocol varies according to the specific analyte with two to six points. Some, such as AFP, use two calibrators, while others, such as thyroxine, use multiple calibrators. The data reduction equation varies accordingly. A least-square equation is used for the two-point curves. A cubic spline is used for the competitive binding assay. In addition, a four-parameter logistic method is also available.

III. SYSTEM PERFORMANCE

The performance of the AIA-1200 system was evaluated for one year in the clinical chemistry laboratory of the Johns Hopkins Hospital. Here, I will summarize our findings.

A. Technical Performance

1. Precision

The intraassay precision (Table 1) was calculated with 20 consecutive, single data points. Three levels of quality control samples were used

Table 1 Intraassay Precision

Analyte	Unit	Level I		Level II		Level III	
		Mean and CV%					
T_4	μg/dl	2.5	6	6.2	5	13.5	4
T_3	μg/l	0.7	15	1.6	10	3.9	6
TSH	mIU/l	0.5	6	7.0	2	36	3
hCG	IU/l	3.2	5	23.2	4	80	4
LH	IU/l	2.1	23	7.6	6	22	3
FSH	IU/l	6.0	5	12.4	4	32.1	4
Prolactin	μg/l	2.3	2	6.8	3	29.4	3
Ferritin	μg/l	78	2	118	2	221	2
CEA	μg/l	4.4	3	17.6	4	43.2	3
AFP	μg/l	19.5	3	72.5	4	200	3
PSA	μg/l	1.7	3	3.4	3	8.0	3

in the determination. The interassay precision (Table 2) was determined by the quality control results over 20 days. Overall, the precisions were acceptable. Only two results exceeded 10%CV. A low T3 sample showed 11–15%CV, and a low LH sample with concentration close to the sensitivity limit of the assay showed 20–23%CV.

2. Sensitivity

The sensitivity is determined by the mean + 2 standard deviations of the values using the zero calibrator (Table 3). Overall, the sensitivity is acceptable. The sensitivity of prostate-specific antigen (PSA) at 0.02 μg/l is sufficiently low to allow using PSA to detect any residual diseases after radical prostatectomy. The sensitivity of TSH is found to be 0.04 mIU/l,

Table 2 Interassay Precision

Analyte	Unit	Level I		Level II		Level III	
		Mean and CV%					
T_4	μg/dl	2.3	8	5.8	8	12.3	8
T_3	μg/l	0.7	11	1.6	6	3.9	4
TSH	mIU/l	0.5	10	7.0	5	35	5
hCG	IU/l	3.2	9	22	8	72	7
LH	IU/l	2.2	20	8.1	6	22	4
FSH	IU/l	5.8	5	12.3	5	30.6	4
Prolactin	μg/l	2.2	4	6.9	3	28.5	4
Ferritin	μg/l	74	5	122	4	225	6
CEA	μg/l	4.2	7	16.5	9	40.3	8
AFP	μg/l	19.6	8	72.2	8	208	8
PSA	μg/l	1.7	8	3.4	10	8.2	6

Table 3 Sensitivity

Analyte	Sensitivity	
T_4	0.5	μg/dl
T_3	0.2	μg/l
TSH	0.04	mIU/l
hCG	0.2	mIU/l
LH	0.6	IU/l
FSH	0.2	IU/l
Prolactin	0.03	μg/l
Ferritin	0.2	μg/l
CEA	0.07	μg/l
AFP	0.2	μg/l
PSA	0.02	μg/l

which is comparable to other ultrasensitive TSH assays. The sensitivity determined by diluting a low-TSH sample was 0.07 mIU/l. The sensitivity determined by using the zero calibrator is the accepted industry standard. However, the practical sensitivity from day to day can be expected to be higher, perhaps twice the minimum detectable amounts. For example, the TSH sensitivity could be 0.08 mIU/l on a daily basis, rather than the 0.04 mIU/l as calculated.

3. Linearity

The linearity of each test was determined by diluting a patient sample with the assay diluent. We were able to verify the linearity up to certain values as shown in Table 4. In all cases, these were the highest values of

Table 4 Linearity

	Linearity		
Analyte	Tested	Claimed	
T_4	16	24	μg/dl
T_3	3.3	6.4	μg/l
TSH	120	100	mIU/l
hCG	340	400	IU/l
Prolactin	125	200	μg/l
LH	54	200	IU/l
FSH	83	300	IU/l
Ferritin	825	1000	μg/l
CEA	67	100	μg/l
AFP	235	400	μg/l
PSA	48	100	μg/l

the available samples tested. The linearity claimed by the manufacturer was also shown for comparison.

4. Method Comparison

Comparison methods used in this study were the TDx and IMx analyzers from Abbott Labs (North Chicago, Illinois) and the Tandem assays from Hybritech Inc. (San Diego, California). The linear regression analysis of the method comparison with the Tosoh method on the *Y* axis and the comparison method on the *X* axis are shown in Table 5. The correlation with the Abbott TDx and IMx assays were acceptable with correlation coefficients between 0.86 and 0.99. The slopes varied from 0.84 to 1.15. The correlation of the Hybritech Tandem assays were acceptable with correlation coefficients between 0.88 and 0.99. The slopes varied from 0.82 to 1.51. The slopes for tumor markers were more variable, depending on the concentration ranges. There were no significant discrepancies.

5. Calibration Curve Stability

The calibration curve stability is important for a random access analyzer to be available 24 h a day. We found that the curve was stable for at least 1 month.

Table 5 Method Comparison

AIA-1200 (*Y*)	Comparison (*X*)	Unit	Slope	Intercept	*r*	*N*
T_4	TDx	μg/dl	0.87	0.46	0.86	173
T_3	TDx	μg/l	0.84	0.3	0.96	30
TSH	IMx	mIU/l	1.03	0.3	0.99	166
hCG	Tandem-E	IU/l	0.91	−0.3	0.99	88
Prolactin	Tandem-E	μg/l	0.82	−0.06	0.99	50
Ferritin	IMx	μg/l	1.15	−12.8	0.99	43
CEA, normal	Tandem-E	μg/l	1.18	0.16	0.95	205
CEA, benign	Tandem-E	μg/l	1.14	0.47	0.97	124
CEA, cancer	Tandem-E	μg/l	1.20	0.74	0.97	243
AFP, normal	Tandem-E	μg/l	0.79	0.56	0.88	207
AFP, benign	Tandem-E	μg/l	1.08	−1.32	0.99	100
AFP, cancer	Tandem-E	μg/l	1.15	−0.74	0.97	159
PSA, normal	Tandem-R	μg/l	1.28	0.15	0.95	201
PSA, benign	Tandem-R	μg/l	1.41	−0.20	0.99	101
PSA, cancer	Tandem-R	μg/l	1.51	0.01	0.99	279

Table 6 Reference Values

Analyte	AIA-1200	Tandem
CEA (μg/l)		
Nonsmoker	<3.1	<2.8
Smoker	<6.2	<6.0
AFP (μg/l)	<6.0	<6.0
PSA (μg/l)		
Male <40 years	<1.8	<1.3
Male >40 years	<3.5	<2.6
Female	<0.1	<0.1

B. Clinical Performance

1. Reference Values

The reference values study were done on a group of healthy volunteers. The reference values were calculated from the mean ± 2 SD of the values. CEA is known to have different reference values for smokers and nonsmokers. The study confirmed the differences. For nonsmokers, the values were 3.1 μg/l for AIA-1200 and 2.8 μg/l for Tandem. For smokers, the values were 6.2 μg/l for AIA-1200 and 6.0 μg/l for Tandem (Table 6). The AFP reference values were 6.0 μg/l for both assays. The PSA values for males under 40 years of age were 1.8 μg/l for AIA-1200 and 1.3 μg/l for Tandem. For males over 40 years of age, the values were 3.5 μg/l for AIA-1200 and 2.6 μg/l for Tandem. The female reference values were less than 0.1 μg/l for both assays.

2. Distribution of Marker Values

The distributions of marker values were shown among healthy subjects, nonmalignant diseases, and malignant diseases for both AIA-1200 and Tandem assays (Tables 7–9). Similar performances were observed between both assays. This was not surprising, since both assays used the same clone of hybridoma to produce monoclonal antibodies. The differences in values may be the results of calibration and other assay parameters.

C. Operational Performance

1. System Operation

The AIA-1200 can be set up in a variety of fashions to meet the user's needs. With the AIA fully turned on and the system utility disks in place, the user can select and set the system specifications. The system specifi-

Table 7 Distribution of CEA Values ($\mu g/l$)

		AIA-1200			Tandem-E		
	Number	0–3.0	3.1–6.0	>6.0	0–3.0	3.1–6.0	>6.0
Healthy							
Nonsmokers	103	88%	10%	2%	93%	6%	1%
Smokers	101	49%	37%	14%	64%	27%	9%
Total	204	69%	23%	7%	79%	16%	5%
Nonmalignant							
Cirrhosis	19	21%	47%	31%	26%	63%	11%
Polyp	20	75%	20%	5%	95%	5%	0%
Pulmonary	19	58%	26%	16%	63%	32%	5%
Pancreatitis	23	48%	35%	18%	65%	26%	8%
Ulcerative colitis	20	45%	30%	25%	65%	10%	25%
Other	21	71%	24%	5%	90%	5%	5%
Total	122	53%	30%	17%	68%	23%	9%
Malignant							
Colorectal	97	13%	16%	70%	21%	16%	63%
Gastric	20	35%	35%	30%	50%	30%	20%
Mammary	47	34%	13%	53%	38%	15%	47%
Ovarian	20	65%	15%	20%	75%	5%	20%
Pancreatic	20	20%	30%	50%	15%	50%	35%
Pulmonary	49	24%	18%	58%	36%	20%	44%
Other	20	50%	25%	25%	60%	30%	10%
Total	273	19%	19%	62%	35%	20%	45%

cations will set the communication format of either the printer, EL-display, or RS-232C interface. The system mode allows the user to set certain functions including automatic reporting, format of sample report, and type of print format. The automatic mode sets the instrument to prompt such functions as data transmission, store statistics, operation name check, system close, and detector standardization acceptance. There is also a special startup parameter that will allow the user to automatically check and prompt detector standardization calibration, assay calibration, and sample program.

Before analytes can be run, the user must check the analyte registration that is preset on the utility disk. There are two files under the analyte registration: system and available analyte lists. The system analyte list allows the addition of new analytes to the existing list and sets the calibration flag. The calibration flag is set for 30 days or the determined stability of the curves. Warning will be given when it is necessary to recalibrate. The available analyte list selects the analytes to be run and sets the priority for each test.

Table 8 Distribution of AFP Values ($\mu g/l$)

		AIA-1200		Tandem-E	
	Number	0–6.0	>6.0	0–6.0	>6.0
Healthy subjects					
Men	104	96%	4%	95%	5%
Women	100	98%	2%	97%	3%
Total	204	97%	3%	96%	4%
Nonmalignant					
Cirrhosis	19	90%	10%	90%	10%
Hepatitis	40	75%	25%	73%	27%
Mammary	10	90%	10%	60%	40%
Pancreatitis	10	100%	0%	100%	0%
Pulmonary	10	80%	20%	60%	40%
Other	10	90%	10%	70%	30%
Carcinoma					
Testicular					
Nonseminoma	50	52%	48%	54%	46%
Seminoma	11	91%	9%	91%	9%
Hepatocellular	51	20%	80%	20%	80%
Gastrointestinal	20	90%	10%	90%	10%
Genitourinary	31	81%	19%	81%	19%
Ovarian	20	85%	15%	85%	15%
Pancreatic	5	100%	0%	100%	0%
Other	20	95%	5%	90%	10%

Next, the user must check and set the four file parameters: calibration file, quality control (QC) material file, assay protocol file, and panel file. The calibration and QC material file define the separate levels for each analyte register and allow the storage of lot number and concentration for each level of calibrator or QC material. The assay protocol file holds the assay parameters for each analyte and allows the editing of the parameters. The panel file allows the user to create and name panels of tests that may be frequently requested together, instead of ordering each test individually. Then it is important to save all new changes on utility disk and system disks. Another good practice is to create backup disks through formatting and copying each disk. This is helpful in case of power failure or cutting off the main power breaker, or damage to current working disks.

Before actually running for the first time or after a long period of nonuse, the user must prepare the AIA-1200 by making fresh diluent, wash, and substrate reagents, following the package inserts. After daily and weekly maintenance, the AIA will need a detector standardization. The detector standardization checks and calibrates the five channels to the reference channel. After the first standardization, the new values are

Table 9 Distribution of PSA Values ($\mu g/l$)

	Number	AIA-1200		Tandem-E	
		0–3.5	>3.5	0–2.6	>2.6
Healthy					
Men <40 years	75	100%	0%	100%	0%
Men >40 years	75	93%	7%	95%	5%
Total men	150	97%	3%	97%	3%
Women	51	100%	0%	100%	0%
Nonmalignant					
Benign Prostatic Hypertrophy	52	46%	54%	46%	54%
Misc. genitourinary	20	80%	20%	80%	20%
Other	30	93%	7%	97%	3%
Malignant					
Prostate					
Stage A	50	56%	44%	60%	40%
Stage B	58	14%	86%	12%	88%
Stage C	50	12%	88%	12%	88%
Stage D	59	2%	98%	2%	98%
Total	217	20%	80%	20%	80%
Other malignant					
Gastrointestinal	20	85%	15%	85%	15%
Bladder	21	86%	14%	86%	14%
Mammary	21	95%	5%	95%	5%
Pulmonary	19	84%	16%	84%	16%
Other	19	95%	5%	95%	5%

compared to the previous values and must be within ±5%. The system has two modes. The first automatically accepts the results. The second allows manual check and acceptance of the results. After a detector standardization, it is necessary to calibrate all assays that are to be performed. This can be set up with one program, initiated, and completed in approximately 1 h. For the most part, it is only necessary to calibrate once a month except for lot changes, lamp replacement, or adjustments. Again, the AIA-1200 has the option of automatic acceptance of the curve or manual acceptance after viewing the data.

Once the AIA-1200 is calibrated, it is ready for patient samples. The user programs the samples that are sequentially numbered. The sample program allows for patient/sample identification up to 10 characters, using letters and/or numbers for positive patient identification. Quality control samples also can be designated as QC. There is a column for either a comment, dilution factor, or priority. The comment can be up to four characters. The dilution factor allows the designation of dilution, and results will automatically be multipled and printed out. The actual dilution must be made manually by the user. The priority selection allows the user to set the priority of the ordered tests instead of the instrument's priority. This can be useful for samples with insufficient quantity. Multiple analytes may be requested per sample as long as the total volume required does not exceed 1.5 ml. The total volume for each sample is printed out on the sample worksheet.

Other programs are available for the AIA-1200. One is group entry, which is used for a large group of samples to be tested for the same analyte(s). The number of samples is entered as a batch. After the first one is programmed, the rest are automatically sequenced. For routine programs that are repeatedly used can be stored on floppy disks and recalled for future use. Finally, the AIA has the ability to be programmed from input online from a host computer via the RC-232C interface.

Next, the user needs to print the programmed samples onto a worksheet. The worksheet prints the order and rack position of each programmed sample. Racks are listed alphabetically with numbered wells for sample cups with 10 wells per rack. It also informs the user of the minimum volume to complete the required tests. Using the worksheet, the user sets up the racks with pipette tips and sample cups, then pours an approximate amount of sample (more than the minimum) into the proper cup. Then the racks are loaded onto the AIA.

The user will need to check the inventory of test cups in the sorter drawer before starting. The sorter drawer holds the inventory of test cups in trays. The trays have a bar code that holds the test code and lot number information. The sorter arm scans the trays, reads the bar code, and counts the number test cup in each tray. The computer has a mapped inventory of each analyte tray and number of test cups per analyte tray. The user must be careful to ensure that test cups are in proper test trays. If the inventory needs to be restocked prior to starting a program, the AIA will take a new inventory after opening the sorter drawer. If the user forgets and starts a program without sufficient test cups, the AIA puts itself into a pause, allowing 2.5 min to replenish the shortage. No assay will start until the pause is released by touching the pause button on the main menu. Those assays that are not restocked will not be run, and a flag will be printed in place of a result.

To initiate assays by selecting the start assay button on the main menu, the AIA computer prompts the user to enter in the sequence number of the last sample that is ready to run. Then it displays a graphic picture of sample and rack placement. This serves as a check for the user. If the set-up racks match the display, select "start." Once a sample is programmed, it can be started at any time. Once the programmed assays are started, the user can continue programming new specimens.

In about an hour, the first set of results will be printed, and thereafter, each result will be printed every 0.5 min until all started specimens are complete. The AIA then gives four options of reporting results. These are master report, preliminary report, analyte report, and final report. The final report is for confirmed test results and once printed cannot be changed or deleted. It also allows transmission to external computer and/or system shutdown archiving.

At the end of the day or shift, one should perform a system close. System close allows the AIA to store and save (archiving) patient data and QC data onto specific data disks for future reference. Also, it will save any new calibration curves and detector standardization on the utilities disk. Then turn the AIA off, discard used pipette tips, empty waste, and discard the disposal bag of used test cups.

2. Maintenance

Maintenance of the AIA-1200 consists of daily, weekly, monthly, quarterly, and as-needed maintenance (Fig. 7). Daily maintenance takes approximately 5 min. Upon turning the AIA on, the first couple of computer screens prompt and aid the checks of fluid volumes, waste volume, air pressure and vacuum gauges, paper supply, automechanics check, and

AIA-1200 PERIODIC MAINTENANCE LOG

MONTH _______ YEAR _____

DAILY	1	2	3	4	5	6	7	8	9	10	11	12	13	14	15	16	17	18	19	20	21	22	23	24	25	26	27	28	29	30	31
Check volumes of diluent, wash and substrate																															
Check expiration dates of all reagents																															
Check and empty as needed the liquid waste reservoir, tip disposal box, test cup waste bag																															
Check air regulator pressure (65 ± 5 psi)																															
Confirm vacuum gauge setting (300-500 mmHg)																															
Check paper supply; refill if necessary																															
Perform SUBSTRATE FLUSH																															
Perform auto mechanics check																															
Check aspiration/dispensing: wash nozzle 1																															
Check aspiration/dispensing: wash nozzle 2																															
Perform temperature controller test																															
WEEKLY	1	2	3	4	5	6	7	8	9	10	11	12	13	14	15	16	17	18	19	20	21	22	23	24	25	26	27	28	29	30	31
SYSTEM OFF: Drain compressor bleed valve/ moisture trap																															
Clean sample level sensor lens																															
Clean wash reservoir filter, PRIME/FLUSH																															
Clean diluent reservoir filter, PRIME/FLUSH																															
Clean wash nozzle 1 filter, check aspiration, dispensing																															
Clean wash nozzle 2 filter, check aspiration, dispensing																															
Clean sample tip probe with H2O, wipe with ethanol																															
Change waste chute liner																															
MONTHLY	1	2	3	4	5	6	7	8	9	10	11	12	13	14	15	16	17	18	19	20	21	22	23	24	25	26	27	28	29	30	31
SYSTEM OFF: Drain vacuum tank																															
SYSTEM OFF: Clean wash station deflector																															
Replace wash reservoir filter, ck aspiration, PRIME/FLUSH																															
Replace diluent reservoir filter																															
Acid wash substrate line (0.1 N HNO3)/ Ethanol rinse																															
Replace substrate in-line filter, SUBSTRATE FLUSH X 2																															
Replace both in-line wash filter cartridges																															
Perform detector standardization																															
Calibrate all assays																															
QUARTERLY	LAST PERFORMED																NEXT DUE														
SYSTEM OFF: Clean test cup pickup seal																															
Clean and polish transport blocks																															
AS NEEDED																															
Clean instrument surfaces after any spills																															
Clean sample racks																															
Acid wash & rinse substrate bottle																															
Wash, bleach, & rinse wash reservoir																															
Wash, bleach, & rinse diluent reservoir																															
Replace both wash nozzle filters																															

Please refer to Section 10 of the Operator's Manual for detailed procedures. rev 4/90

Figure 7 Periodic maintenance log.

flushing the substrate line. The wash nozzles must be checked for proper dispensing and aspiration. This may add a little more time unless one can reach the nozzles without lifting up the entire instrument top. It takes another menu screen to check and record the various temperatures.

Weekly maintenance adds another 15 min to daily maintenance. The instrument has to be off to bleed the air compressor. The rest of the maintenance consists of cleaning sample level sensor, sample tip probe, and wash and diluent filters followed by flushes. The wash nozzles are replaced, then checked for dispensing and aspiration. The waste chute liner should be changed, thus reducing the chance of a blockage of test cups leaving the system.

Monthly maintenance takes approximately 30 min to complete and includes a detector standardization. It does not include calibration of all analytes that must be done following a detector standardization. While the instrument is off, the wash-station deflector is removed and cleaned, and the vacuum tank is drained. Wash and diluent filter and in-line filters are replaced, followed by flushes of the lines. Old filters need to be thoroughly clean and then can be reused. The substrate line is given an acid wash to avoid bacterial contamination of the lines. Afterward, the in-line filter needs to be replaced, followed by two flushes of substrate solution.

Quarterly maintenance consists of two parts, one quick and easy and one long. The quick one is the cleaning of the test-cup pickup seal, which takes about 2 min while the instrument is off. The long one is the cleaning and polishing of the transport blocks and takes approximately 30 min. As tedious as it may be, it is necessary to keep the transport blocks cleaned and polished because of the way the instrument keeps track of the blocks.

As-needed maintenance consists of commonsense items such as cleaning up spills in the instrument, cleaning sample racks, and the washing and bleaching of the wash and diluent bottles. In addition, wash the substrate bottles with acid if one suspects contamination.

3. Reliability

Overall, the AIA-1200 has proven to be a dependable instrument and one that has been easy to fix for the few problems it had. All problems have been resolved by the user or with Tosoh phone assistance. Depending on the type and location of the error, the system may be able to complete samples that were in process. The samples that were unfinished or never started needed to be restarted. The AIA-1200 has an emergency stop button, which shuts down the instrument to allow correction of the problem but saves all programmed samples. After the instrument has been restarted, the saved program is ready to restart without having to reprogram. We have used the emergency button for transport block error, sampling rack error, and sorter malfunction error. The first two errors were caused by an obstruction in the areas related to the error code and the last by the sorter head not being homed properly. The AIA-1200 has a code of errors that are printed and/or flashed on the computer screen that give a brief idea of the problem. In the AIA-1200 manual is a list of the error codes, probable cause and how to resolve the error, or when to call Tosoh.

There were other errors or malfunctions that did not affect the AIA-1200's overall ability to run. These small malfunctions have been a dirty liquid level sensor, even after cleaning it, high pressure in the regulator gauge causing a "fountain" of diluent, and an occasional pipette tip that did not attach. The liquid sensor and regulator gauge were replaced by Tosoh field service. Pipet tips that do not attach mean that the sample must be reprogrammed and restarted.

4. Impact of Automation

A fully automated, random access immunoassay system can impact a clinical laboratory in two main areas: turnaround time, and technologist's time of testing. The turnaround time should improve since testing can be performed continuously. In theory, there is no batching of the testing. In practice, small batches can be performed on the system. Faster turnaround time means that test results are available earlier. This may allow diagnosis or decision for further intervention of the disease process to be made earlier. It may shorten the patient's stay in the hospital.

In a study designed to simulate the workload in our laboratory, we collected the patient specimens for 1 week (n = 847). Testing was performed on the AIA-1200 analyzer according to the time of arrival in the laboratory. The average turnaround time for the current batch operation on the routine methodologies was 27.8 h. By performing testing during the day shift using the AIA-1200 analyzer, the turnaround time was improved to 5.4 h. The turnaround time was further improved to 2.5 h if testing was performed around the clock (Fig. 8A).

The second impact of automation is the reduction of actual technical time required to perform the testing. The AIA-1200 analyzer has long-term calibration stability, prepackaged reagents, and fully automated operation. It is therefore possible to set up the system, load the samples, and walk away until results become available. In practice, an operator is needed if testing is to be performed continuously. The operator will also verify results as they become available. Nevertheless, the overall technical time required for performing such a system should be much less than performing manual, semiautomated, or batch immunoassay systems. During the same 1-week study, we estimated that the actual technical time using the AIA-1200 analyzer was 10.9 h as compared to 67.8 h using the current methologies. The net saving was 56.9 h per week (Fig. 8B).

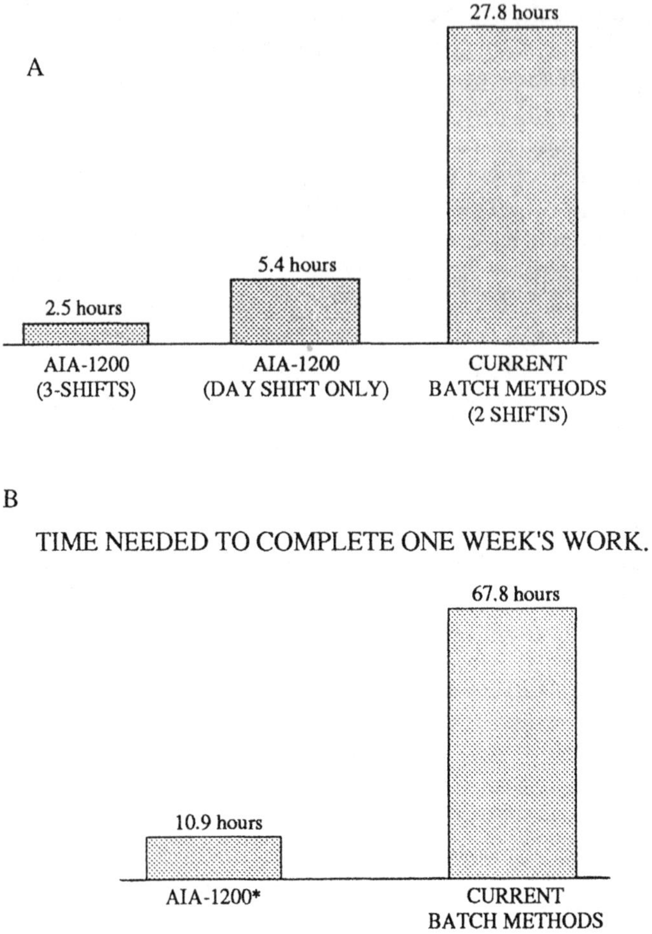

Figure 8 Comparison of the turnaround (A) and technical (B) time using the AIA-1200 analyzer and by the current batch methods.

In the future, automation of the sample handling and processing will enhance the system. Bar coding of patient sample and the ability of sampling directly through the primary blood collection tube should be given priority in the overall improvement of the AIA-1200 immunoassay system.

IV. CONCLUSION

The AIA-1200 immunoassay system is a fully automated, random access analyzer using prepackaged reagents. Each reagent pack contains magnetized beads coated with specific antibodies and alkaline phosphatase conjugated to antibody or antigen. The system performs well technically, and the patient results compared favorably with other assays currently used in our laboratory. The major advantages for this system are the ability to improve the turnaround time and to reduce the technical time required to perform the testing. In the future, automation of the sample handling will further improve the total testing process.

CHAPTER 11

Amerlite Immunoassay System

James D. Faix
Division of Laboratory Medicine,
Department of Pathology,
Beth Israel Hospital, Boston, Massachusetts

I. INTRODUCTION

Enzymes were the first widely used alternatives to radioisotopes in nonisotopic immunoassays. Either antigen or antibody can be labeled by chemical conjugation with an enzyme. The immunoassay format in which detection occurs on a solid phase (usually a microtiter plate well) by the addition of substrate (usually chromogenic) has been termed enzyme-linked immunosorbent assay or ELISA. Although alternative approaches (such as homogeneous enzyme immunoassay) have been developed, the traditional ELISA configuration continues to be popular. Many modifications have been made to enhance sensitivity and specificity. These include the use of various solid phases, monoclonal antibodies, different enzyme labels and substrates, coenzymes such as the avidin-biotin complex, and coupled secondary enzyme systems.

The two enzymes most frequently used in ELISA are horseradish peroxidase (HRP) and alkaline phosphatase, both of which can be easily coupled to either antigen or antibody without any significant loss of either enzyme activity or immunologic properties. The most commonly used chromogenic substrates have been *o*-phenylenediamine dihydrochloride (OPD) for HRP and *p*-nitrophenyl phosphate (PNPP) for alkaline phosphatase. Because product color development is difficult to standardize and also subject to various interferences, precision and sensitivity are important considerations. Furthermore, most ELISA readers demonstrate limited linearity in the higher optical density range (Catty and Raykundalia, 1989).

For these reasons, alternatives to chromogenic substrates have been studied to optimize the end-point determination in ELISA procedures. Fluorogenic substrates have been used, but they share some of the disadvantages of chromogenic substrates. Another approach has been the use of chemiluminescent substrates. This chapter describes the first automated immunoassay system that utilized this approach. It was developed by scientists at the University of Birmingham and the Wolfson Research Laboratories in Birmingham, U.K., and has been marketed by Amersham Diagnostics under the tradename Amerlite.

II. SYSTEM DESCRIPTION

A. Instrumentation

Amerlite is a semiautomated immunoassay system in which all of the individual steps are (or can be) automated but in which the operator must occasionally (and briefly) intervene. It uses a 96-well microtiter plate format and the system includes the following instrumentation:

1. microtiter plate shaker (with one speed, automatic heating to 37°C, programmable timer and capacity for four plates)
2. microtiter plate washer (with built-in pump and 12-aspirator manifold)
3. luminometer

There is also a work station consisting of a plate holder and pipettes and dispensors for manual pipetting of samples and reagents. An optional automated sampler is available. The entire system is illustrated in Fig. 1.

Since a luminometer is basically a photomultiplier tube, much early work in chemiluminescence and bioluminescence utilized either fluorometers (with the excitation lamp switched off) or liquid scintillation counters. There are now many custom-designed luminometers available. Amersham manufactures a luminometer that has been optimized for use with the Amerlite assays, called the Amerlite Analyzer. This is an automated bench-top luminometer that uses a microtiter plate transport mechanism to position each well under a photomultiplier tube. The transport mechanism is mounted in a light-tight box, and opaque microtiter plates are used to eliminate carryover. The photomultiplier tube is very sensitive and can detect 1 fmol of ATP in a standard firefly luciferase assay (Bronstein and Kricka, 1990). The luminometer accepts an entire microtiter plate (one at a time). It is controlled by a microprocessor, and a dual

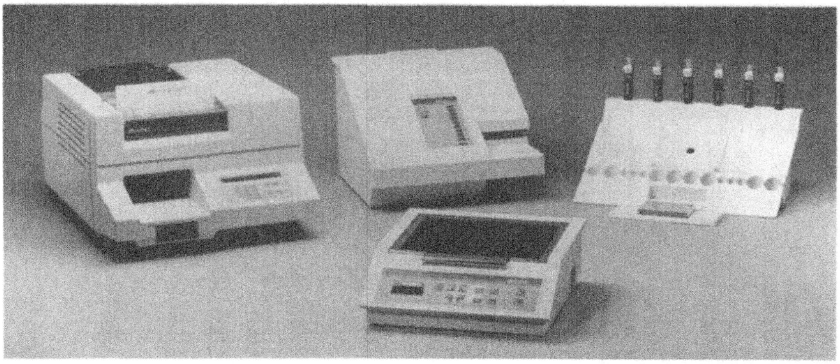

Figure 1 The Amerlite immunoassay system.

disk drive allows for data reduction and storage. All operations are performed via a touch-pad keyboard with a user-friendly alphanumeric display. A Hewlett-Packard ink-jet printer is mounted as part of the analyzer. Reading of one complete microtiter plate (including data reduction and printing of results) takes approximately 2 min.

B. Method and Principle

Chemiluminescence is the production of light (instead of heat) as a consequence of a chemical reaction (usually oxidation). Fireflies produce their familiar glow of light through the ATP-dependent oxidative decarboxylation of luciferin. (The term "bioluminescence" has been applied to chemiluminescence occuring in living organisms.) This reaction is catalyzed by firefly luciferase and has been used to develop bioluminescent immunoassays. However, the limited availability of luciferin has led to the use of more readily available luminescent compounds, which are oxidized as indicators in chemiluminescent immunoassay systems.

Two major approaches to chemiluminescent immunoassay have been taken. Amerlite is a conventional ELISA in which the enzyme is HRP and the detection is achieved by measuring the light produced as a consequence of HRP-catalyzed oxidation of luminol (Thorpe and Kricka, 1986). The CIBA Corning Magic Lite system (described in Chapter 18) employs an acridinium ester as a direct label. Detection is achieved by measuring the light produced as a consequence of its oxidation by hydrogen peroxide (Weeks and Woodhead, 1984). Recently, a third approach, using enzymatically activated (or "triggered") dioxetanes, has been described (Bronstein *et al.*, 1989).

The exact mechanism of light production during the HRP-catalyzed oxidation of luminol is unknown, but the generally accepted sequence of reactions is summarized below (Thorpe and Kricka, 1986):

$$\text{Peroxidase} + H_2O_2 \longrightarrow \text{Compound I} + H_2O$$

$$\underset{\text{(luminol)}}{\text{Compound I} + LH^-} \longrightarrow \underset{\text{(luminol radical)}}{\text{Compound II} + L^- + H_2O}$$

$$\text{Compound II} + LH^- \longrightarrow \text{Peroxidase} + L^-$$

$$L^- + O_2 \longrightarrow \underset{\text{(superoxide radical)}}{L + O_2^-}$$

$$L^- + O_2^- \longrightarrow \underset{\text{(luminol endoperoxide)}}{LO_2^{2-}}$$

$$LO_2^{2-} \longrightarrow \underset{\text{(excited 3-aminophthalate dianion)}}{N_2 + AP^{*2-}}$$

$$AP^{*2-} \longrightarrow \text{LIGHT} + \text{3-aminophthalate dianion}$$

The oxidation of acridinium esters is simpler, with multiple bond cleavage forming a dioxetanone intermediate that decomposes spontaneously with the emission of light. Although acridinium esters are much more highly luminescent than luminol, chemiluminescent reactions in general are not as efficient as fluorescence or radioactivity and tend to decay very rapidly. The multistep nature of the HRP-catalyzed reaction actually provided an opportunity to optimize the efficiency of the light production, increasing its intensity and slowing its decay significantly.

This was accomplished by the use of various enhancers. Although many agents were tried, synthetic luciferin initially produced the greatest effect (Whitehead *et al.*, 1983). Subsequently, related 6-hydroxybenzothiazole derivatives (Thorpe *et al.*, 1985a) and also *para*-substituted phenols (Thorpe *et al.*, 1985b) produced even greater enhancement, and the reaction was adapted to a microtiter plate format (Thorpe *et al.*, 1985c). The mechanism of the enhancement is not well understood. Enhanced light emission has a spectrum similar to that of the unenhanced reaction, so it is unlikely that enhancers form complexes with luminol. They may accelerate one or more of the steps in the reaction prior to the emission of light.

The currently available Amerlite assays all employ *para*-substituted phenols as enhancers. As shown in Fig. 2, they increase the intensity of the light production and cause it to be emitted as a continuous glow, rather than a flash of light. This simplifies the design of automated instrumentation (eliminating the need for injection of hydrogen peroxide immediately in front of the detector) and also allows measurement without the need for critical timing. The Amerlite assays can be read at any time between 2 and 20 min after addition of luminol, hydrogen peroxide, and enhancers (this cocktail is referred to as the signal reagent). In addition, since light emission from the unenhanced reaction is of low intensity and the enhancers are very specific for the HRP-catalyzed reaction (Thorpe and Kricka, 1986), nonspecific interferences are eliminated.

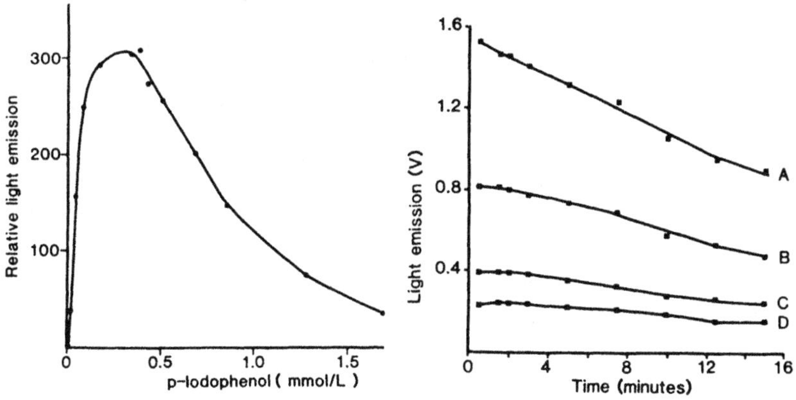

Figure 2 (*left*) Increase in light emission from HRP-catalyzed oxidation of luminol by addition of *p*-iodophenol. (*right*) Kinetics of *p*-iodophenol enhanced light emission in an immunoassay for factor VIII-related antigen. Standard A, 2.0; B, 1.0; C, 0.5; D, 0.25 IU/ml. Reproduced with permission from Thorpe *et al.* (1985c).

In the procedure for noncompetitive immunoassay using the Amerlite system, solid-phase antibody binds protein antigen present in the sample and the familiar "sandwich" is formed with HRP-labeled antibody, which can either be added simultaneously (one-step) or sequentially (two-step). After the final incubation and washing, signal reagent is added. Following a brief incubation, the emitted light can be measured. Currently, the following assays are available using this approach: thyroid-stimulating hormone (TSH), follicule-stimulating hormone (FSH), luteinizing hormone (LH), prolactin, human chorionic gonadotropin (hCG), carcinoembryonic antigen, alpha-fetoprotein (AFP), and ferritin. A similar noncompetitive assay using solid-phase antigen is also available to measure anti-rubella, anti-HBV, and anti-HIV antibodies.

In the procedure for competitive immunoassay using the Amerlite system, samples are pipetted into wells coated with anti-mouse immunoglobulin. HRP-labeled antigen and murine monoclonal primary antibody are added and during the assay incubation, the solid-phase heterologous antibody binds the murine primary antibody for which labeled antigen competes with antigen from the sample. This format (as opposed to direct coating of the wells with primary antibody) has been shown to optimize the kinetics of the immune reaction, increasing the precision and dynamic range of the assay (Hubi *et al.*, 1988). After washing, signal reagent is added and light can be measured. Currently, the following assays are available using this format: T_4, T_3, T_3 uptake, free T_4, free T_3, thyroxine-binding globulin (TBG), estradiol, progesterone, cortisol, and digoxin.

III. PERFORMANCE

A. Technical

Published reports during the development of the technology utilized in the Amerlite assays compared luminescent and colorimetric end-point determinations using commercial kits employing an HRP ELISA format. Similar results were seen with assays for rubella antibodies (Thorpe *et al.*, 1984a), T_4 (Thorpe *et al.*, 1984b), IgE (Thorpe *et al.*, 1985d), hCG, digoxin, and factor VIII-related antigen (Thorpe *et al.*, 1985b). Since the introduction of the Amerlite system, published evaluations of AFP (John *et al.*, 1986a), TSH (John *et al.*, 1986b), T_4, TBG (Wood *et al.*, 1988), cortisol (Westerhuis, 1988), ferritin, free T_4 (Armbruster *et al.*, 1989) and hCG (Banfi *et al.*, 1989) have documented technical performance comparable to either in-house or commercial radioimmunoassay. Although deviation from expected TSH results was reported in one study as samples were diluted to levels less than 0.5 mIU/l (Parnham and Tarbit, 1987) and Amerlite TSH precision profiles revealed less sensitivity than that estimated by replicate analysis of the zero standard (McConway *et al.*, 1989), another study found that the Amerlite TSH precision profile compared favorably with almost all of the other nine assays evaluated in the hyperthyroid range (Thonnart *et al.*, 1988). Overall, interassay precision in Amerlite assays ranges from 5 to 12% and good linearity is present with both competitive and noncompetitive assays. Agreement with radioimmunoassay and other nonisotopic assays is good, with *r* values ranging from 0.87 to 0.98.

B. Clinical

Published reports of extensive clinical evaluations of the Amerlite system have been limited to thyroid disease. Early versions of the TSH assay produced anecdotal falsely elevated results (Dilley and Clarke, 1988) and discrepancies dependent upon the time of signal reading (Edwards *et al.*, 1988), but these problems were addressed by Amersham. Reporting on 19 months of routine use of the TSH assay, Squire and Gimlette (1988) cited only 10 falsely elevated results out of a total of 10,800 patients (0.09%). Amerlite TSH compared favorably with nine other assays when receiver-operating characteristic curves were evaluated for diagnosis of hyperthyroidism in a population of 600 patients, of whom 217 were judged to be hyperthyroid (Thonnart *et al.*, 1988). Amerlite TSH successfully identified thyroid status in 93 unselected patients (Parnham and Tarbit, 1987) and in larger groups of hyperthyroid, hypothyroid, sick euthyroid, and pregnant patients (Squire and Gimlette, 1987). Also, Amerlite T4 and TBG assays correctly identified thyroid status in 165 unselected thyroid outpatients (Wood *et al.*, 1988).

The Amerlite free T_4 assay was demonstrated to have diagnostic sensitivities of 97% for hyperthyroidism and 88% for hypothyroidism in a population of 497 patients of which 65% were euthyroid, 22% hyperthyroid, and 13% hypothyroid (Perdrisot *et al.*, 1989). The assay employs an analogue that binds poorly to albumin (Midgley *et al.*, 1987) and has been found to be more accurate in familial dysalbuminemic hyperthyroxinemia than other analogue assays (Sapin *et al.*, 1988, 1989) and a kinetic two-step method (Seghers *et al.*, 1988). Assaying 2000 consecutive patients attending a primary care center, abnormally high or low results were obtained in several cases, but these specimens were normal when reassayed after use of a polyethylene glycol precipitation step suggested by Amersham to eliminate anti-T_4 antibody interference (Lindstedt *et al.*, 1988).

C. Operational

Each test kit contains strips of coated wells, liquid standards, assay reagent and/or conjugate, and assay identification labels to place on assembled plates during assays. The conjugate may be supplied ready-to-use or as a concentrate that needs to be diluted in supplied conjugate buffer. Kits are stored at refrigerator temperature.

Separately supplied by Amersham are 2-l bottles of borate buffer for plate washing that may be stored at room temperature and signal reagent. The signal reagent is supplied as 30-ml bottles of hydrogen peroxide (which can be stored at room temperature in the dark) and separately foil-sealed tablets of luminol and enhancers (which must be stored at refrigerator temperature). Just prior to performing an assay, signal reagent must be prepared by adding one of each tablet to a bottle of hydrogen peroxide. The tablets easily dissolve within 5 min. Each bottle contains enough signal reagent for one full plate.

All reagents have long shelf-lives (between 6 months and 1 year), which is a characteristic feature of nonisotopic immunoassay reagents.

The microtiter plates must be assembled using strips of 12 rows, which are stored in sealed plastic sleeves. The required number of strips are removed and placed in plastic strip holders, which can each hold up to eight strips. Those with fewer than 12 rows can be filled with blank wells and the unused assay wells stored in a supplied plastic tube. In this way, optimal use of the test kit can be made.

Pipetting must be done with great care, especially for small sample volumes (e.g., 10 μl). Manual pipetting of samples is therefore difficult and tedious. Reagent pipetting with repeating dispensers is relatively easy, but the use of an automated pipetting station is mandatory for large workloads.

All incubations take place at 37°C in the plate shaker, which can accommodate up to four plates at a time. The shaker is covered, but each plate must also be covered with individual lids. Different incubation periods can be separately programmed very easily and the digital timer will keep track of elapsed time after the alarm sounds. Incubations are either 60, 30, or 15 min.

After the final incubation, the plates are washed one at a time in the plate washer. The plate washer is sturdy and dependable, but care must be taken that the strips are properly seated in the strip holder as the washer prongs pass close to the well surface. The washing will continue as programmed if the prongs jam, causing flooding.

After the final wash, signal reagent is dispensed and, any time between 2 and 20 min later, the plate is read in the luminometer. A minor problem is the seating of the plate in the transport mechanism, which contains a snap-locked cover. Positioning the plate so that the cover can be closed properly takes a little practice. Also, since the transport mechanism moves in and out of the analyzer through a closed port, carriage damage can occur if the cover is not properly closed over the plate.

The analyzer performs a curve fit and prints both a calculated curve-fit factor and a light index, which is the light emitted by the standard with the highest luminescence. If either of these is unacceptable, the assay will be rejected. The most common causes of assay rejection are pipetting the wrong standards and failing to prepare the signal reagent properly. The user may edit the standard curve by omitting a calibrator. The data reduction is otherwise controlled by the analyzer and can not be changed online by the user. Also, the "raw data" printed by the analyzer consist of the luminescence only as a percentage of that of the highest standard. These limitations may be a disadvantage to the user who wishes to experiment with alternative methods of data reduction or other adaptations of the assay procedure.

A calibration may be stored and subsequent assays run using only four of the six standards as singlets. The user may also choose to run the entire assay as singlets. Reference ranges and quality control target ranges may also be stored in the analyzer and up to 1 month worth of data may be printed separately at any time. A separate port of the RS232C configuration allows for interfacing with an external computer as well.

There is no preventative maintenance required by the user other than keeping the instruments clean with a soft cloth moistened in mild detergent solution. Amersham regularly calibrates the luminometer. User satisfaction with the system has been reported as excellent (Alpert, 1989).

D. Economics

The current list price for the Amerlite instrumentation is approximately $35,000. Most clinical laboratories may prefer to lease it from Amersham. The exact cost of the reagents under such circumstances are, of course, subject to negotiation and dependent on volume. However, it is fair to say that, although Amerlite may cost more per reportable test than comparable manual radioimmunoassay methods, it will probably be less expensive than other automated systems.

IV. CONCLUSION

The Amerlite system offers all of the advantages of a nonisotopic immunoassay methodology. The ELISA technology is robust and the Amerlite version offers many advantages over chromogenic alternatives. The ability to initiate the reaction outside of the luminometer (and reread the wells) offers advantages in terms of automated light detection over other chemiluminescent immunoassays. From the perspective of automation, Amerlite is obviously not a completely automated system. However, if an automated sample pipettor is used, all of the labor-intensive steps involved in traditional immunoassay have been automated. This approach will appeal to laboratories that wish to maintain flexibility. A completely automated instrument employing the Amerlite ELISA technology is under development at Amersham. The intense and prolonged nature of the emitted light also allows for the use of photographic film to detect reactions, and this may have future applications for simplified screening assays.

REFERENCES

Alpert N. L. (1989). Luminescence immunoassay system. *Clin. Instrument Systems* **10**(4), 1–8.

Armbruster, D. A., Jirinzu, D. C., and Williams, J. V. (1989). Evaluation of enhanced luminescence immunoenzymometric assays (LIA) for ferritin and free T4. *J. Clin. Lab. Anal.* **3**, 78–83.

Banfi, G., Casari, E., Murone, M., and Bonini, P. A. (1989). Three nonisotopic methods for human choriogonadotropin evaluated. *Clin. Chem.* **35**, 1545–1546.

Bronstein, I., and Kricka, L. J. (1990). Instrumentation for luminescent assays. *Am. Clin. Lab.* **9**, 33–37.

Bronstein, I., Voyta, J. C., Thorpe, G. H. G., Kricka, L. J., and Armstrong, G. (1989). Chemiluminescent assay of alkaline phosphatase applied in an ultrasensitive enzyme immunoassay of thyrotropin. *Clin. Chem.* **35**, 1441–1446.

Catty, D., and Raykundalia, C. (1989). ELISA and related enzyme immunoassays. *In* "Antibodies Volume II, A Practical Approach" (D. Catty, ed.), pp. 97–154. IRL Press, Oxford, England.

Dilley, C. M., and Clarke, A. (1988). The Amerlite thyrotrophin (TSH) assay (letter). *Ann. Clin. Biochem.* **25,** 194–198.
Edwards, W., Anderson, I., Clark, N., and Grieg, M. (1988). Inaccuracies in plasma thyrotropin concentrations with the Amersham "Amerlite" (monoclonal) assay. *Clin. Chem.,* **34,** 2161–2162.
Hubi, W., Dazenbichler, G., Meissner, D., and Thiele, H. J. (1988). An improved solid-phase enzyme and luminescent immunoassay system for steroid hormones and digoxin. *Clin. Chem.* **34,** 2521–2523.
John, R., Henley, R., and Shankland, D. (1986a). Evaluation of an enhanced luminescence assay for alpha-fetoprotein. *Clin. Chem.* **32,** 2066–2069.
John, R., Henley, R., Chang, D., and McGregor, A. M. (1986b). Enhanced luminescence immunoassay: Evaluation of a new, more sensitive thyrotropin assay. *Clin. Chem.* **32,** 2171–2183.
Lindstedt, G., Lungberg, P. A., Johansson, P. M., Eggertsen, R., Petersen, K., and Nystrom, E. (1988). Interference in a luminometric enzyme-labelled analog assay for free T_4. *Clin. Chem.* **34,** 2581–2582.
McConway, M. G., Chapman, R. S., Beastall, G. H., Brown, E., Tillman, J. A., Bonar, J. A., Hutchinson, A., Allison, T., Finlayson, J., Weston, R., Beckett, G. J., Carter, G. D., Carlyle, E., Herbertson, R., Blundell, G., Edwards, W., Glen, A. C. A., and Reid, A. (1989). How sensitive are immunometric assays for thyrotropin? *Clin. Chem.* **35,** 289–291.
Midgley, J. E. M., Moon, C. R., and Wilkins, T. A. (1987). Validity of analog free thyroxin immunoassays. Part II. *Clin. Chem.* **33,** 2145–2148.
Parnham, A. J., and Tarbit, I. F. (1987). "Delfia" and "Amerlite": Two sensitive nonisotopic immunoassay systems for assay of thyrotropin compared. *Clin. Chem.* **33,** 1421–2424.
Perdrisot, R., Bounaud, M. P., Bounaud, J. Y., and Jallet, P. (1989). Four nonisotopic immunoassays of free thyroxin evaluated. *Clin. Chem.* **35,** 115–120.
Sapin, R., Gasser, F., and Chambron, J. (1989). One-step enzyme immunoassay for free thyroxin: Results with dysalbuminemic sera and one serum containing autoantibodies. *Clin. Chem.* **35,** 888–889.
Sapin, R., Gasser, F., and Schlienger, J. L. (1988). Free thyroxin in familial dysalbuminemic hyperthyroxinemia, as measured by five assays. *Clin. Chem.* **34,** 598–599.
Seghers, J., De Nayer, P., and Beckers, C. (1988). Clinical evaluation of Amerlite's one-step immunoassay for determining free thyroxin. *Clin. Chem.* **34,** 2160.
Squire, C. R., and Gimlette, T. M. (1987). Assessment of an enhanced chemiluminescent immunometric assay for TSH in 1127 patients. *Ann. Clin. Biochem.* **24,** 419–425.
Squire, C. R., and Gimlette, T. M. (1988). The Amerlite thyrotropin (TSH) assay (reply). *Ann. Clin. Biochem.* **25,** 195.
Thonnart, B., Messian, O., Colas Linhart, N., and Bok, B. (1988). Ten highly sensitive thyrotropin assays compared by receiver-operating characteristic curves analysis: Results of a prospective multicenter study. *Clin. Chem.* **34,** 691–695.
Thorpe, G. H. G., and Kricka, L. J. (1986). Enhanced chemiluminescent reactions catalyzed by horseradish peroxidase. *Methods Enzymol.* **133,** 331–353.
Thorpe, G. H. G., Haggart, R., Kricka, L. J., and Whitehead, T. P. (1984a). Enhanced luminescent enzyme immunoassays for rubella antibody, immunoglobulin E and digoxin. *Biochem. Biophys. Res. Commun.* **119,** 481–487.
Thorpe, G. H. G., Gillespie, E., Haggart, R., Kricka, L. J., and Whitehead, T. P. (1984b). An immunoassay for serum thyroxine employing enhanced luminescent quantitation of horseradish peroxidase conjugates. *In* "Analytical Applications of Bioluminescence and Chemiluminescence" (L. J. Kricka, P. E. Stanley, G. H. G. Thorpe and T. P. Whitehead, eds.), pp. 243–248. Academic Press, Orlando, Florida.
Thorpe, G. H. G., Kricka, L. J., Gillespie, E., Moseley, S., Amess, R., Baggett, N., and Whitehead, T. P. (1985a). Enhancement of the horseradish peroxidase-catalyzed chemilu-

minescent oxidation of cyclic diacyl hydrazides by 6-hydroxybenzothiazoles. *Analyt. Biochem.* **145,** 96–100.

Thorpe, G. H. G., Kricka, L. J., Moseley, S. B., and Whitehead, T. P. (1985b). Phenols as enhances of the chemiluminescent horseradish peroxidase-luminol-hydrogen peroxide reaction: Application in luminescence-monitored enzyme immunoassays. *Clin. Chem.* **31,** 1335–1341.

Thorpe, G. H. G., Moseley, S. B., Kricka, L. J., Stott, R. A., and Whitehead, T. P. (1985c). Enhanced luminescence determination of horseradish peroxidase conjugates. Application of benzothiazole derivatives as enhancers in luminescence assays on microtitre plates. *Anal. Chim. Acta* **170,** 101–107.

Thorpe, G. H. G., Williams, L. A., Kricka, L. J., Whitehead, T. P., Evans, H., and Stanworth, D. R. (1985d). A rapid luminescently monitored enzyme immunoassay for IgE. *J. Immunol. Methods.* **79,** 57–63.

Weeks, I., and Woodhead, J. S. (1984). Chemiluminescence immunoassay. *J. Clin. Immunoassay* **7,** 82–89.

Westerhuis, L. W. J. J. M. (1988). Measurement of cortisol with EMIT and Amerlite immunoassays. *Clin. Chem.* **34,** 2374.

Whitehead, T. P., Thorpe, G. H. G., Carter, T. J. N., Groucutt, C., and Kricka, L. J. (1983). Enhanced luminescence procedure for sensitive determination of peroxidase-labelled conjugates in immunoassay. *Nature* **305,** 158–159.

Wood, W. G., Rohde, C., and Jacobs, A. (1988). A comparison of commercially available luminescence enhanced enzyme immunoassays with in-house non-radioisotopic assays for thyroxine binding globulin and total thyroxine. *J. Clin. Chem. Clin. Biochem.* **26,** 135–140.

CHAPTER 12

COBAS-FARA II Analyzer

Barbara M. Goldsmith
Clinical Chemistry, St. Christopher's Hospital for Children, and Department of Pediatrics, Temple University School of Medicine, Philadelphia, Pennsylvania

I. GENERAL DESCRIPTION

The COBAS-FARA II, manufactured by Roche Diagnostic systems, is a robotic centrifugal chemistry analyzer. This instrument is a sequential discrete and batch parallel analyzer capable of stat and routine programming, with an analysis rate of up to 400 tests per hour. The five measurement modes on the analyzer include absorbance, fluorescence polarization, fluorescence intensity, turbidimetry, and nephelometry; the sixth, an ion-selective electrode module, is optional.

Two robotic pipettor arms (*XYZ* axis) are programmed to select and load several reagents, samples, diluent and pretreatment solutions into a 30-place disposable plastic cuvette rotor. Prior to transfer of sample and reagents into the cuvette, the rotor is spun briefly to verify the optical quality of the cuvette wheel. Each cuvette has two compartments, one for sample and the other for reagents. After rotor acceleration and braking, the contents in the two compartments mix. Additional reagents are added, the rotor accelerates and mixes, and the second reaction starts.

Reagents and sample volumes are controlled by two positive-displacement Hamilton syringes. Temperature is controlled to ±0.1°C over a range of 20–50°C by hot and cold airflow.

A rack system consisting of separate racks for samples, reagents, and calibrators is assembled on the analyzer. Each rack is labeled with bar codes and read by a rack reader. Samples are placed in translucent polyethylene sample cups with lids that prevent evaporation of sample. A sample probe penetrates the top of the lid and aspirates sample. After sample delivery into the cuvette, the probe is rinsed in the wash tower.

The analyzer contains a pulsed, high-intensity xenon flash lamp with a holographic grating monochromator that has a spectral range of 285–750 nm. Optical system specifications state that the wavelength accuracy is ±1 nm with a spectral half band width of 5.5 nm at 500 nm. The linear absorbance range at 340 nm is 0–3.0 Å with a photometric accuracy as low as ±0.5% of the value or 0.0001 Å (whichever is greater). The polarizer is stepper motor controlled and a semiconductor photodiode is the detector.

Absorbance measurements are made by placing cuvettes in a position horizontal to the light path. Pulsed light sends flashing light to a concave mirror behind the bulb, which directs the light toward collimating lenses and then toward an input slit. This focuses light on the monochromator. Light of a preselected wavelength is reflected from the grating, and passes through an output slit and onto a beam splitter. Ninety percent of the light emitted from the beam splitter passes through the photometer lens, through the cuvette, and through another lens in the photometer. Light then passes through four bandpass filters to eliminate stray light, reaches the photodiode, and is converted to an electronic signal. The signal passes to an analog/digital converter and the absorbance measurement is recorded.

For fluorescence polarization, the light passes through the grating monochromator as just described. Monochromatic light is horizontally polarized by an excitation polarizing filter. This results in parallel polarized light. The fluorescent tracer reagent in the cuvette emits light at a longer wavelength, which is detected by the photodiode located at a 90° angle to the excitation light. Depolarization is calculated from measurements of parallel and perpendicular light intensities as the emitted light passes through a polarization wheel before reaching the photodiode detector. The electronic signal from the photodiode passes through an analog/digital converter and is then converted into millipolarization units.

Fluorescent and nephelometric measurements use the same mechanism for pulsing and reflecting light as described above. The emitted and scattered light, respectively, is detected at a 90° angle by the photomultiplier tube.

II. PROGRAMMING

A 9-in cathode ray tube (CRT) within the instrument displays characters and graphics simultaneously. Four main headings (Routine, Stat, Program, and Info) contain submenus under which all functions can be accessed (COBAS-FARA II Operator's Manual).

Tests can be done in Routine and Stat modes, with the Stat work list processed first. Work lists are designed by assigning tests or profiles to samples. Samples are entered as numbers corresponding to the position number on a sample rack.

Test parameters are programmed by the user. These define the manner in which an assay is analyzed, calculated, and calibrated. The user is given choices from which to select the measurement, reaction, and calibration modes, as well as the wavelength, temperature, incubation times, number of readings, etc. for each assay. Up to three reagents can be used per assay. Calibration curves are stored in memory. An example of a test parameter list for phenobarbital using Roche Diagnostics fluorescence polarization reagents is given in Table 1.

Under Info, the user can access test results, patient reports, calibration information, quality control data, work lists, and system diagnostics. In this program, test parameters can be temporarily modified. Some examples of why this offers advantages are (1) the operator can change a calculation step from endpoint to kinetic, (2) the calibration curve can be recalculated based on a different calibration mode, and (3) results can be recalculated if the reagent blank is removed from the calculation.

Table 1 Phenobarbital Program Parameters

1. Units (12 = μg/ml)	12
2. Calculation factor	1
3. Standard 1 conc.	0.0
	2.5
	7.5
	15
	30
	60
4. Standard 2 conc.	0
5. Standard 3 conc.	0
6. Limit	25
7. Temperature	25°C
8. Type of analysis	7.6
9. Wavelength	487.1
10. Sample volume	2 μl
11. Diluent volume	50 μl
12. Reagent volume	200 μl
13. Incubation time	10s
14. Start reagent volume	30 μl
15. Time of first reading	30s
16. Time interval	10s
17. Number of readings	1.13
18. Blanking mode	0
19. Printout mode	2

III. APPLICATIONS

A. Assays

A great advantage of this analyzer is its flexibility. Assays can be customized through a large number of programming options. This allows for reagent flexibility, and enables the use of a wide range of manufacturers reagents as well as "homemade" reagents. For example, in a research application the FARA II has been used to measure DNA in *in vitro* cell culture media using the fluorescence measurement mode (Mate *et al.*, 1990b). Roche Diagnostics manufactures a number of general chemistry reagents that can be adapted to the FARA II analyzer. One study that evaluated the precision of enzyme and colorimetric chemistries by implementing the NCCLS protocol showed intra- and interprecision to be less than 4% (Mate *et al.*, 1990a).

B. Calculations

The calculation of a result is dependent upon the calculation step (end point, kinetic, kinetic search) and the calibration mode. There are seven calibration modes: (1) factor, (2) slope average, (3) linear regression, (4) linear interpolation, (5) logit/log 4, (6) logit/log 5, and (7) exponential 5. The first three calibration modes are used when the observed signal change and the concentration of the analyte follow a linear relationship. The others calculate results in which there is no linear relationship (i.e., therapeutic drugs, or specific protein quantitations using nephelometry or turbidimetry).

C. Flags

Test flags are printed to the right of or in place of a result when a result check fails. Result checks follow test file specifications; if more than one of the result checks fail, the highest priority flag is printed. There is an extensive list of flags and messages provided by the manufacturer, which allows troubleshooting by the operator.

D. Maintenance

Daily maintenance involves inspecting the sample needle and reagent probe, checking the sample syringe for air bubbles, the flow of the diluent stream, and the action of the robotic arms, and cleaning the optical lenses.

Rack reader and CRT checks are performed weekly. In addition, a sample precision test (a minimum of 15 sample cups with potassium dichromate solution), which checks pipetting precision, is done weekly. Twice a month the Teflon tips on the sample and reagent syringes are replaced. Monthly maintenance consists of replacing the sample needle and cleaning the fluid system with an alcohol flush. A reagent precision test is also performed using a pipetting test solution.

E. Quality Control

Up to three quality control levels can be programmed per test file. Quality control parameters include the level, the position at which the controls are located on the calibrator/control rack, the assigned value, and the low and high limits. There are two quality control subdirectories: (1) daily reports, which store the current statistics and the last four values for the day, and (2) monthly reports, with statistics for all days on which at least one control was run. Flagged controls are not stored in the quality control file. The system requires that the controls be rerun or that the test parameters be converted to accept the out-of-range control.

IV. EVALUATION OF THE ANALYZER

Roche Diagnostics has marketed therapeutic drug reagents that use the fluorescent polarization. We evaluated eight therapeutic drugs using Roche Diagnostics COBAS-FP reagents on the FARA II analyzer. The evaluation consisted of an intraprecision study (Table 2) using COBAS-FP TDM controls (75 control samples per level of control), an interprecision study (Table 3) (five replicates of three control levels over 5 days), standard curve stability over a 35-day period, and a correlation study where samples were run on the FARA II and the Abbott TDx. The TDx uses fluorescence polarization for measuring therapeutic drug concentrations.

The seven drugs evaluated were theophylline, carbamazepine, tobramycin, phenytoin, valproic acid, primidone, and phenobarbital. Intra- and interprecision data showed coefficients of variation of 5% or less. Correlation data between the FARA II and the TDx are presented in Table 4. There was a high correlation between assay methods for each of the seven drugs.

Other published studies yielded similar findings (Cheng *et al.*, 1989; Farrenkopf, 1989), where there is good agreement between fluorescent polarization assays. However, in one study (Trundle *et al.*, 1990) a method bias on the FARA II was seen in six out of 12 drugs evaluated when the

Table 2 Intraprecision Study

Drug	*N*	Mean	SD	SE	% CV
Theophylline					
Level I	75	5.10	0.183	0.021	3.59
Level II	75	13.59	0.313	0.313	2.30
Level III	75	22.55	0.459	0.459	2.04
Carbamazepine					
Level I	75	3.22	0.147	0.017	4.56
Level II	75	8.31	0.306	0.035	3.69
Level III	75	15.79	0.547	0.063	3.47
Tobramycin					
Level I	75	1.99	0.124	0.041	6.23
Level II	75	5.15	0.189	0.022	3.68
Level III	75	7.33	0.211	0.024	2.89
Phenytoin					
Level I	75	4.698	0.139	0.016	2.96
Level II	75	12.469	0.646	0.075	5.18
Level III	75	20.188	0.958	0.111	4.74
Phenobarbital					
Level I	75	12.474	1.382	0.160	11.08
Level II	75	27.678	0.882	0.102	3.19
Level III	75	41.162	1.219	0.141	2.96
Primidone					
Level I	75	3.851	0.535	0.062	13.89
Level II	75	7.689	0.302	0.035	3.93
Level III	75	12.684	0.482	0.056	3.80

bias was calculated as a percent difference from the assigned values. Interference studies evaluating the effect of bilirubin, hemoglobin, and Intralipid on the COBAS-FP assays showed less interference on the FARA II than observed on the TDx, Stratus II, or Cobas-Bio analyzers (Cole *et al.*, 1990).

Table 3 5-Day Interprecision Study

	Level I			Level II			Level III		
Drug	Mean	SD	% CV	Mean	SD	% CV	Mean	SD	% CV
Theophylline	5.07	0.18	3.6	13.66	0.30	2.2	22.61	0.41	1.8
Carbamazepine	3.25	0.14	4.2	8.49	0.20	2.4	16.14	0.60	3.7
Tobramycin	1.90	0.04	2.0	5.00	0.07	1.5	7.08	0.19	2.7
Phenytoin	4.62	0.11	2.4	12.34	0.25	2.0	20.06	0.59	2.9
Phenobarbital	12.60	0.36	2.8	27.62	0.62	2.3	41.58	0.98	2.4
Primidone	3.92	0.11	2.7	7.80	0.28	3.6	12.86	0.30	2.4

Table 4 Correlation between FARA II and TDx Analyzers

Drug	*N*	Slope	Y Intercept	*r*
Theophylline	100	1.0296	0.1674	0.9964
Carbamazepine	100	0.9311	0.5332	0.9697
Tobramycin	101	0.8784	0.0257	0.9960
Phenytoin	108	0.9946	1.0693	0.9937
Valproic acid	100	0.9584	2.0470	0.9919
Primidone	84	1.0540	−0.0234	0.9904
Phenobarbital	100	1.0230	−0.6979	0.9930

V. SUMMARY

Since the FARA II analyzer can be programmed to use small reagent volumes, it is cost-effective. In our experience, the only significant problems we encountered were electronic. A stable electric current is required to avert such problems.

The FARA II is a flexible analyzer that is readily adaptable to a variety of applications for the clinical and research laboratories.

REFERENCES

Cheng, C., Farrenkopf, B., Jerome, H., and Kaufman, R. A. (1989). TDM assays by fluorescence polarization on the COBAS FARA II™: Determination of serum NAPA, theophylline and phenytoin. *Clin. Chem.* **35,** 1178.

COBAS FARA II Operator's Manual, Roche Diagnostic Systems, October 1989.

Cole, R., Bradley, H., and Trundle, D. (1990). Comparison of interferences in 12 drug methods on four instruments: FARA II. TDx, Stratus II, and COBAS-BIO. *Clin. Chem.* **36:**1111.

Farrenkopf, B. C., Mylott, G., Awdziej, T., and Kaufman, R. A. (1989). TDM assays by fluorescence polarization on the COBAS FARA II™ analyzer: Determination of serum amikacin, gentamicin and tobramycin. *Clin. Chem.* **35,** 1178.

Maclin, E., Young, D. S. (1987). Automation in the clinical laboratory. *In* "Fundamentals of Clinical Chemistry" (N. W. Tietz, ed.), 3rd ed., pp. 177–178. W. B. Saunders, Philadelphia.

Mate, A., Little, J., Pignatello, M., *et al.* (1990a). An evaluation of precision on the Roche Cobas FARA II centrifugal analyzer according to NCCLS guidelines EP-5. *Clin. Chem.* **36:**1201.

Mate, A., Little, J., and Lipman, J. M. (1990b). An application of the Roche COBAS FARA II centrifugal analyzer for the microdetermination of DNA using Hoescht 33258. *Clin. Chem.* **36,** 1176.

Trundle, D., Cole, R., and Bradley, H. (1990). Evaluation of analytical performance of polarization fluorescence methods for twelve drugs on the FARA II. *Clin. Chem.* **36,** 1201.

CHAPTER 13

CyberFluor Immunoassay System

Graham Ellis
Department of Clinical Biochemistry,
The Hospital for Sick Children,
and Department of Clinical Biochemistry,
University of Toronto, Toronto, Ontario, Canada

I. INTRODUCTION

During the 1960s and 1970s, radioimmunoassays made the routine measurement of drugs and hormones possible. The inherent specificity of a good antibody was combined with the sensitivity of detection of a radioisotope. In order to match this sensitivity without using radioisotopes, labels are needed that can be detected at low concentration and incorporated into systems with good signal-to-noise characteristics. Enzyme labels have these properties (especially those with high turnover numbers acting on fluorogenic or chemiluminescent substrates). Alternately, labels that have intrinsic properties of chemiluminescence or fluorescence may be used. The sensitivity and specificity of fluorescence measurements are very much influenced by the fluor chosen and by the presence in biological materials of fluorescent interfering materials such as drugs or natural products. Clinical time-resolved fluorescence systems (Diamandis, 1988; Hemmilä, 1988) often employ lanthanide-based fluors that have longer Stokes shifts than those of interfering materials. (The Stokes shift is the difference in wavelength between emitted and exciting wavelength). Time resolution (measurement of the long-lived fluorescence of the specific fluor at a defined time after an excitation pulse) also increases specificity and signal-to-noise ratio. Because most fluorescent interferences have a shorter life than those of the lanthanide fluors, the time between excitation and the start of measurement can be increased to eliminate the interference from short-lived fluors. Many manual and automated immunoassay systems incorporate antibody or ligand bound to solid phase (e.g., bead, tube, or microtiter well). This makes the assay technically easier to perform in manual systems, but it also permits easier multiple washing steps to remove interferences and also improve signal-to-noise ratio. The CyberFluor immunoassay system uses time-resolved fluorescence with a microtiter plate format to produce an analytical system that has sensitivity similar to or better than radioimmunoassay (RIA) (Diamandis, 1988).

II. SYSTEM DESCRIPTION

A. Instrumentation

1. CyberFluor 615 Immunoanalyzer

This is a time-resolved pulsed-laser-based fluorometer designed to read the fluorescence of a fluor captured on the plastic surface of microtiter plates following an immunoassay (Fig. 1). The instrument can be loaded with up to four microtiter plates that may be from the same or different assays, but each plate must contain 6–12 wells comprising an appropriate standard curve for the assay on that plate. Each plate may consist of up to 96 wells arranged in up to eight strips of 12 wells. Standards and unknowns are always run in duplicate. The immunoanalyzer has a built-in IBM compatible 640-KB RAM computer with key pad or keyboard interface and dual 720-KB 3.5 inch microfloppy disc drives. After the plates are loaded on the instrument, the operator keys in the plate number, assay type, and the number of wells to be read on each plate. Each plate is moved in turn to the optical compartment of the instrument, where each well is successively illuminated by a 3- to 4-ns pulse of light from the laser at 337.1 nm. The resulting fluorescence intensity of the illuminated area in the well is measured at 615 nm between 200 and 600 μs after the light pulse. The mean fluorescence determined from 16 firings of the laser at approximately 50-ms intervals is taken as the "raw" fluorescence of the well. The "raw" fluorescence is corrected for laser intensity, which is measured directly by a phototube during each firing of the laser. A full microtiter plate of 96 wells is read in approximately 2.5 min. After each plate has been read, the standard fluorescence count data are fitted to a standard curve that can be "fine-tuned" by the operator to eliminate any undesirable counts on the rare occasions that this is necessary. When the standard curve is accepted, the unknowns are calculated and printed out.

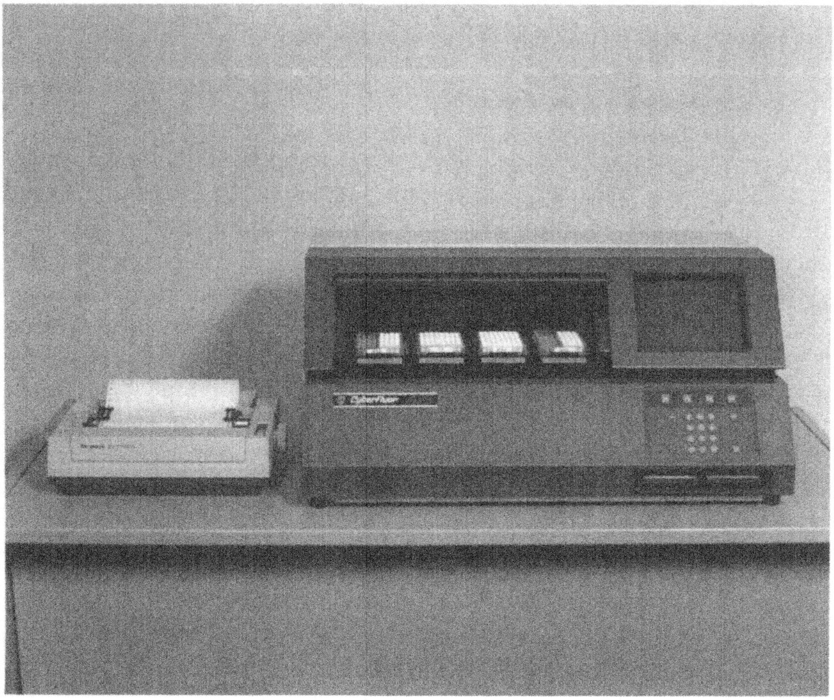

Figure 1 The CyberFluor 615 immunoanalyzer.

2. CyberFluor Strip Washer

This is a plate washer that can be programmed by a magnetic card to perform a prescribed series of washes to each strip of wells on the microtiter plate. Normally wells are washed four times on each of two occasions for each assay (after the incubation of serum and immunoassay reagents and after incubation with the EuroFluor S reagent). The washer permits the wells to be in contact with the wash solution for a fixed time, and effectively removes most of the wash solution at the end of each wash.

3. CyberFluor Strip Dryer

The fluor used in the CyberFluor system is quenched by water and so in early protocols the microtiter plate was dried prior to reading. The inverted microtiter plate was placed in the dryer with 96 nozzles through which a built-in fan supplied air flow. The drying time was 10 min. Subsequent protocols incorporate the addition of a solution (EuroFluor S Reading Solution) that causes dissociation of the antibody/ligand complex and solubilizes the fluor. The fluorescence is then read in solution. The Strip Dryer is not required for the new protocols.

4. Automated Sample Handling

Several automated sample handlers have been tested by CyberFluor for use with their system. Models tested include the Tecan Robotic Sample Processor Series 5000 (Tecan US Ltd., Hillsborough, North Carolina 27278), the Kemble Kemtek 1000 and 700 Sample Processors (Kemble Instruments, Burgess Hill, West Sussex, RH15 8QY, U.K.), and the Hamilton Microlab 2000 Fluid Processing System (Hamilton Company, Reno, Nevada 89520-0012). Protocols have been developed to optimize the use of CyberFluor reagents with these systems (e.g., to minimize carryover, minimize reagent usage, add reagents at the optimal time, etc.). Each system has an optional bar-code reader for patient sample identification. By applying an adhesive bar-code label to each plate, positive identification of the sample and the plate on which it is dispensed can be assured. A customized interface and software package are required to transfer the data between the immunoanalyzer and the computer of the automated sample handler or the lab information system.

B. Reagents

1. The Fluorescent Label EuroFluor S and Its Properties

The CyberFluor system uses a Europium chelate of BCPDA [4,7-bis-(chlorosulfophenyl)-1,10phenanthroline-2,9-dicarboxylic acid] as its fluor. In the format used with many of the assays, approximately 450 molecules of the fluor are attached to approximately three thyroglobulin moieties that are linked to a single molecule of streptavidin (Morton and Diamandis, 1990). This configuration provides a great increase in fluorescence associated with each streptavidin molecule compared with simply linking one molecule of the fluor to each streptavidin molecule and gives sensitivity comparable to that achieved by the use of radioisotopes. The EuroFluor S–streptavidin complex binds avidly to biotin moieties on biotinylated antibodies, with low nonspecific binding.

2. Assay Principle

The system is suitable for large or small molecules. The assay format for large molecules is a sandwich-type format, whereas that for small molecules is one of competition.

a. Sandwich-Type Format (Fig. 2) CyberFluor FIAgen test kits include microtiter plates coated with an antibody to the antigen that is to be

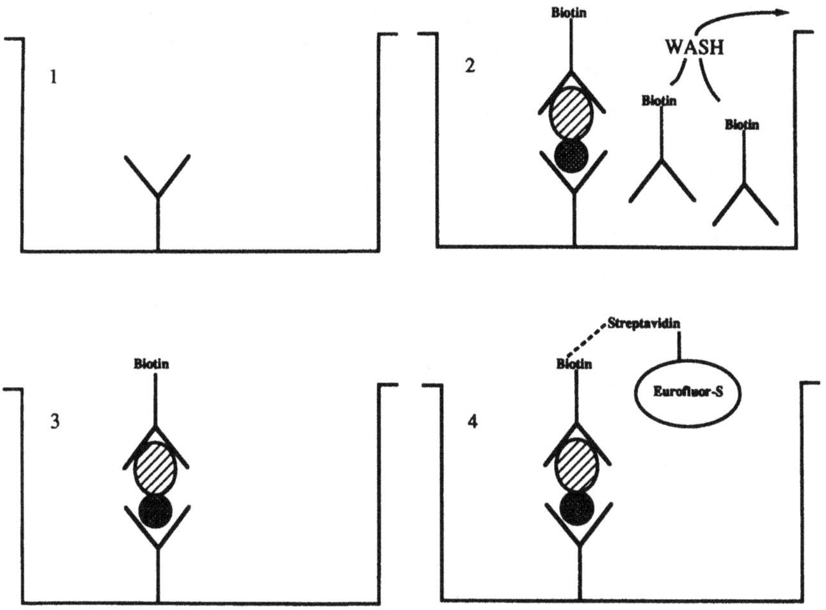

Figure 2 Principle of a sandwich-type assay on the CyberFluor system. Plates are precoated with antibody to the analyte of interest (panel 1). During incubation, the analyte and excess biotinylated antibody (directed against a second epitope) form a sandwich with the immobilized antibody and the excess biotinylated antibody is washed away (panels 2–3). EuroFluor S–streptavidin reagent binds to the biotinylated complex and after a second wash to remove excess reagent, the bound Eurofluor S remains and gives the fluorescence (panel 4).

measured. The sample containing the antigen is added followed by a buffer containing an excess of a biotinylated antibody directed against an alternate epitope of the antigen. Antibody pairs are selected that do not hinder each other for binding to the antigen. After a suitable reaction time (2–4 h, at room temperature on a shaker), buffer, sample, and excess biotinylated antibody are aspirated and the plate is washed four times with a wash solution containing a mild detergent. The wells that have samples containing the antigen have antigen bound to their plastic surface and biotinylated antibody bound to that antigen. The amount of biotinylated antibody increases with increasing antigen concentration. EuroFluor S–streptavidin reagent is then added. The plates are incubated at room temperature for 30–45 min during which the EuroFluor S–streptavidin reagent binds to the biotinylated antibody on the plate. Excess reagent is aspirated and the plate is washed four times with wash solution. Traces of residual wash solution are expelled by hitting the plate vigorously on a porous surface. The remaining traces of moisture were removed on the

CyberFluor dryer in protocols developed by CyberFluor prior to 1991. In recent protocols, the dryer is not used. Instead, EuroFluor S Reading Solution is added to solubilize the fluor and the plates are shaken for 15 min. The fluorescence is then read and the unknowns are calculated against the standard curve.

b. Competition-Type Format (Fig. 3) With this format, FIAgen kits contain plates coated with an analog of the analyte that is to be measured. The analog is selected to compete with this analyte for the binding of a biotinylated antibody. The sample containing the analyte is placed in the sample well followed by buffer containing a biotinylated antibody. During an incubation (1–2 h with shaking), in the absence of the analyte to be measured, a high proportion of the biotinylated antibody binds to the analog on the plate. Conversely, if there is a large amount of analyte present, it binds to the biotinylated antibody, preventing the antibody from binding to the analog on the plate. Buffer containing unbound biotinylated antibody and any excess of analyte from the sample is aspirated and the plate is washed four times with the wash solution. EuroFluor S–streptavidin reagent is then added and the plate is incubated for 30–45 min at room temperature with shaking, during which time the EuroFluor S binds to the biotinylated antibody. The excess reagents are aspirated and the plate is washed four times with wash solution. It is then either dried or EuroFluor S Reading Solution is added with a 15-min incubation on the shaker. The plate is read on the immunoanalyzer as before.

III. PERFORMANCE

A. Technical

1. Accuracy

Accuracy is difficult to assess in immunoassays, especially those for protein hormones. Using standard material provided by CyberFluor, we have confirmed recovery of 89–117% for growth hormone (GH), follicle-stimulating hormone (FSH), and luteinizing hormone (LH) assays. Data filed by CyberFluor with their Food and Drug Administration (FDA) application for other tests also show good recovery. Precision is shown in Table 1.

2. Nonspecific Binding

The microtiter format coupled with effective washing procedures and the use of the Eurofluor S–streptavidin label gives very low nonspecific binding. This is readily apparent in sandwich-format assays where the fluorescence of the zero standard is approximately 0.1–0.6% of the highest standard.

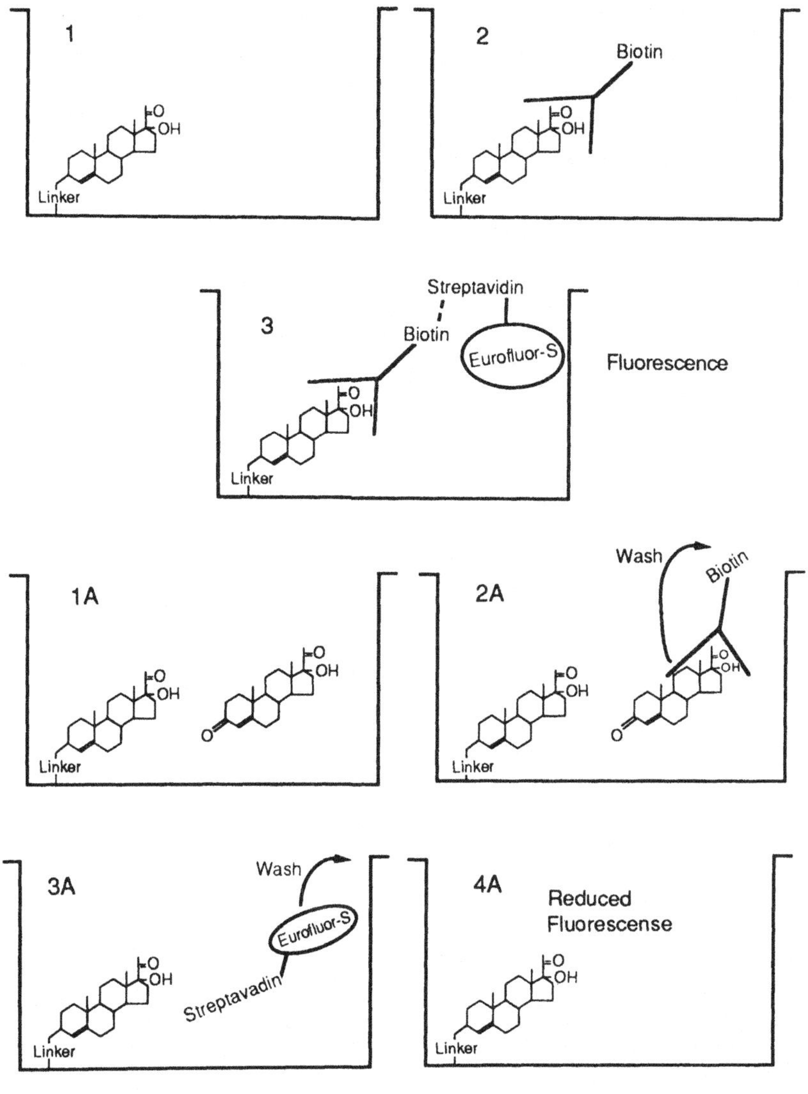

Figure 3 Principle of a competition-type assay on the CyberFluor system. In the absence of analyte (panels 1–3), biotinylated antibody can easily bind to the steroid analog in the well. After washing away excess antibody, Eurofluor S–streptavidin reagent binds to this bound antibody. After a second wash to remove excess reagent, the bound Eurofluor S remains and gives the fluorescence. When analyte is present from the sample (panels 1A–4A), competition occurs and the final fluorescence is reduced.

Table 1 Between-Batch Precision with the CyberFluor System[a]

	Low level		Medium level		High level	
	CV (%)	At mean value	CV (%)	At mean value	CV (%)	At mean value
Cortisol (μg/dl)	7.3	(10.7)	8.9	(18.2)	8.2	(40.4)
Chorionic gonadotropin (hCG, IU/l)	9.2	(2.5)	5.6	(37.2)	5.6	(543.3)
Ferritin (μg/l)	9.9	(72.1)	8.7	(140.5)	10.0	(316.0)
Follitropin[b] (FSH, IU/l)	6.3	(4.9)	7.1	(11.2)	11.1	(25.0)
Growth hormone[b] (GH μg/l)	13.6	(2.6)	7.1	(5.6)	6.1	(13.4)
Lutropin[b] (LH, IU/l)	8.1	(6.8)	9.9	(41.9)	10.4	(102.7)
Prolactin (μg/l)	7.0	(17.1)	9.1	(24.0)	3.7	(55.3)
T_3 uptake	5.7	(21.3)	3.8	(30.0)	3.5	(36.0)
Thyroxine binding globulin (TBG, mg/l)	6.5	(24.8)	5.8	(30.0)	3.9	(34.8)
Thyroxine (T_4, μg/dl)	11.6	(3.1)	9.3	(7.6)	5.5	(16.7)
Thyrotropin (TSH, mIU/l)	7.9	(1.8)	8.7	(9.0)	7.0	(18.6)

[a] Data from CyberFluor package insert obtained in clinical trials, except for assays marked *b*.
[b] Data obtained at our hospital (n = 15) with manual pipetting of serum and reagents.

3. Sensitivity

The low nonspecific binding, coupled with the sensitivity of time-resolved fluorescence measurement, yields excellent sensitivity, particularly for assays that are in sandwich-type format. Two standard deviations of the zero calibrator are <0.1 μg/l for GH, 0.03 mIU/l for TSH (manufacturer's data), 0.1 IU/l (68/907) for LH (manufacturer's data), and 0.1 IU/l for FSH (manufacturer's data). Comparable data for competitive assays are 5 μg/l for T_4, and cortisol.

4. Linearity

The CyberFluor 615 immunoanalyzer can be set to two sensitivity ranges. The more sensitive scale is achieved by increasing the photomultiplier tube voltage. This setting "PMT High" is used most often. With assays in which large concentrations of EuroFluor S are used, the photomultiplier tube could lose linearity, and the PMT setting is set to "PMT Low". At each setting, the instrument detection system covers 3.5 orders of magnitude above the minimum detectable signal. Assay linearity is dependent upon assay type. Typically assays are linear (after appropriate curve fitting and interpolation) for one to two orders of magnitude above the detection limit for competition assays and two to four orders of magnitude for sandwich assays.

5. Beginning and End of Plate Effects

The CyberFluor system of coated wells differs from the RIA system of coated test tubes in one important respect that is not immediately apparent. For any given RIA tube, the coating of the tube by antibody and the subsequent reaction with antigen from the standard or patient sample and label binding must be constant for a given amount of analyte. However, the evenness of coating or uniformity of the reaction with the sample is not critical because the gamma counter responds to all the radioactivity in the bottom 2–3 cm of the tube. In contrast, the CyberFluor immunoanalyzer laser illuminates a part of the base of the well, and the fluorescence is measured from that area. Effectively the measurement is one of surface fluorescence density. The area is only part of that to which antibody is bound in sandwich-type assays. If sample is added to one well and left for a period of time before further reagent is added, the high-affinity antibody may rapidly remove analyte on the wetted area. This could happen at the beginning of a plate while samples are prepared for later wells. In contrast, the last well of the plate could receive sample, followed rapidly by reagent, and the well area over which the analyte could react with antibody could be larger, and ultimately the fluorescence density of the laser-illuminated area could be lower for the same analyte concentration. It is for this reason that in order to minimize this effect, CyberFluor recommends addition of reagent to each strip of 12 wells after sample addition. The effect is antibody- and analyte-dependent, but clearly wells should not be left for long periods with sample present, without reagent. Because reagent and sample are added almost simultaneously with automated sample preparation and because antibody is the last addition in competition-type assays, this is only a potential problem with sandwich-type assays done manually (M. J. Khosravi, personal communication). Use of the EuroFluor S Reading Solution to solubilize the fluor improves precision by eliminating any uneven distribution of fluorescence in the well.

B. Clinical Correlation

All CyberFluor assays correlate with other immunoassays, and at least two such correlations are submitted for FDA approval with each assay. When immunoassays assays fail to agree, it is often difficult to define the erroneous assay unless it has a defined cross-reactivity problem [e.g., an LH assay with known human chorionic gonadotropin (hCG) cross-reactivity would be assumed to be in error if it gave higher results in a pregnant patient than those obtained by a more specific assay] or if one assay is clearly less sensitive than the other and most of the discrepant results are at the sensitivity limit of the less sensitive assay. When we compared the CyberFluor LH assay with RIA from Ciba Corning Canada Inc., Richmond Hill, Ontario, we found fairly good correlation except at the lower values that were at the sensitivity limit for the RIA (Ellis *et al.*, 1989). We saw similar results when we compared our in-house RIA for GH with the CyberFluor assay (Kahan *et al.*, 1990). In general, as might be expected, the CyberFluor assays tend to correlate better with two-site immunoradiometric assays than with RIAs. The CyberFluor LH assay, like many RIAs, has high hCG cross-reactivity, but in patients with precocious puberty, CyberFluor LH correlated better with the clinical condition of the patient than the Corning RIA, presumably because the latter detected LH species lacking bioactivity (Ellis *et al.*, 1989). The exquisite sensitivity of the LH assay on the CyberFluor system may permit the detection of early puberty by observation of the pulsatile release of small quantities of LH from the pubertal pituitary (F. J. Holland, personal communication; see also Haavisto *et al.*, 1990). We have assessed the CyberFluor GH assay (Kahan *et al.*, 1990) and find that it gives clinically useful information. Most of the CyberFluor assays were developed by Diamandis and Khosravi and colleagues. In many of their published descriptions they have included clinical correlates, although many of their clinical assignments were determined by biochemical testing rather than by review of patients' medical records (Khosravi and Diamandis, 1987; Diamandis *et al.*, 1988; Khosravi *et al.*, 1988a,b; Khosravi and Diamandis, 1989; Khosravi and Sudsbury, 1989; Papanastasiou-Diamandi *et al.*, 1989a,b; Reichstein *et al.*, 1989; Tan *et al.*, 1989; Kahan *et al.*, 1990; Shankaran *et al.*, 1990; Tan *et al.*, 1990).

C. Operational

1. General

Many radioimmunoassay laboratories are staffed by technologists who are very experienced in rapid, manual pipetting of multiple samples and solutions. Some technologists prefer to do these assays rather than to load automated high-throughput analyzers. Because of the non-stat nature of the majority of endocrinology tests, work flow is often run in batch mode. In this environment, it is relatively easy to change from RIA to the CyberFluor system (or to those similar, e.g., Delfia, Chapter 14, or Amerlite, Chapter 11).

The microtiter format is at first alien to the technologist who is used to 12 × 175 mm plastic tubes. But the advantages of wells that no longer require further marking of "tube number," and the small sample and reagent volumes, especially in pediatrics, soon become apparent. There is initial concern about specimen integrity because of possible transfer of sample to adjacent wells over the small barrier of the microtiter well during shaking. However, in reviewing many printouts, we have not seen any evidence that this occurs in routine use. As with RIA, there are various timed incubation steps in CyberFluor protocols during which other assays may be set up, or specimen receiving or reporting done.

2. Throughput

All assays can be completed in a half work day. Throughput is limited by:

a. The speed with which the technologist or sample preparation unit can pipette standards and samples into the microtiter wells. In our lab, with microsamples and careful confirmation of sample identification, this takes 20–30 min per plate of 96 wells (e.g., 6 standards in duplicate and 42 samples or controls in duplicate). All plates require a standard curve, and CyberFluor recommends duplicate pipetting of standards and unknowns. Thus, the throughput of manual pipetting is about 80–90 samples/h before it is reduced by the operator's fatigue. With automated sample preparation, the rate will range from approximately 168 to 336 patient or control samples per hour.

b. Assays require the use of a plate shaker, so throughput is affected by the number of shakers available. The number of plate washers and dryers available is less likely to affect throughput.

c. The speed with which plates can be read is rapid compared with that at which RIA tubes may be counted. Each plate of 96 wells can be read in 2.5 min. With a slow printer, printout would take a further 5 min. A faster printer or downloading to disk or host computer speeds up this step to about 4 min per plate of 42 unknown samples in duplicate, giving a throughput of 630 patient or control samples per hour, if the laboratory can prepare samples at this rate.

3. Reliability of the CF 615 Immunoanalyzer

The instrument in our laboratory has been very reliable. The transport mechanism has jammed on two or three occasions over a 2-year period when inexperienced operators have misloaded plates. The information in the computer was affected after a period of intermittent mains electricity instability that probably produced spikes of high voltage. The laser thyrotron tube was replaced. Similar reliability has been found in most other installations. The downtime has typically been less than 2–3 days per year (information from CyberFluor, Inc.).

4. The Plate Washer and Shaker

Effective shaking and plate washing are critical to the assays. The plate washer should be cleaned weekly to maintain its effectiveness.

5. Stability of the Fluor

The fluor is extremely resistant to photobleaching. A strip of 10 wells was repeatedly read on the CyberFluor 615 analyzer. After being read 50 times, the fluorescence was 87% of that initially read.

6. Coating of the Microtiter Plates

The CyberFluor methodology depends upon effective coating of the microtiter plates with excess antibody (in the case of sandwich assays) or with a limiting quantity of analog (in competition assays). All wells in the plate must be coated to the same extent for good precision. We have generally found this to be so, but unequal coating (or bad pipetting) necessitates reassay of one or two samples per plate because of unsatisfactory duplicates. This frequency is similar to that seen in other immunoassays. We concur with the recommendation of CyberFluor, Inc., that assays be run in duplicate.

7. Maintenance

Each day a single plate prepared for instrument quality control is read. Results are compared with those of the previous day and should be within 1–2% of those values. The time taken is approximately 5 min. The analyzer has built-in diagnostics that facilitate trouble-shooting. It is recommended that these are run at each daily startup. The 615 immunoanalyzer requires periodic dusting, but there are no parts in the instrument that require service by the user. As mentioned previously, the washer head requires weekly cleaning.

D. Economic Factors

The 1990 list price of the CyberFluor system including the immunoanalyzer, shaker, and printer is CDN $45,350 (approximately US $38,548). The list price of kits comprising two or ten 96-well coated plates and all reagents for the assay is CDN $350 or 1344 (approximately US $297 or 1142). With six standards and six quality control (QC) samples and 36 patient samples in duplicate per plate, the reagent cost is CDN $4.86–3.73 (US $4.13–3.17) per patient result. Quantity discounts and reagent leasing arrangements are also available.

IV. CONCLUSIONS

The CyberFluor immunoassay system uses time-resolved fluorescence to quantify a europium chelate label (EuroFluor S) that becomes bound to microtiter wells during incubations. The technology is very sensitive and can be applied to large molecules (e.g., protein hormones) in a sandwich-type format and to small molecules (e.g., thyroxine, cortisol) in competition-type format. The system uses automated washing of the microtiter plate, which is then read in a dedicated analyzer. Automated sample handling is an option for labs with very large work load. The assay protocols are similar to those of RIA (sample preparation, incubation, separation step, "counting" fluorescence) and are easily adopted by technologists who are experienced in RIA procedures. Precision is similar to RIA, and results correlate well with RIA or immunoradiometric assay procedures. Overall throughput is higher than that of many dedicated immunoassay analyzers because reading is so rapid after batches have been prepared and incubated.

ACKNOWLEDGMENTS

Our evaluation of the CyberFluor instrument was supported by a grant from CyberFluor, Inc.

REFERENCES

Diamandis, E. P. (1988). Immunoassays with time-resolved fluorescence spectroscopy: Principles and applications. *Clin. Biochem.* **21,** 139–150.

Diamandis, E. P., Bhayana, V., Conway, K., Reichstein, E., and Papanastasiou-Diamandi, A. (1988). Time-resolved fluoroimmunoassay of cortisol in serum with a europium chelate as label. *Clin. Biochem.* **21,** 291–296.

Ellis, G., Holland, F. J., and Makela, S. K. (1989). Comparison of luteinizing hormone (LH, lutropin) immunoreactivity in serum by RIA and time-resolved fluorescence. Findings in serum from normal children and those treated with LHRH analogs. *Clin. Chem.* **35,** 1150 (Abstr.).

Haavisto, A. M., Dunkel, L., Pettersson, K., and Huhtaniemi, I. (1990). LH measurements by *in vitro* bioassay and a highly sensitive immunofluorometric assay improve the distinction between boys with constitutional delay of puberty and hypogonadotropic hypogonadism. *Pediatr. Res.* **27,** 211–214.

Hemmilä, I. (1988). Lanthanides as probes for time-resolved fluorimetric immunoassays. *Scand. J. Clin. Lab. Invest.* **48,** 389–400.

Kahan, I., Papanastasiou-Diamandi, A., D'Costa, M., and Diamandis, E. P. (1989). Measurement of serum prolactin by a simple and rapid time-resolved immunofluorometric assay. *Clin. Chem. Enzyme Commun.* **1,** 293–303.

Kahan, I., Papanastasiou-Diamandi, A., Ellis, G., Makela, S., McLaurin, J., D'Costa, M., and Diamandis, E. P. (1990). Sensitive time-resolved fluorescence immunoassay of somatotropin in serum. *Clin. Chem.* **36,** 503–508.

Khosravi, M. J., and Diamandis, E. P. (1987). Immunofluorometry of choriogonadotropin by time-resolved fluorescence spectroscopy, with a new europium chelate as label. *Clin. Chem.* **33,** 1994–1999.

Khosravi, M. J., and Diamandis, E. P. (1989). Time-resolved immunofluorometry of follitropin in serum. *Clin. Chem.* **35,** 181.

Khosravi, M. J., and Sudsbury, R. (1989). Ultra-specific time-resolved immunofluorometric assay of lutropin in serum. *Clin. Chem.* **35,** 2251.

Khosravi, M. J., Morton, R. C., and Diamandis, E. P. (1988a). Sensitive, rapid procedure for time-resolved immunofluorometry of lutropin. *Clin. Chem.* **34,** 1640–1644.

Khosravi, M. J., Chan, M. A., Bellem, A. C., and Diamandis, E. P. (1988b). A sensitive time-resolved immunofluorometric assay of ferritin in serum with monoclonal antibodies. *Clin. Chim. Acta.* **175,** 267–276.

Morton, R. C., and Diamandis, E. P. (1990). A streptavidin-based macromolecular complex labelled with a europium chelator suitable for time-resolved fluorescence immunoassay applications. *Anal. Chem.* **62,** 1841–1845.

Papanastasiou-Diamandi, A., Bhayana, V., and Diamandis, E. P. (1989a). A simple time-resolved fluoroimmunoassay of total thyroxine in serum. *Ann. Clin. Biochem.* **26,** 238–243.

Papanastasiou-Diamandi, A., Conway, K., and Diamandis, E. P. (1989b). Digoxin immunoassay with monoclonal and polyclonal antibodies using time-resolved fluorometry. *J. Pharm. Sci.* **78,** 617–621.

Reichstein, E., Morton, R., and Diamandis, E. P. (1989). Sensitive time-resolved immunofluorometric assay of thyrotropin in serum. *Clin. Biochem.* **22,** 23–29.

Shankaran, P., Reichstein, E., Khosravi, M. J., and Diamandis, E. P. (1990). Detection of Immunoglobulins G and M to rubella virus by time-resolved immunofluorometry. *J. Clin. Microbiol.* **28,** 573–579.

Tan, Y. K., Khosravi, M. J., and Diamandis, E. P. (1989). Time-resolved immunofluorometric assay for thyroxine-binding globulin in serum. *J. Immunoassay* **10,** 413–428.

Tan, Y. K., Bhayana, V., Papanastasiou-Diamandi, A., and Khosravi, M. J. (1990). Triiodothyronine uptake measurement in serum by time-resolved fluorescence immunofluorometry. *J. Immunoassay* **11**(2), 123–138.

CHAPTER 14

DELFIA (Dissociation-Enhanced Lanthanide Fluoroimmunoassay) Analyzer

James D. Faix
Department of Pathology, Division of Laboratory Medicine,
Beth Israel Hospital, Harvard Medical School, Boston, Massachusetts

I. INTRODUCTION

Fluorescence is the emission of light by an excited molecule as it returns to a lower energy level. The ability to be excited by radiation (such as ultraviolet light) and to emit characteristic visible light during relaxation is primarily a property of complex and unsymmetrical compounds. The most familiar fluorochrome in the clinical laboratory is probably fluorescein isothiocyanate (FITC). Tests that use fluorochrome-conjugated antibodies are generally referred to as immunofluorescent tests.

Since their introduction by Coons *et al.* (1942), direct and indirect immunofluorescent tests have been widely used in immunology and microbiology to identify antigens and antibodies. Most of these tests utilize fluorescence microscopy, but solid-phase applications have been developed and these have been adapted to produce quantitative noncompetitive immunoassays to measure plasma proteins. FITC-conjugated antigens have been used in competitive fluorescence polarization immunoassays to measure small molecules, and many enzyme immunoassays now employ fluorogenic substrates. However, despite its superior specific activity (in terms of potential signal emitted per mole of label), FITC has not been

Immunoassay Automation: A Practical Guide

widely used to replace radioisotopes as direct labels in conventional immunoassays.

The relative unpopularity of FITC (and alternative organic fluorochromes such as rhodamine and umbelliferone) as nonisotopic labels has been attributed to the high background. This is caused by light scattering and, in addition, the autofluorescence of various serum constituents under the conditions used to measure these fluorochromes (Soini and Hemmila, 1979). Such interferences could be reduced by sample pretreatment, gating, and optical filters, but it was not until the application of time-resolved fluorometry using unique chelates of fluorescent metal ions that these background problems were successfully eliminated from conventional fluoroimmunoassay techniques (Hemmila, 1985).

This chapter describes the first automated immunoassay system that utilized this approach. It was developed by scientists at the Wallac Biochemical Laboratory (a division of LKB, Inc.) in Turku, Finland, in association with the Department of Molecular Endocrinology at the Middlesex Hospital in Middlesex, U.K.. The system was named DELFIA for "dissociation-enhanced lanthanide fluoroimmunoassay."

II. SYSTEM DESCRIPTION

A. Instrumentation

DELFIA is a semiautomated immunoassay system in which all of the individual steps are (or can be) automated but in which the operator must occasionally (and briefly) intervene. It uses a 96-well microtiter plate format and includes the following instrumentation:

1. Microtiter plate shaker (with two speeds and capacity for four plates)
2. Microtiter plate washer (with built-in pump, 12-needle manifold, automatic prewash program, and individual assay-specific wash programs)
3. Automated liquid dispensers for reagents (either preadjusted or user-adjusted)
4. Push-button or foot-pedal operated microtiter plate pipetting guide
5. Automated time-resolving fluorometer

An automated disk puncher is also available to punch out sample disks from dried blood spots for neonatal screening.

Time-resolving fluorometers are similar to conventional fluorometers except that the excitation is a brief flash in comparison to the lifetime of the emitted signal and the photomultiplier tube is gated so that detection of the emitted signal occurs only during a specified time after excitation. The signal is usually integrated over many flashes so that the signal-to-noise ratio is enhanced (Soini and Kojola, 1983). The Arcus, which was introduced by Wallac in 1984, is no longer manufactured and has been recently replaced by a more compact plate fluorometer (which does not have its own "name"). The current complete system is illustrated in Fig. 1.

The DELFIA plate fluorometer is an automated bench-top instrument that uses a pulsed xenon flash at 340 nm and electronic gating to detect the resulting fluorescence at 613 nm between 400 and 800 μs after the excitation flash. This sequence of events is shown in Fig. 2 and is repeated approximately 1000 times per second for each sample. Both excitation and emission peaks are isolated with interference filters and a diode detector controls the excitation voltage pulse.

In addition to the wide Stokes shift (see below), the delay in detection efficiently removes the interference caused by background fluorescence and scattered light, which is short-lived, allowing only the long-lived fluorescence specifically related to the assay label to be detected. In the Arcus, the excitation enters the well through the side and the emitted fluorescence is measured through the bottom. The plate fluorometer does not measure fluorescence at a right angle from excitation but from the bottom of the well with excitation occurring above. However, the sensitiv-

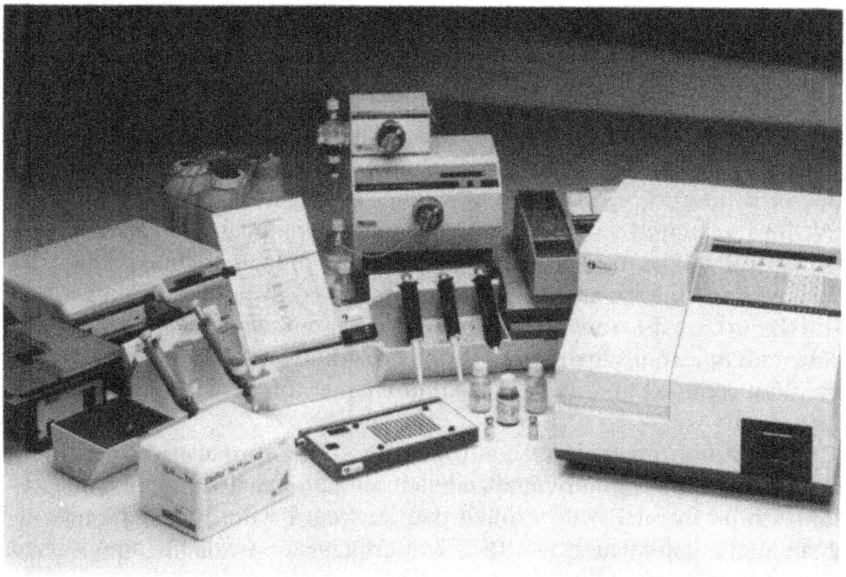

Figure 1 The DELFIA immunoassay system.

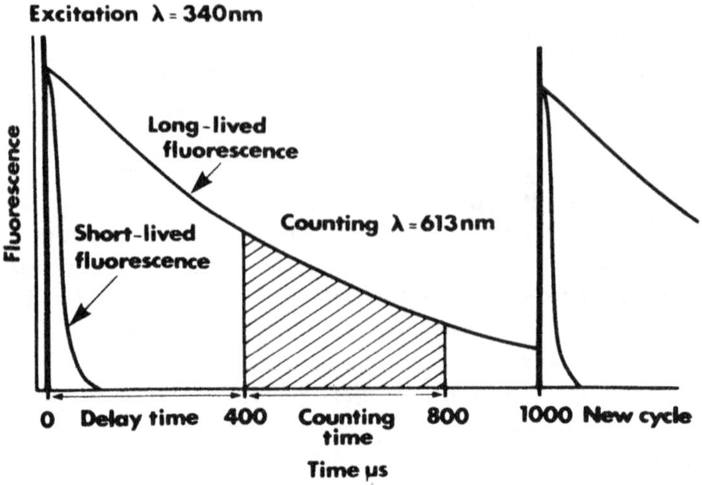

Figure 2 Principle of time-resolved fluorescence. Pulsed excitation lasts less than 1 μs. Detection of the emitted signal occurs only during a specified time after excitation, removing background fluorescence (which is short-lived). Note also the wide Stokes shift. Reproduced with permission from Soini and Lovgren (1988).

ity and dynamic range of the two instruments are the same. The detection limit for a b-ketone chelate of europium (the chelate measured in the system) is 10^{-14} mol/l (Soini and Lovgren, 1987).

The Arcus has an automated sample changer that shuttles racks of 12 microtiter plate wells through the reading sequence. There is space for 30 racks (or 360 mitrotiter plate wells), which would require approximately 6 min to be read. The plate fluorometer accepts an entire microtiter plate (one at a time) in a plate carrier where it is held in place by a spring. Reading (accomplished by moving the plate carrier in an $X-Y$ plane) is still 1 s per well but the total measurement time is 3 min per plate. Although the total reading time for a comparable number of wells is slightly longer than with the Arcus, the rows no longer need to be removed from the microtiter plate and placed in separate racks to be read. Overall "hands-on" time is therefore reduced and there is also no chance for error in terms of rack placement.

Both fluorometers are controlled by a microprocessor, and a dual disk drive allows for individualized data reduction and storage. All operations are performed with a touch pad keyboard with a user-friendly alphanumeric display and two RS-232 interfaces are available. One is used for a printer and the other can be used for an interface with a separate data analysis or laboratory information system. Although the "Arcus" had a manual filter changer to allow for excitation wavelengths other than that used for europium, this is more easily done with the plate fluorometer, enhancing user-specific applications and anticipating dual-label DELFIA assays.

Another automated immunoassay system employing time-resolving fluorometry is the CyberFluor system, which uses a different europium chelate as the nonisotopic label. The Cyberfluor time-resolving fluorometer cannot be used with the DELFIA assays because it measures fluorescence from a solid phase rather than in solution (see Chapter 13).

B. Method and Principle

The DELFIA assays all employ chelates of the lanthanide series of metal ions as direct labels in either competitive or noncompetitive immunoassays. These elements are all trivalent metal ions with an unfilled 4*f* electron shell, which can hold up to 14 electrons. Their inorganic salts are only weakly fluorescent. When chelated to an organic ligand, however, their fluorescence is greatly increased.

The organic ligand initially absorbs the excitation wavelength (and emits some short-lived fluorescence and phosphorescence) but much of the excitation is tranferred to the 4*f* energy level of the lanthanide ion. As the excited metal ion deactivates, fluorescence is emitted. This intermolecular transfer of energy is responsible for both the large Stokes shift (the difference between the excitation and emission wavelength) and the long decay time of the metal ion fluorescence.

The elements of the lanthanide series vary in their ability to display this feature. Lanthanum itself and several others are not suitable, either because the energy level of the 4*f* electron shell is not close to organic ligand donor levels or because significant nonradiative deactivation occurs. The most useful lanthanides are samarium (Sm^{+3}), europium (Eu^{+3}), terbium (Tb^{+3}), and dysprosium (Dy^{+3}), and, of these, europium has the widest Stokes shift and strongest fluorescence intensity (shown in Fig. 3).

To be suitable as a direct label, of course, the organic chelate of europium needed to be not only strongly fluorescent but also capable of being covalently linked to antigen and/or antibody in a stable manner. No organic chelate suitable for both these purposes was identified when the DELFIA system was being developed. Therefore, two different chelates were used.

For linking purposes, europium is chelated with an activated *N*-benzyl derivative of a polyaminopolycarboxylate, usually ethylenediamine tetraacetic acid (EDTA). Initially, diazotized aminophenyl-EDTA was used, but replacing the diazo with an isothiocyanato group allowed

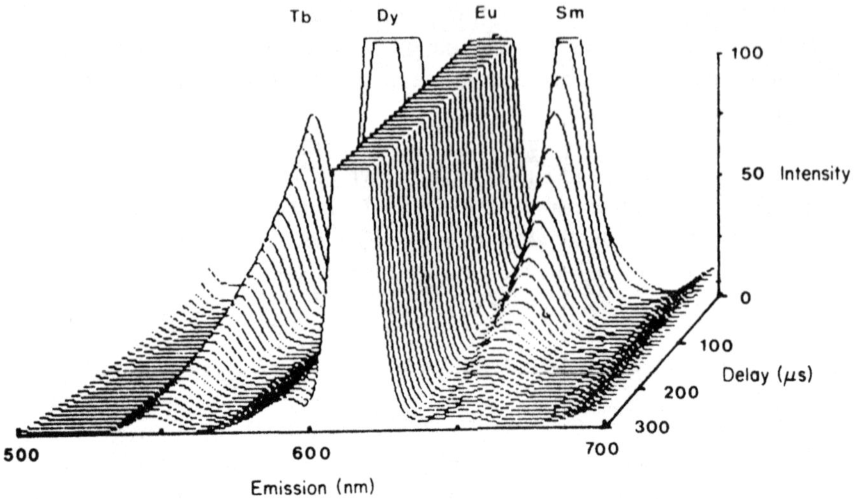

Figure 3 Emission intensity and decay profile of diketone chelates of terbium (Tb), dysprosium (Dy), europium (Eu), and samarium (Sm). Europium has the greatest emission intensity and the longest decay time. Reproduced with permission from Hemmila (1988).

for a significantly higher labeling ratio (Hemmila *et al.*, 1984). Although isothiocyanatophenyl-EDTA has been used in most of the DELFIA assays, alternative chelates are now being used as well (Mukkala *et al.*, 1989). The linkage of chelated europium to protein is stable, but most of these chelates are not very fluorescent. Therefore, after the immunoassay is carried out (see below), the europium is dissociated from these chelates by lowering the pH. A new chelate is formed with diketone 2-naphthoyltrifluoroacetone in the presence of a synergistic agent (trioctylphosphine oxide) and detergent (Triton X-100) to prevent quenching. The cocktail containing these agents is referred to as the enhancement solution.

The first major clinical applications of the DELFIA technique were noncompetitive immunoassays of protein antigens. The procedure is outlined for TSH in Fig. 4. Wells coated with antibody are washed and samples are pipetted. Solid-phase antibody binds protein antigen present in the sample and the familiar "sandwich" is formed with EDTA–europium–labeled antibody, which can either be added simultaneously ("one-step") as shown or sequentially after an initial incubation and washing ("two-step"). Most of the assays use the latter procedure. After the final incubation and washing, enhancement solution is added to dissociate and rechelate the solid-phase bound europium. After a brief incubation, the fluorescence can be measured. The amount of fluorescence is directly

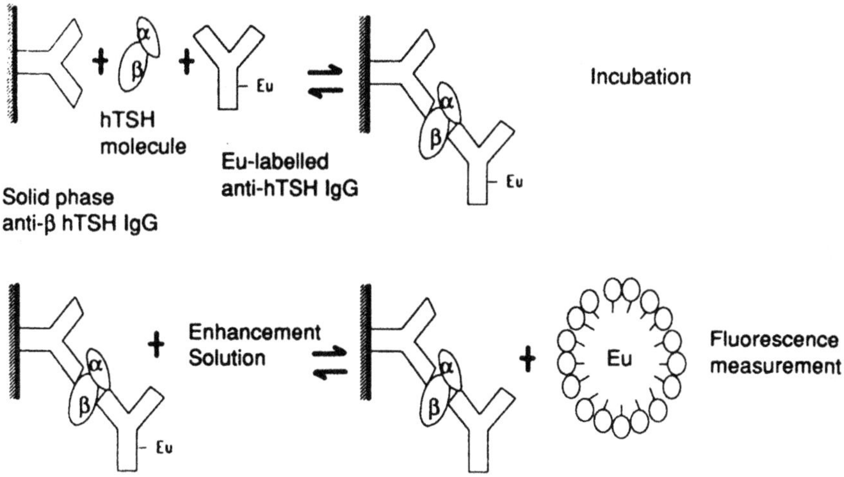

Figure 4 Noncompetitive immunoassay of TSH using the DELFIA approach (see text).

proportional to the concentration of the protein antigen and is typically linear over a very wide dynamic range.

Currently, the following assays are available using this approach: alpha-fetoprotein (AFP), sex hormone binding globulin (SHBG), thyroid-stimulating hormone (TSH), follicle-stimulating hormone (FSH), luteinizing hormone (LH), prolactin, human chorionic gonadotropin (hCG), immunoglobulin E (IgE), ferritin, carcinoembryonic antigen (CEA), CA-50, and hepatitis B surface antigen (HBsAg). An additional LH assay ("hLH Spec") has only minimal cross-reactivity with hCG.

Small molecules that are inappropriate for noncompetitive assays were initially difficult to label with EDTA–europium chelates. Therefore, the first DELFIA competitive immunoassays employed labeled antibodies, as outlined for T_4 in Fig. 5 (top). Wells coated with T_4 bound to a carrier protein are washed and samples are pipetted. EDTA–europium–labeled antibody is added, and during the assay incubation, the solid-phase antigen competes with the antigen from the sample for antibody binding sites. After incubation and washing, enhancement solution is added to dissociate and rechelate the solid-phase bound europium. The amount of fluorescence is inversely proportional to the amount of antigen present in the sample.

Subsequently, more conventional DELFIA competitive immunoassays were introduced, as outlined for T_4 in Fig. 5 (bottom). Wells coated with anti-mouse immunoglobulin are washed and samples are pipetted. A

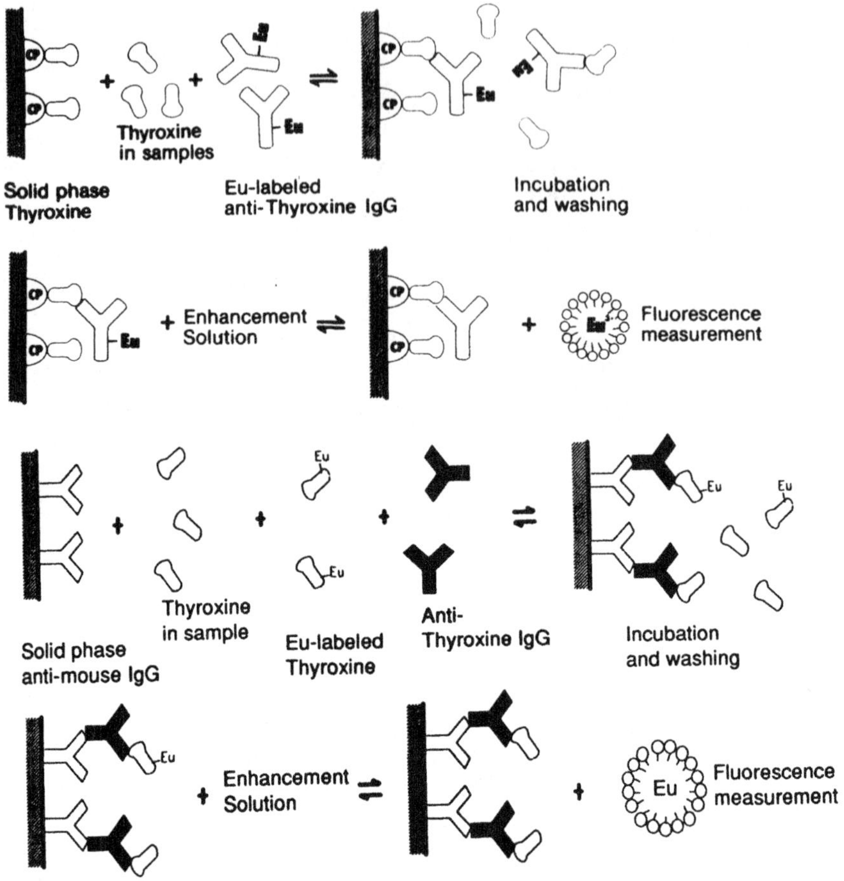

Figure 5 Competitive immunoassay of T_4 using the DELFIA approach. The first generation of competitive assays employed a labeled-antibody format (top). Subsequently more conventional competitive assays using labeled antigen (bottom) were introduced (see text).

mixture of europium-chelate–labeled T4 and murine monoclonal anti-T_4 antibody is added, and during the assay incubation, the solid-phase heterologous antibody binds the murine anti-T_4 antibody for which labeled T_4 competes with T_4 from the sample. After washing, enhancement solution is added and fluorescence can be measured.

The differences between the two DELFIA approaches to competitive immunoassay are discussed below. Currently, assays for digoxin and cortisol are available using the original competitive format; assays for T_4, T_3, thyroxine-binding globulin (TBG), progesterone, and estradiol are available using the labeled antigen format. A two-step, nonanalogue assay for free T_4 using europium-labeled T_4 is also available.

III. PERFORMANCE

A. Technical

The initial applications of time-resolved fluoroimmunoassay were in virology, including attempts to measure virus in stool specimens and nasopharyngeal secretions. The first detailed report (Meurman *et al.*, 1982) described an assay to measure anti-rubella antibodies, using polystyrene beads coated with rubella antigen and anti-human IgG antibody labeled with aminophenyl-EDTA–europium via the diazo reaction. The following year, a noncompetitive assay to measure HbsAg using primary antibody coated on polystyrene tubes (Siitari *et al.*, 1983) was published. With the report of a noncompetitive assay for phospholipase A2 using the microtiter strip format and isothiocyanato-EDTA–europium–labeled secondary antibody (Eskola *et al.*, 1983), all of the important features of the DELFIA system had been described and, in 1984, the DELFIA trademark was established. Monoclonal TSH and LH noncompetitive assays and competitive assays for cortisol and testosterone were developed (Lovgren *et al.*, 1984; Bertoft *et al.*, 1984). Since then, many additional assays (and applications) have been reported and marketed.

Published evaluations of the TSH (Kaihola *et al.*, 1985; Paterson *et al.*, 1985; Savaser *et al.*, 1987), hCG (Pettersson *et al.*, 1983; Stenman *et al.*, 1983; Savaser *et al.*, 1987; Banfi *et al.*, 1989), SHBG (Thomas *et al.*, 1987), ferritin (Koskinen *et al.*, 1989), and AFP (Suonpaa *et al.*, 1985; Savaser *et al.*, 1987) noncompetitive assays have documented technical performance comparable to either in-house or commercial radioimmunoassay. Overall, interassay precision ranges from 5 to 12%, and excellent linearity is present over wide dynamic ranges. Correlation with radioimmunoassay is excellent (with r values ranging from 0.96 to 0.99), although the DELFIA assays generally produce slightly lower results. No "high-dose hook" is present with either ferritin or hCG, although the two-step procedure is recommended for both assays.

Because native antibody activity is retained even at labeling ratios of up to 20 Eu^{+3}/IgG, the DELFIA noncompetitive assays are very sensitive. No deviation from linearity is present in the TSH assay when specimens are diluted into the hyperthyroid range (Parnham and Tarbit, 1987). In a study designed to assess the analytical performance of 10 immunometric assays for TSH in this range, the DELFIA assay demonstrated the greatest sensitivity, whether determined by replicate analysis of the zero standard or by precision profile (McConway *et al.*, 1989). A modification of the DELFIA TSH assay, in which biotinylated second antibody is subsequently interacted with europium-labeled avidin or streptavidin, has demonstrated even greater sensitivity (Hemmila *et al.*, 1989). The hCG assay is also sensitive to less than 1 mIU/ml, as determined by precision profile (Pettersson *et al.*, 1983).

In contrast, however, the evolution of the DELFIA competitive assays has been somewhat problematic. The original format was the previously described labeled-antibody technique. Ovalbumin and bovine thyroglobulin were commonly used to make protein derivatives of antigens, which were coated on the microtiter wells. Optimization of this format necessitated relatively low concentrations of solid-phase antigen, making the requirement for reproducible coating of the wells mucn more important than for the noncompetitive assays (where primary antibody is present on the solid phase in great excess). Since labeled antibody was also present in small amounts, the immune reactions did not always come to equilibrium within the incubation periods chosen.

Furthermore, conventional ways to displace protein-bound hormones in the patient samples could not be used in the DELFIA assays. Low pH would cause dissociation of europium from the labeled antibody as well; attempts to use other agents (such as 8-anilino-1-naphthalene) were unsuccessful. Consequently, a novel displacement approach, using trichloroacetic acid at neutral pH, was used (Eskola *et al.*, 1985).

Despite published reports of excellent linearity (approximately 100% recoveries) and good correlation with conventional competitive radioimmunoassays (*r* values ranged from 0.93 to 0.98), problems with precision prevented wide acceptance of the competitive DELFIA assays. Although reported interassay precision was occasionally excellent, such as 5–6% CV for digoxin (Helsingius *et al.*, 1986), ranges of 6–18% for testosterone (Lovgren *et al.*, 1984) and 5–28% for cortisol (Eskola *et al.*, 1985) were more typical. The consistency of the coating of the wells with limited amounts of antigen and the potential imprecision of the pipetting steps probably accounted for most of this problem.

In an attempt to improve the assays, a more conventional competitive approach (using europium-labeled antigen derivatives and wells coated with primary antibody) was studied but initially judged "not acceptable" (Lovgren, 1987). Since then, however, changes in format and reagent have allowed this approach to be successful. The wells are now coated with heterologous anti-immunoglobulin, and primary antibody is added separately, along with sample and labeled antigen. This format (as opposed to direct coating of the wells with primary antibody) has been shown to optimize the kinetics of the immune reaction, increasing the precision (Hubi *et al.*, 1988). In addition, alternative europium chelates and antigen derivatives have been developed (Hemmila *et al.*, 1988). Most of the DELFIA competitive assays now utilize this new approach, and data included in the product inserts claim that interassay precision is less than 10%. It is important to note, however, that extensive evaluations have not yet been published.

B. Clinical

DELFIA TSH compared favorably with nine other assays when receiver-operating characteristic curves were evaluated for diagnosis of hyperthyroidism in a population of 600 patients, of whom 217 were judged to be hyperthyroid (Thonnart *et al.*, 1988). In smaller studies, DELFIA TSH correctly identified thyroid status in 93 unselected patients (Parnham and Tarbit, 1987) and in 157 patients, of which 76 had clinically defined thyroid disease (Paterson *et al.*, 1985).

The DELFIA neonatal TSH assay (which uses dried blood spots) was evaluated in a study of 11,531 samples from newborns (Torresani and Scherz, 1986). Testing was done in parallel in each of two screening laboratories and DELFIA was compared to radioimmunoassay. The correlation was excellent and the incidence of false positive results after single TSH determination by DELFIA assay (using an overnight incubation) was very low (0.16%). Higher false positive rates may be found with the 4-h incubation alternative (Wong and Demshar, 1989).

DELFIA hCG has been shown to be comparable to radioimmunoassay in the diagnosis of pregnancy (Stenman *et al.*, 1983) and useful in the monitoring of patients following *in vitro* fertilization (Alfthan *et al.*, 1988) and abortion (Makinen *et al.*, 1987). Using DELFIA reagents, investigators detected small changes in hCG in nonpregnant women and men (Stenman *et al.*, 1987) and in FSH and LH during female puberty (Apter *et al.*, 1989).

The DELFIA LH assay has been shown to correlate with LH bioactivity better than radioimmunoassay in a variety of clinical conditions with decreased gonadotropin secretion (Jaakkola *et al.*, 1990). Good agreement between FSH bioactivity and both DELFIA and radioimmunoassay was observed, but the discrepancies seen between the LH assays prompted the authors to question the validity of previous clinical investigations using radioimmunoassays.

The DELFIA free T4 assay is the only nonisotopic two-step free T4 immunoassay currently available. It correctly classified hyperthyroid and hypothyroid patients when compared with a two-step radioimmunoassay and correlated well with an equilibrium dialysis method in 138 patients with nonthyroidal illness and in 36 pregnant women (Nuutila *et al.*, 1990). Although there is controversy concerning the reliability of immunoassays for free T4, many investigators believe that two-step assays provide more accurate results than one-step analogue immunoassays.

C. Operational

Each DELFIA test kit contains eight strips of coated wells, standards, labeled antibody (or antibody and labeled antigen), assay buffer, wash concentrate, and enhancement solution. Kits are stored at refrigerator temperature. Since none of the kit components are available separately in bulk packaging (or in larger-sized kits), excessive storage space may be required.

The strips of coated wells are already in the strip frame and constitute a full 96-well microtiter plate. If fewer wells are needed, strips must be removed and stored sealed in the foil package. One minor disadvantage is that the individual strips can not be divided (and replaced by blank wells) if fewer than 12 wells are needed to complete the final strip. The plate must be washed prior to the pipetting of samples and reagents with Tris-HCl–buffered (pH 7.8) salt solution. Wash concentrate diluted in distilled water is stable at room temperature for up to 2 weeks. This same wash solution is used to wash the plates after the assay incubations.

With a very few exceptions, the standards and stock reagents are liquid and need no reconstitution. Most of the stock antigen and/or antibody reagents are also liquid. These must be diluted in assay buffer (Tris-HCl–buffered salt solution with bovine protein, detergents, and assay-specific displacement agents). Assay reagents must be diluted immediately prior to the assay. Otherwise, all reagents have long shelf-lives (between 6 months and 1 year), which is a characteristic feature of nonisotopic immunoassay reagents.

Pipetting must be done with care, although most of the sample volumes are 25 μl or greater. Manual pipetting of samples can be tedious. The DELFIA Plateguide can help, but the use of an automated pipetting station is mandatory for large workloads. The DELFIA plate dispensor automates the pipetting of the assay reagents. A separate dispensor with separate tubing automates the addition of the enhancement solution. An automated pipettor can be used instead to add the assay reagents, but the addition of the enhancement solution (which is a critical step in the assay) should probably be done only with the dedicated DELFIA dispensor, since any contamination of this instrument with europium must be avoided. Although dust in the laboratory may contain variable amounts of europium, the most common cause of high backgrounds is contamination of the enhancement solution dispensor with europium-labeled reagent.

Almost all incubations take place on the DELFIA plate shaker, which can accommodate up to four plates at a time. Each plate must be covered with plastic strips. There are many different assay incubation times, ranging from 2 to 4 h. Rapid procedures are available for hCG and LH. Rarely, overnight incubation (without shaking) at 4°C may be utilized. Otherwise, almost all incubations take place at room temperature. The only exceptions are the HBsAg incubations and the second incubation in the free T_4 assay, which take place (without shaking) at 40° and 4°C, respectively.

After the final incubation, the plates are washed one at a time in the plate washer. The plate washer has stored protocols for each assay. If the plate is not properly aligned, the washer will stop and display an error message, avoiding flooding. After the final wash, enhancement solution is dispensed and the plate is placed on the shaker for 5 min (an alternative slower speed is used). After an additional 5- to 10-min wait, the plate is read in the fluorometer.

The fluorometer performs a curve fit and prints both raw data and calculated dose for all samples, as well as replicate precision. Reference ranges may be included in the printout, and data from the run may be automatically stored on diskette. Data files may be made by the user by means of the fluorometer keyboard. A separate port of the RS232C configuration allows for interfacing with an external computer. A separate software system (MultiCalc) is available for alternative data evaluation and quality control management as well. The user may program the fluorometer's parameters (flash cycle, delay, window and dead times, excitation and emission filters, etc.) for research protocols.

There is no preventative maintenance required by the user other than keeping the instruments clean with a soft cloth moistened in mild detergent solution. User satisfaction with the system has been reported as excellent (Alpert, 1988).

D. Economics

The current list price for the DELFIA instrumentation is approximately $34,000. Most clinical laboratories may prefer to lease it from Pharmacia. The exact costs of the reagents under such circumstances are, of course, subject to negotiation and dependent on volume. However, it is fair to say that although DELFIA may cost slightly more per reportable test than comparable manual radioimmunoassay methods, it will probably be less expensive than other automated systems.

IV. CONCLUSION

The DELFIA system offers all of the advantages of a nonisotopic immunoassay methodology. From the perspective of automation, DELFIA is obviously not a completely automated system. However, if an automated sample pipettor is used, all of the labor-intensive steps involved in traditional immunoassay have been automated. This approach will appeal to laboratories that wish to maintain flexibility. Also, DELFIA europium-labeling kits are available so that investigators may easily use the system for customized applications.

The DELFIA technology is sensitive and robust. Using separate europium- and terbium-labeled beta chain-specific monoclonal antibodies, a simultaneous dual assay for FSH and LH has been described (Hemmila *et al.*, 1987). Homogeneous assays, based on quenching of europium-labeled antigen by antibody, have also been developed (Hemmila *et al.*, 1988). Other innovative applications, such as fluorescence microscopy (Soini *et al.*, 1988), cytotoxicity (Granberg *et al.*, 1988), and DNA hybridization (Dahlen *et al.*, 1988), suggest that the future usefulness of lanthanides in clinical laboratory medicine may extend beyond immunoassay.

REFERENCES

Alfthan, H., Schroder, J., Fraser, R., Koskimies, A., Halila, H., and Stenman, U.-H. (1988). Choriogonadotropin and its b subunit separated by hydrophobic-interaction chromatography and quantified in serum during pregnancy by time-resolved immunofluorometric assays. *Clin. Chem.* **34,** 1758–1762.

Alpert, N. (1988). Time-resolved fluorescence immunoassay. *Clinical Instrument Systems* **9**(2), 1–6.

Apter, D., Cacciatore, B., Alfthan, H., and Stenman, U.-H. (1989). Serum luteinizing hormone concentrations increase 100-fold in females from 7 years of age to adulthood, as measured by time-resolved immunofluorometric assay. *J. Clin. Endocrinol. Metab.* **68,** 53–57.

Banfi, G., Casari, E., Murone, M., and Bonini, P. A. (1989). Three nonisotopic methods for human choriogonadotropin evaluated. *Clin. Chem.* **35,** 1545–1546.

Bertoft, E., Eskola, J. U., Nanto, V., and Lovgren, T. (1984). Competitive solid-phase immunoassay of testosterone using time-resolved fluorescence. *FEBS Lett.* **173,** 213–216.

Coons, A. H., Creech, H. J., Jones, R. N., and Berliner, E. (1942). The demonstration of pneumococcal antigens in tissues by the use of fluorescent antibody. *J. Immunol.* **45,** 159–170.

Dahlen, P., Hurskainen, P., Lovgren, T., and Hyypia, T. (1988). Time-resolved fluorometry for the identification of viral DNA in clinical specimens. *J. Clin. Microbiol.* **26,** 2434–2436.

Eskola, J. U., Nanto, V., Meurling, L., and Lovgren, T. N.-E. (1985). Direct solid-phase time-resolved immunofluorometric assay of cortisol in serum. *Clin. Chem.* **31,** 1731–1734.

Eskola, J. U., Nevalainen, T. J., and Lovgren, T. N.-E. (1983). Time-resolved fluoroimmunoassay of human pancreatic phospholipase A2. *Clin. Chem.* **29,** 1777–1780.

Granberg, C., Blomberg, K., Hemmila, I., and Lovgren, T. (1988). Determination of cytotoxic T lymphocyte activity by time-resolved fluorometry using europium-labelled concanavalin A-stimulated cells as targets. *J. Immunol. Methods* **114,** 191–195.

Helsingius, P., Hemmila, I., and Lovgren, T. (1986). Solid-phase immunoassay of digoxin by measuring time-resolved fluorescence. *Clin. Chem.* **32,** 1767–1769.

Hemmila, I. (1985). Fluoroimmunoassays and immunofluorometric assays. *Clin. Chem.* **31,** 359–370.

Hemmila, I. (1988). Lanthanides as probes for time-resolved fluorometric immunoassays. *Scand. J. Clin. Lab. Invest.* **48,** 389–400.

Hemmila, I., Dakubu, S., Mukkala, V.-M., Siitari, H., and Lovgren, T. (1984). Europium as a label in time-resolved immunofluorometric assays. *Anal. Biochem.* **137,** 335–343.

Hemmila, I., Heikkila, J., and Leivo, P. (1989). Direct and indirect immunofluorometry of thyrotropin. *Clin. Chem.* **35,** 1206.

Hemmila, I., Holttinen, S., Pettersson, K., and Lovgren, T. (1987). Double-label time-resolved fluoroimmunoassay of lutropin and follitropin in serum. *Clin. Chem.* **33,** 2281–2283.

Hemmila, I., Malmainen, O., Mikola, H., and Lovgren, T. (1988). Homogeneous time-resolved fluoroimmunoassay of thyroxin in serum. *Clin. Chem.* **34,** 2320–2322.

Hubi, W., Dazenbichler, G., Meissner, D., and Thiele, H. J. (1988). An improved solid-phase enzyme and luminescent system for steroid hormones and digoxin. *Clin. Chem.* **34,** 2521–2523.

Jaakkola, T., Ding, Y-Q., Kellokumpu-Lehtinen, P., Valavaara, R., Martikainen, H., Tapanainen, J., Rönnberg, L., and Huhtaniemi, I. (1990). The ratios of serum bioactive/immunoreactive luteinizing hormone and follicle-stimulating hormone in various clinical conditions with increased and decreased gonadotropin secretion: reevaluation by a highly sensitive immunometric assay. *J. Clin. Endocrinol. Metab.* **70,** 1496–1505.

Kaihola, H.-L., Irjala, K., Viikari, J., and Nanto, V. (1985). Determination of thyrotropin in serum by time-resolved fluoroimmunoassay evaluated. *Clin. Chem.* **31,** 1706–1709.

Koskinen, P., and Irjala, K. (1989). Commercially available dissociation-enhanced lanthanide fluoroimmunoassay kit evaluated for quantifying ferritin in serum. *Clin. Chem.* **35,** 327–328.

Lovgren, T. N.-E. (1987). Time-resolved fluoroimmunoassay of steroid hormones. *J. Steroid Biochem.* **27,** 47–51.

Lovgren, T., Hemmila, I., Pettersson, K., Eskola, J. U., and Bertoft, E. (1984). Determination of hormones by time-resolved fluoroimmunoassay. *Talanta* **31,** 909–916.

Makinen, J., Anttila, L., Irjala, K., Salmi, T., and Kaihola, H.-L. (1987). Serum hCG levels measured by time resolved fluoroimmunoassay in first-trimester pregnancy and after pregnancy termination. *Eur. J. Obstet. Gynecol. Reprod. Biol.* **26,** 219–224.

McConway, M. G., Chapman, R. S., Beastall, G. H., Brown, E., Tillman, J. A., Bonar, J. A., Hutchison, A., Allison, T., Finlayson, J., Weston, R., Beckett, G. J., Carter, G. D., Carlyle, E., Herbertson, R., Blundell, G., Edwards, W., Glen, A. C. A., and Reid, A. (1989). How sensitive are immunometric assays for thyrotropin? *Clin. Chem.* **35,** 289–291.

Meurman, O. H., Hemilla, I. A., Lovgren, T. N.-E., and Halonen, P. E. (1982). Time-resolved fluoroimmunoassay: A new test for *Rubella* antibodies. *J. Clin. Microbiol.* **16,** 920–925.

Mukkala, V.-M., Mikola, H., and Hemmila, I. (1989). The synthesis and use of activated *N*-benzyl derivatives of diethylenetriamine tetraacetic acids: Alternative reagents for labeling of antibodies with metal ions. *Anal. Biochem.* **176,** 319–325.

Nuutila, P., Koskinen, P., Irjala, K., Linko, L., Kaihola, H-L., Eskola, J. U., Erkkola, R., Seppälä, P., and Viikari, J. (1990). Two new two-step immunoassays for free thyroxin evaluated: solid-phase radioimmunoassay and time-resolved fluoroimmunoassay. *Clin. Chem.* **36,** 1355–1360.

Parnham, A. J., and Tarbit, I. F. (1987). "Delfia" and "Amerlite": Two sensitive nonisotopic immunoassay systems for assay of thyrotropin compared. *Clin. Chem.* **33,** 1421–1424.

Paterson, N., Biggart, E. M., Chapman, R. S., and Beastall, G. H. (1985). Evaluation of a time-resolved immunofluorometric assay for serum thyroid stimulating hormone. *Ann. Clin. Biochem.* **22,** 606–611.

Pettersson, K., Siitari, H., Soini, E., Lovgren, T., Hanninen, V., Tanner, P., and Stenman, U.-H. (1983). Time-resolved fluoroimmunoassay of human choriogonadotropin. *Clin. Chem.* **29,** 60–64.

Savaser, A. N., Hosten, N., Schulz, E., Jorno, L., and Felix, R. (1987). Fluoroimmunoassay: An alternative to radioimmunoassay? *Eur. J. Nucl. Med.* **13,** 397–401.

Siitari, H., Hemmila, I., Soini, E., Lovgren, T., and Koistinen, V. (1983). Detection of hepatitis B surface antigen using time-resolved fluoroimmunoassay. *Nature* **301,** 258–260.

Soini, E., and Hemmila, I. (1979). Fluoroimmunoassay: Present status and key problems. *Clin. Chem.* **25,** 353–361.

Soini, E., and Kojola, H. (1983). Time resolved fluorometer for lanthanide chelates—A new generation of nonisotopic immunoassays. *Clin. Chem.* **29,** 65–68.

Soini, E., and Lovgren, T. (1987). Time-resolved fluorescence of lanthanide probes and applications in biotechnology. *CRC Crit. Rev. Anal. Chem.* **18,** 105–154.

Soini, E., and Lovgren, T. (1988). Time-resolved fluoroimmunoassay. *In* "Nonisotopic Immunoassay" (T. T. Ngo, ed.), pp. 231–243. Plenum Press, New York.

Soini, E. J., Pelliniemi, L. J., Hemmila, I. A., Mukkala, V.-M., Kankare, J. J., and Frojdman, K. (1988). Lanthanide chelates as new fluorochrome labels for cytochemistry. *J. Histochem. Cytochem.* **36,** 1449–1451.

Stenman, U.-H., Alfthan, H., Ranta, T., Vartiainen, E., Jalkanen, J., and Seppala, M. (1987). Serum levels of human chorionic gonadotropin in nonpregnant women and men are modulated by gonadotropin-releasing hormone and sex steroids. *J. Clin. Endocrinol. Metab.* **64,** 730–736.

Stenman, U.-H., Myllynen, L., Alfthan, H., and Seppala, M. (1983). Ultrarapid and highly sensitive time-resolved fluoroimmunometric assay for chorionic gonadotropin. *Lancet* **September 17**: 647–649.

Suonpaa, M. U., Lavi, J. T., Hemmila, I. A., and Lovgren, T. N.-E. (1985). A new sensitive assay of human alpha-fetoprotein using time-resolved fluorescence and monoclonal antibodies. *Clin. Chim. Acta* **145,** 341–348.

Thomas, C. M. G., van der Berg, R. J., and Segers, M. F. G. (1987). Precision of assays for sex-hormone binding globulin: an I-IRMA and two Eu-IFMA kits compared. *Clin. Chem.* **33,** 2120.

Thonnart, B., Messian, O., Colas Linhart, N., and Bok, B. (1988). Ten highly sensitive thyrotropin assays compared by receiver-operating characteristic curves analysis: Results of a prospective multicenter study. *Clin. Chem.* **34,** 691–695.

Torresani, T. E., and Scherz, R. (1986). Thyroid screening of neonates without use of radioactivity: Evaluation of time-resolved fluoroimmunoassay of thyrotropin. *Clin. Chem.* **32,** 1013–1015.

Wong, S. T., and Demshar, H. P. (1989). Decreasing false positive results when using the Pharmacia Wallac "DELFIA" neonatal TSH kit. *Infant Screening* **12,** 9.

CHAPTER 15

The Eclipse ICA: An Immunoassay and Clinical Chemistry System

Walter C. Mahoney[1]
Biotope, Inc., Redmond, Washington

Kent E. Opheim
Children's Hospital and Medical Center, Department of Laboratories, Seattle, Washington

Tom M. Fleck, Paula A. Schueler, David L. Enfield, and John T. Kingsley
Biotope, Inc., Redmond, Washington

I. INTRODUCTION

Diagnostic testing continues to evolve toward greater automation, higher throughput, and broader applicability. Systems found in the clinical laboratory range from devices that measure the results of simple spot tests to large, fully automated systems capable of yielding over 1000 clinical answers per hour. Most diagnostic instrumentation has two major components, a sample preparation or sample addition section and an analytical section. In the first of these sections, or "front end" of the analyzer, samples and reagents are typically added to a consumable, and any sample pretreatment or dilution steps are executed. This portion of the analyzer is

[1] Current address: Boehringer Mannheim Research and Development, Indianapolis, Indiana 46250-0457.

Immunoassay Automation: A Practical Guide

usually equipped with a pipetting device and a washing station to reduce pipette induced cross-contamination of samples. In the analytical portion of the instrument, or "back end" of the analyzer, the tests are incubated and mixed, separation steps occur if necessary, and the measurement is performed. These instrument systems can generally be subdivided further into those systems that perform chemistry tests [glucose, cholesterol, blood urea nitrogen (BUN), etc.] and those that perform immunoassays (TSH, digoxin, etc.). Few instruments have the capability of running both types of tests. This has been due principally to the technical inability to deal with a mix of chemistry tests and immunoassays on instruments designed principally to perform chemistry tests without diminishing current levels of performance.

II. INSTRUMENT CONCEPT

The Eclipse ICA analyzer is a table-top, random access, fully automated centrifugal immunoassay and chemistry system (Fig. 1). The system was

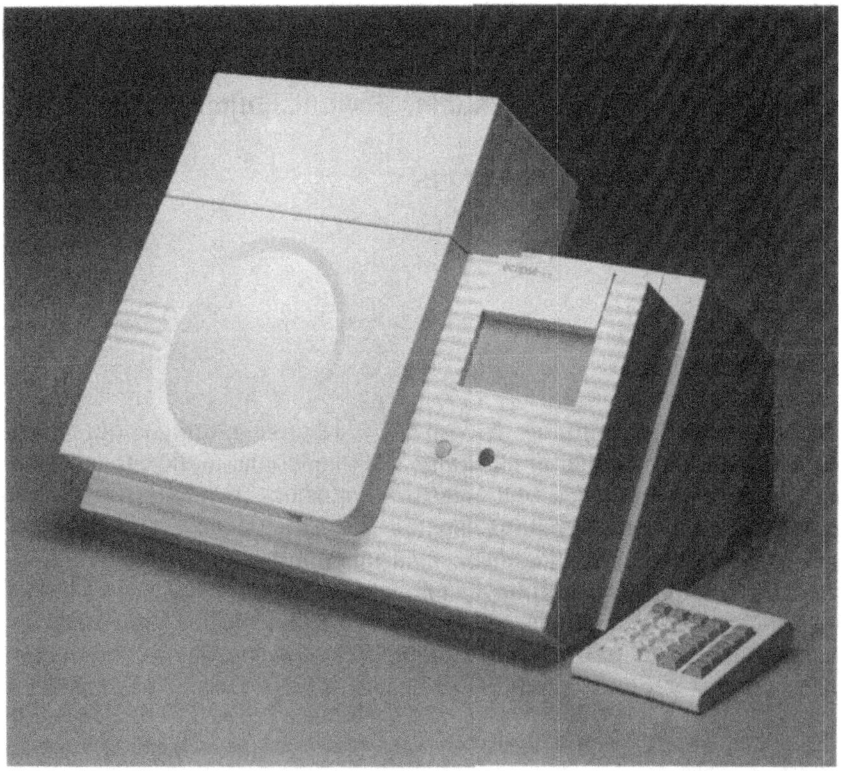

Figure 1 The Eclipse ICA instrument and keypad.

Table 1 Assays Currently Available on the Eclipse ICA System

Test	Method	Status	Sample type[a]
Glucose	End point	FDA 510K approved	WB,S,P
Cholesterol	End point	FDA 510K approved	WB,S,P
Triglycerides	End point	FDA 510K approved	WB,S,P
BUN	Rate (340 n*M*)	FDA 510K approved	WB,S,P
HDL cholesterol	End point	Under development	ND
Potassium	End point	Under development	ND
TSH	Fluorescence rate	FDA 510K approved	WB,S,P
Digoxin	Fluorescence rate	FDA 510K approved	S,P
Theophylline	Fluorescence rate	Under development	ND
T_4	Fluorescence rate	Under development	ND

[a] WB, whole blood; P, plasma; S, serum; ND, not determined.

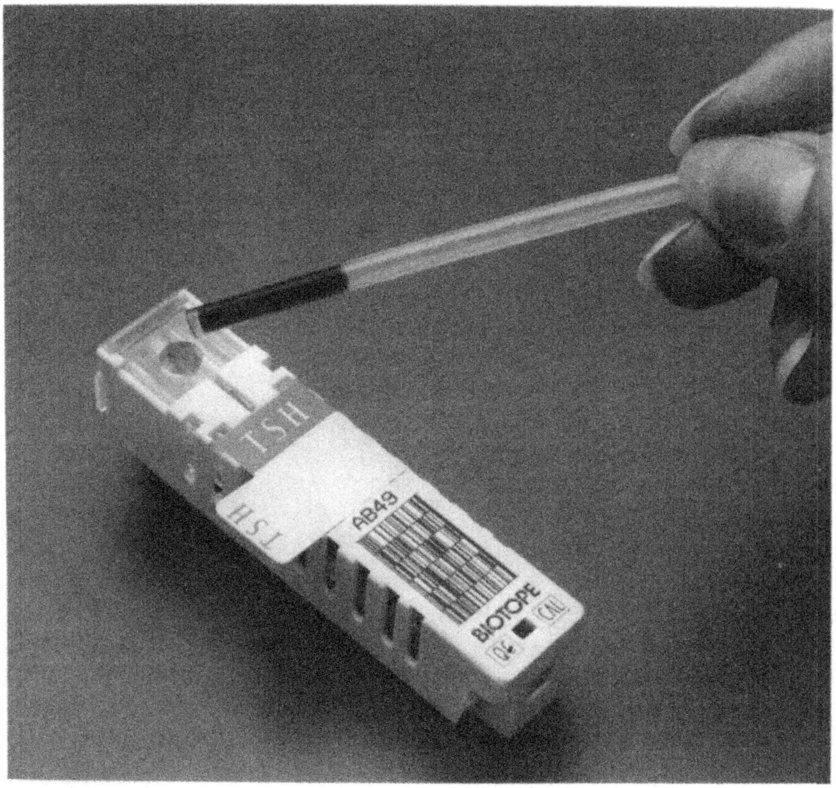

Figure 2 Addition of an imprecise sample to a TSH Eclipse ICA cassette.

designed to yield high precision and accuracy on both chemistry tests and immunoassays. The system can accommodate 16 tests per run with a maximum run time of approximately 17 min. Currently, FDA 510K approved tests include blood urea nitrogen (BUN), cholesterol, triglycerides, glucose, digoxin, and thyroid-stimulating hormone (TSH) (Table 1). The system is free of resident buffers, pipetters, and liquid waste. The core of the technology underlying the Eclipse system is embodied in the consumable, a disposable, self-contained device that includes all of the reagents necessary to perform an assay (Fig. 2). All pipetting, mixing, incubation, washing, and sample measurement take place within this cassette. As such, tasks generally relegated to either the front end (sample preparation) or back end (analysis) of other instrument systems have been combined in the cassette, with the elimination of precision pipetting by the operator. This also eliminates any instrument-induced cross-contamination of samples. No lengthy and error-prone centrifugation, separation, or sample pretreatment steps are required. Once blood is drawn from a patient and added to the cassette, the Eclipse system will generate immunoassay and clinical chemistry results in 17 min or less.

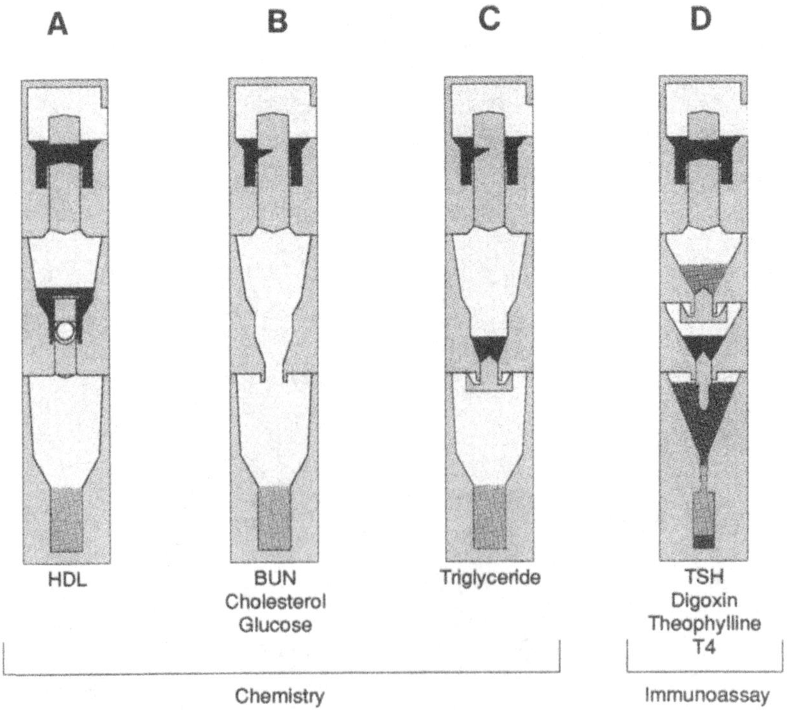

Figure 3 The four Eclipse cassette configurations. Cassettes A, B, and C are used for chemistry tests, and cassette D for all immunoassay tests.

For the tests listed in Table 1, the system currently provides sensitivity and performance equivalent to existing technologies, has a throughput of 50–90 tests per hour, and possesses random access, batch, and panel capabilities.

The system was designed specifically for the small hospital and large physician group practices. Since immunoassays have multiple steps requiring numerous precise operations and are difficult to automate, most immunoassay testing today is still performed in the clinical laboratories by highly trained technologists. The Eclipse system is intended to be a cost-effective alternative to sending assay samples to reference laboratories. Clinical testing done in real time, during the normal course of a patient visit, should improve the quality of patient care.

III. THE CASSETTE

The test cassettes are composed of a series of chambers separated by centrifugally activated valves, much like a multiple-stage rocket (Fig. 3).

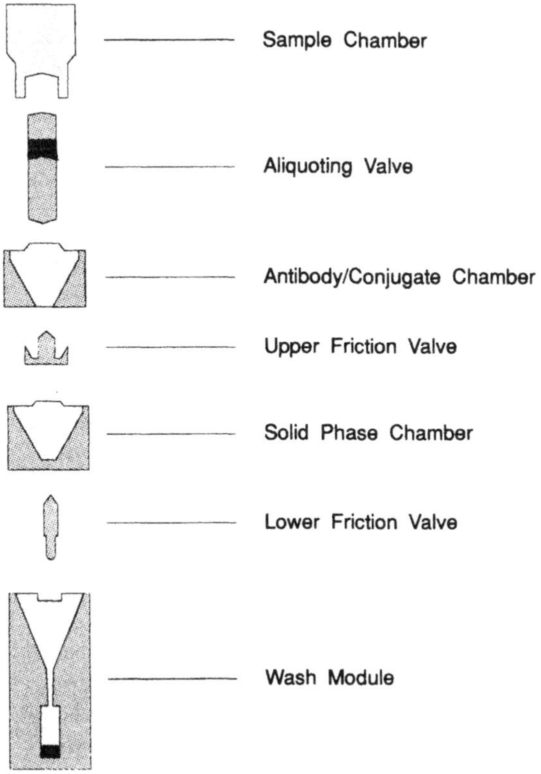

Figure 4 Exploded view of the immunoassay cassette.

The valves, triggered to release at specific preset centrifugal forces, control the movement of materials through the cassette chambers. Currently, there are four variations of the test cassette, three different configurations for chemistry tests (Fig. 3A, B, C), and a single immunoassay cassette (Fig. 3D). These cassette variations currently allow the running of single-reagent clinical chemistry tests (cholesterol, glucose, etc.) (Fig. 3B), dual reagent clinical chemistry tests (triglycerides, creatine, etc.) (Fig. 3C), tests requiring an intermediate precipitation step (HDL-cholesterol and potassium) (Fig. 3A), and immunoassays (Fig. 3D).

The immunoassay cassette, which is the most complex of the cassette configurations utilizes four chambers and three valves (Fig. 4):

Cassette portion	Contents/Function
Sample chamber	Receives sample, pellets cells, precisely delivers a portion of sample
Aliquoting valve	Meters a portion of the sample in the sample chamber and transfers it to the antibody/conjugate chamber
Antibody/conjugate chamber	Contains antibody or antiserum and/or enzyme–hapten conjugate or enzyme–antibody conjugate, an incubation site for sequential sandwich assays
Upper friction valve	Separates antibody/conjugate chamber from the solid-phase chamber
Solid-phase chamber	Contains antibody or antiserum covalently immobilized to 1.1 μm bromostyrene particles, the second incubation site for sequential sandwich assays, the incubation site of simultaneous sandwich or simultaneous competitive immunoassays
Lower friction valve	Separates solid-phase chamber from the wash/detection chambers
Wash module	Contains water layer followed by an oil layer
Detection area	Contains enzyme substrate and buffer in a medium of the correct density to remain below the oil

A. The Sample Chamber

The sample delivery module is the uppermost portion of the test cassette. This component has the capacity to transfer a precise sample volume to the next (antibody/conjugate) chamber. The sample chamber has three major portions: the body, the cap, and the valve. The sample chamber is assembled by first inserting the valve into the chamber body, followed by pressing the cap onto the chamber body. A small volume of a wax blend is then added to the area between the valve and the body. When the wax hardens, the valve is ready to use. The valve itself has a molded cavity, which fills with a precise amount of sample, ready for delivery. The sample size is controlled by the volume of the molded cavity. Valves currently in use are designed to deliver either 5 or 50 μl. These valves are capable of very precise deliveries. For example, the sample volumes delivered by the 5- and 50-μl valves have coefficients of variation of 1.25 and 0.51%, respectively. During the run, sample delivery occurs when the accumulated force applied to the valve is sufficient to cause the wax to fail under the strain. As the wax fails, the valve moves downward. This brings the metered sample into the next chamber. The taper curving outward at the top of the valve not only stops the movement of the valve but, in concert with the wax blend, reseals the valve, thus preventing the entry of any additional sample into the antibody/conjugate chamber.

IV. IMMUNOASSAY TEST PROCEDURE

Two types of immunoassay format are available, sandwich and competitive. As an example, the four major steps in performing a sandwich TSH assay, as shown in Fig. 5, will be described briefly. To perform the test, the user selects a test cassette filled with TSH-specific reagents (Fig. 6) and dispenses a patient's sample into the sample chamber (Fig. 2). An important aspect of the consumable is that the volume of the sample introduced need not be precise. The cassette itself is able to transfer a precise portion of the sample into the antibody/conjugate chamber of the consumable. For the majority of the tests this sample can be whole blood, serum, or plasma. The cassette itself is filled by the manufacturer with all of the required reagents. In the instrument, the cassette is identified by way of a bar code that contains the test type, calibration-specific information, lot number, and expiration date. After snapping the cassette lid closed, the cassette is loaded onto the instrument rotor, which then operates according to a preset program.

The sequence of events which occur in a TSH immunoassay are summarized in Fig. 7 (steps 1–10). The instrument starts with a brief spin at 150 rpm during which the bar code on each cassette is read. The speed of the rotor then increases to 1800 rpm. This speed is maintained for 3 min. During this portion of the cycle, the test cassette is warmed to 37°C (±0.1°C). Additionally, if the sample is whole blood, the cells are pelleted to an area in the sample chamber below that of the aliquoting valve cavity. This allows the molded cavity to fill with a cell-free sample for the delivery to the antibody/conjugate chamber. Following the 1800 rpm portion of the cycle, the rotor quickly accelerates to 3600 rpm and holds that speed for

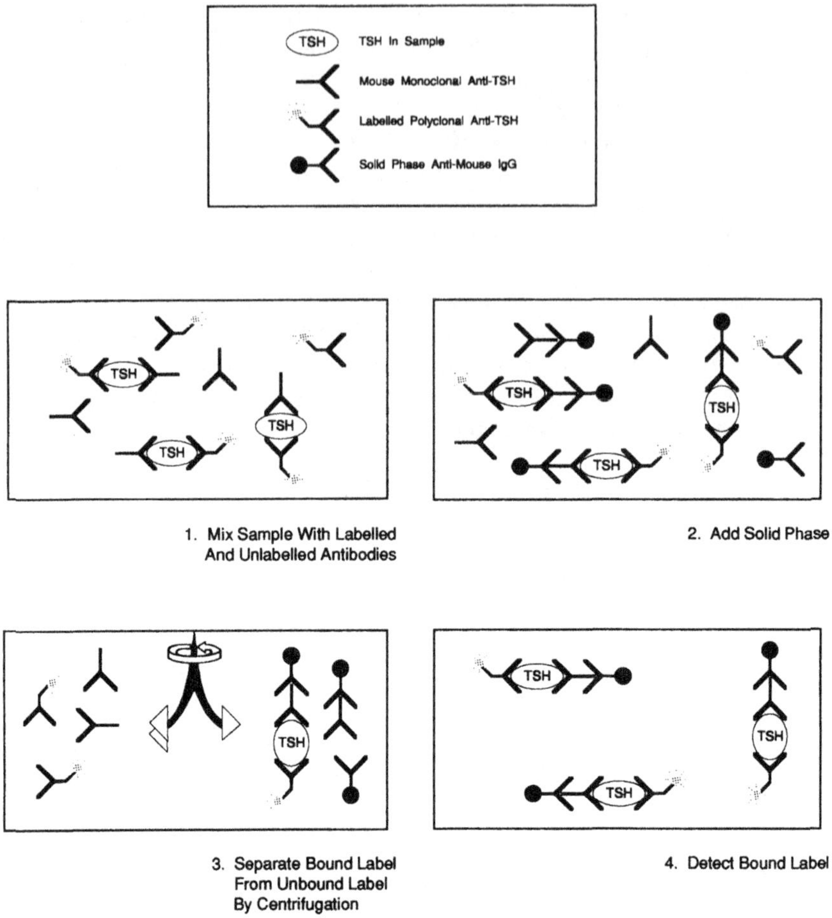

Figure 5 Major steps in performing an Eclipse TSH immunoassay. Step 1: The sample is mixed with a monoclonal anti-TSH antibody and a polyclonal goat anti-TSH antiserum that has been conjugated to calf intestinal alkaline phosphatase. Step 2: Particles containing immobilized goat anti-mouse antiserum are added to the reaction mixture to capture the mouse monoclonal antibody. Step 3: The particles are collected. Step 4: The alkaline phosphatase activity associated with the particles is measured.

12 s. Reaching this point, the aliquoting valve delivers a sample to the antibody/conjugate chamber. In the case of a sequential TSH assay, the antibody/conjugate chamber contains a polyclonal anti-TSH antiserum covalently coupled to calf intestinal alkaline phosphatase, and a monoclonal anti-TSH antibody. The sample is incubated with these reagents for 8 min, while mixing back and forth continuously, with some

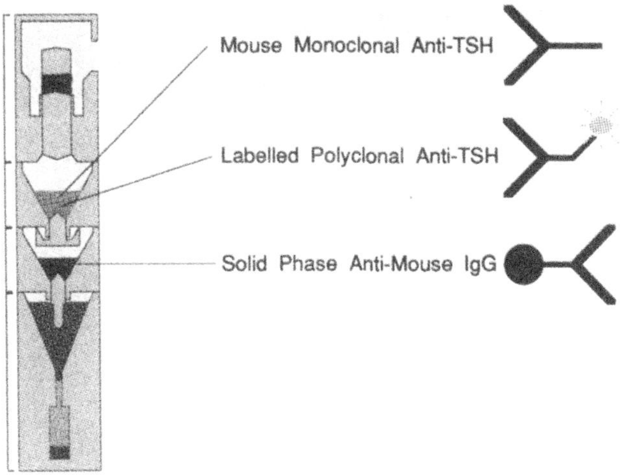

Figure 6 Position of the TSH immunoassay specific components in the Eclipse TSH cassette.

precessional positional change. Subsequently, the instrument accelerates to 4300 rpm and holds that speed for 10 s. This accomplishes the release of the upper friction valve, transferring the reaction mixture to the solid-phase chamber. The solid-phase chamber contains approximately 100 μg of goat anti-mouse IgG antiserum covalently bound to spherical 1.1-μm bromostyrene particles (Fig. 8). The instrument re-initiates mixing for an additional 2 minutes allowing the monoclonal antibody to be captured by the anti-mouse-IgG particles. At the end of the incubation the instrument accelerates to 6000 rpm releasing the lower friction valve. The particles travel from the solid-phase chamber through the water wash and the oil layer to the substrate, leaving any unbound lower-density material stranded at the oil–water interface. The bound conjugate reaches the substrate layer, triggering an enzymatic reaction that is read as the rate of change of fluorescence. The determined slope measurement is interpolated using a stored standard curve, which converts the slope value to an analyte concentration, which is subsequently printed. With a simultaneous sandwich immunoassay, the upper friction valve is set to deliver simultaneously with the aliquoting valve. This allows incubation of sample, antibody or antiserum, solid phase, and conjugate together in the solid-phase chamber for the full incubation period.

The Eclipse digoxin immunoassay is a simultaneous competitive immunoassay. In this assay the conjugate (digoxigenin-calf intestinal alkaline phosphatase) is placed in the antibody/conjugate chamber and the particles, which have sheep anti-digoxin antiserum covalently coupled to

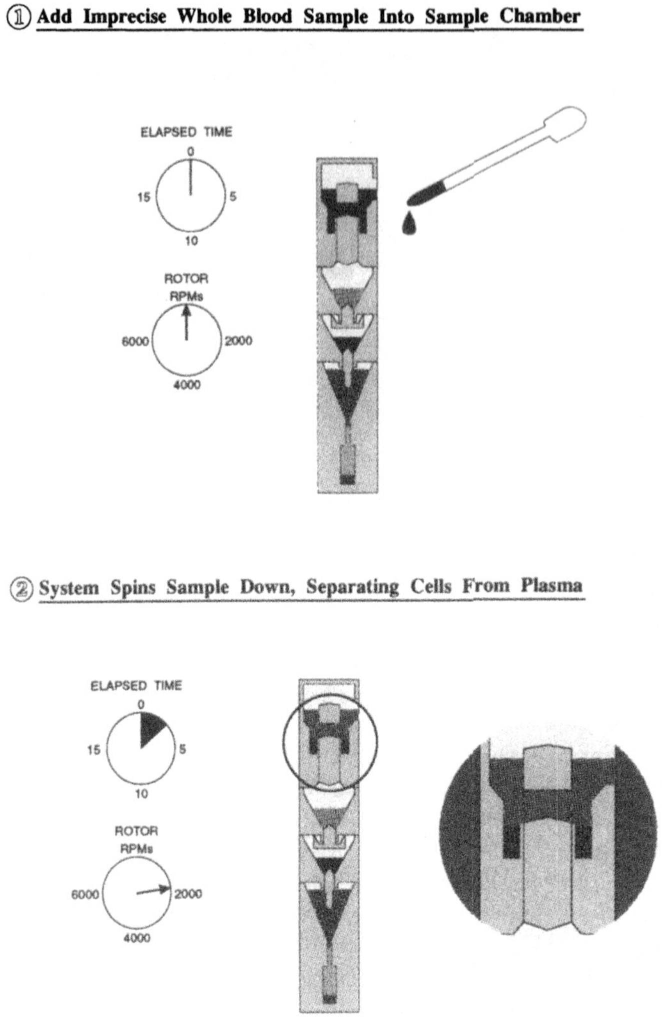

Figure 7 The major steps involved in an automated whole-blood Eclipse TSH immunoassay.

the particle surface, are placed in the solid-phase chamber. The only difference between this format and that described above for the sequential TSH immunoassay is that at 3600 rpm the aliquoting valve and the upper friction valve release concurrently. This combines the sample, digoxigenin-alkaline phosphatase conjugate, and antibody together in the solid-phase chamber, where the entire incubation phase of the assay transpires. At the end of the incubation phase, the instrument accelerates to

③ Aliquoting Valve Releases To Deliver a Precise Plasma Sample Into Antibody Chamber

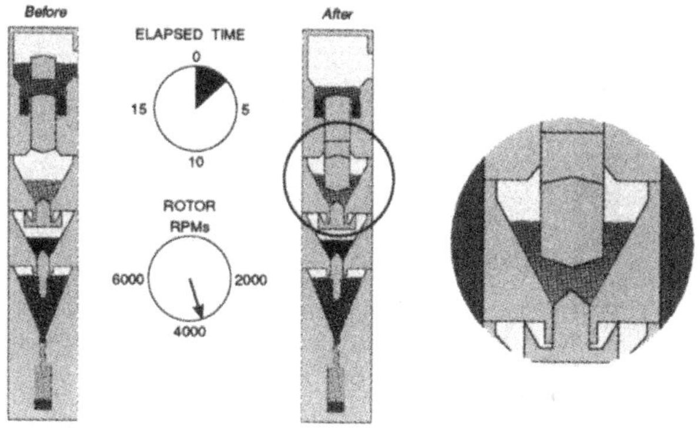

④ Sample Is Mixed With Antibody Mixture

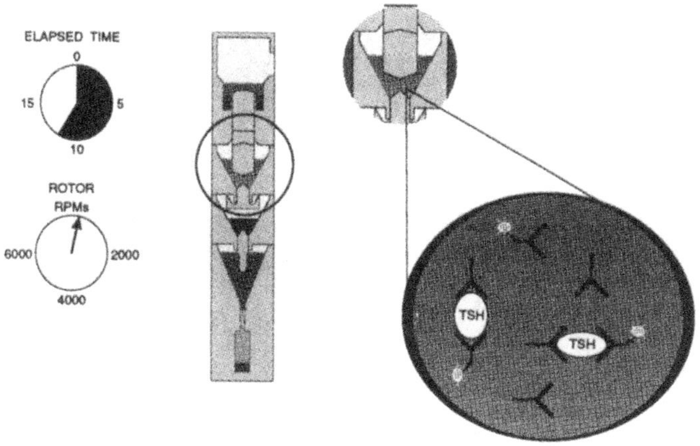

Figure 7 Continued

6000 rpm, releasing the lower friction valve, which ultimately allows the bound conjugate access to the substrate.

A. Random Access

All assays, chemistry tests, and immunoassays operate independently under the command of the same programmed instructions; the instrument

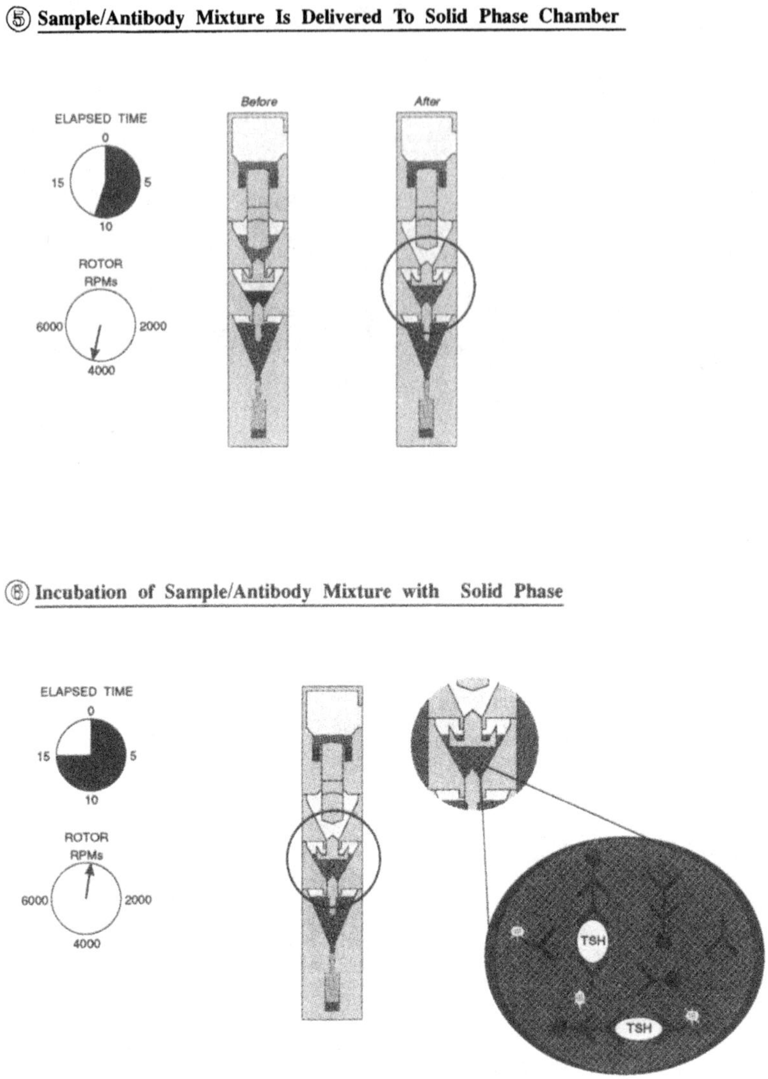

Figure 7 Continued

program is the same regardless of the sample mix. The feature that permits each assay to function independently and permit random access in the Eclipse system, is the order and timing of the valve releases and the time the chemistries and immunoassays are read.

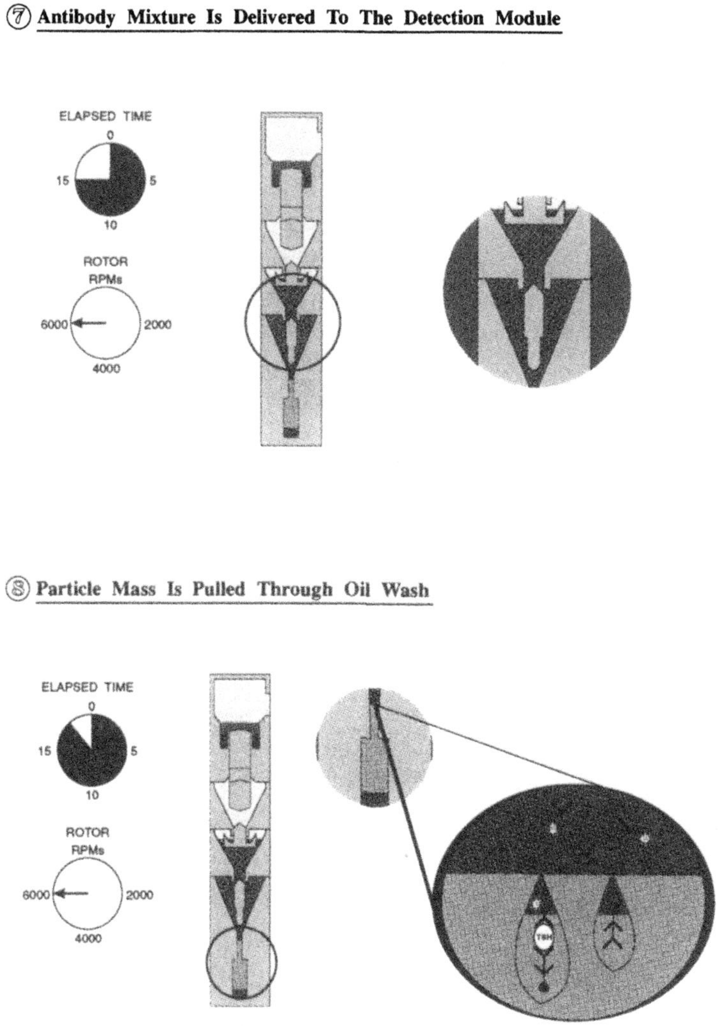

Figure 7 Continued

B. Calibration/Quality Control

Assay calibration is determined at the factory and the analyte concentration curve parameters are encoded in the bar code. When a test is run the bar code is read and the resulting test result is interpolated from the stored

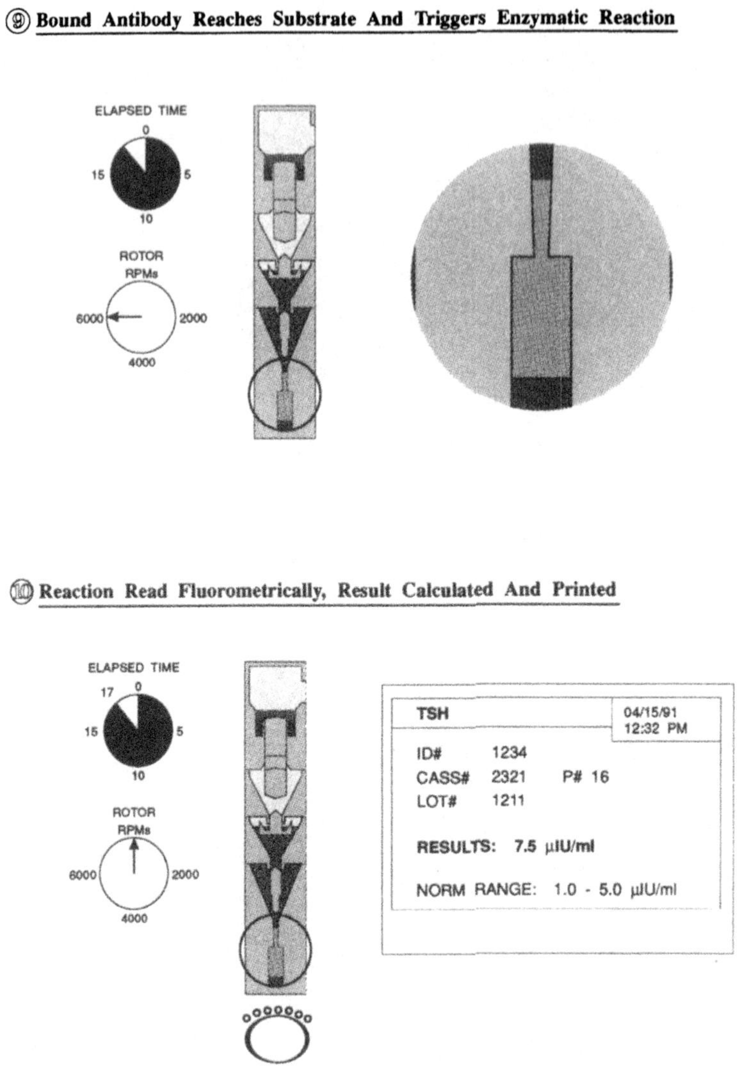

Figure 7 Continued

curve. The chemistry tests are all linear and the data are plotted by least squares regression. The immunoassays employ a four- parameter logistic equation to fit a line to the standard curve data. In each case, the calibration curves can be adjusted by running a single calibrator, which defines for the system the response value for a set analyte concentration. A single-point curve adjustment is accomplished by adding the appropriate

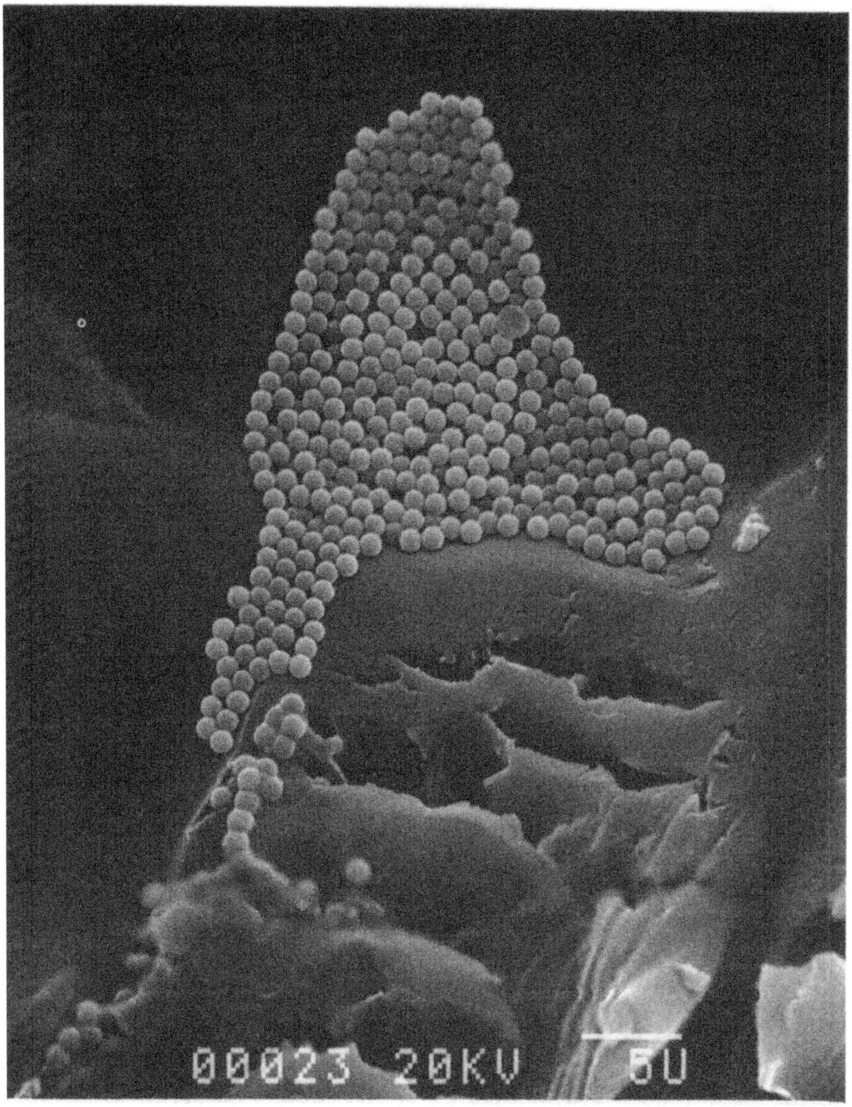

Figure 8 Photomicrograph of the 1.1-μm bromostyrene particles with immobilized sheep anti-digoxin antiserum. The magnification is 8000 times.

calibrator to the test cassette, filling in the "Cal" box on the cassette label, and subsequently, running the test.

The Eclipse system also has the capacity to maintain and print quality control (QC) records in a number of different formats, all selectable by the laboratorian. When a control sample is run, filling in the "QC" box on the cassette label will enable the system's computer to store the data and perform several statistical tests on the results.

V. INSTRUMENTATION

The instrument is a compact, high-speed centrifugal analyzer (Fig. 1). It contains a fully programmable computer, 512 KB of high-speed dynamic RAM memory, a $3\frac{1}{2}$-in 1.44-MB high-density floppy drive, a colorimeter, a spectrofluorophotometer, a bar-code reader, two data input/output (I/O) ports, a printer, and a user-interactive touch-screen graphic display. Since all of the system software is stored on a $3\frac{1}{2}$-in diskette, the user can quickly and inexpensively make on-site enhancements to the software for new assays. The instrument occupies less than 3 sq ft of bench space.

The instrument has been designed with several unique features that assist the user in performing immunoassays and clinical chemistry tests. The Eclipse analyzer is designed for use by individuals with no formal laboratory training. In order to facilitate loading and unloading of test cassettes, the centrifuge is positioned at a 55° angle. In addition, the rotor includes a self-balancing feature, which allows users to load cassettes without regard to the number of samples or the rotor position. A boom above the rotor carries both a bar-code reader and a detector that can determine whether sufficient amount of a patient sample has been added to the cassette. The instrument can maintain temperature control at $37 \pm 0.1°C$. Temperature probes are placed throughout the instrument and case. A temperature algorithm uses the sensor information to regulate the various heaters. Detection in the optics portion of the instrument is by a silicon photodiode, which has five decades of dynamic range. The lamps for absorbance and fluorescence are incandescent halogen and have an expected life of 2 years under normal use. The instrument is equipped with a filter wheel that moves different bandpass filters in place as required by the assay. Currently, absorbance measurements can be taken at 340, 405, 500, 540, and 623 nm. Fluorescence, is measured using excitation and emission wavelengths of 365 and 465 nm, respectively. All fluorescence measurements are normalized using on-rotor quinine sulfate standards, correcting the data as necessary for anomalies in fluorescence signal due to variations in lamp voltage, temperature, etc.

VI. WASHING TECHNOLOGY

One of the technologies basic to the operation of the Eclipse immunoassays is the oil wash. Passing particles through a substance to accomplish a wash prior to the entry into the detection zone has been used in research laboratories before (Bennett and Branton, 1977). These separations, which have mostly employed radioactive tracers, involved passage through an aqueous medium and have exploited varying densities of the separation media, such as sucrose or cesium chloride gradients. The Eclipse system uses a silicone oil with a specific gravity of 1.08. Since the particles employed have a specific gravity of 1.5, they move through the oil layer when exposed to centrifugal force. No measurable enzyme activity is lost during the passage through the oil into the substrate. The buffered substrate has a specific gravity of 1.22, generated by the addition of sucrose to the buffer. Once the particles enter the substrate, 4-methylumbelliferyl phosphate, in a diethanolamine buffer, is cleaved to 4-methylumbelliferone by the conjugated alkaline phosphatase with the generation of fluorescence. The rate of the fluorescence generation is measured during the linear portion of the reaction (e.g., 25–125 s at 5-s intervals for digoxin) and a slope is calculated. The slope is interpolated from the standard curve to yield the concentration of the analyte of interest.

VII. ASSAY PROTOCOL

All assays are performed as follows:

1. The Eclipse ICA analyzer should be in the standby mode.

2. Remove the specific assay cassette pouch from the refrigerator. Prepare the cassette for sample addition by carefully removing it from the protective pouch.

3. Pipette 250–300 μl of patient sample into the sample port (in the case of a whole blood specimen, mix it gently several times before sampling). All tests require the same sample size.

4. Snap the cover into the sample port to seal the cassette.

5. Open the door to the Eclipse ICA analyzer and position the cassette(s) in the instrument rotor.

7. Close the door.

8. Press "RUN" to initiate the assay.

9. The results will be printed on the paper tape within 17 min.

A. TSH Assay Performance

The Eclipse TSH immunoassay is a sequential sandwich immunoassay that employs three antibodies: a monoclonal anti-TSH, a goat anti-TSH polyclonal antiserum that has been conjugated to calf intestinal alkaline

Table 2 TSH immunoassay Precision

Sample	Replicates	Mean (μIU/ml)	Standard deviation (μIU/ml)	Coefficient of variation (%)
Within-run				
Level I	14	1.09	0.06	5.83
Level II	14	10.30	0.66	6.42
Level III	14	19.65	0.93	4.75
Between-run				
Level I		0.82	0.07	8.62
Level II		9.92	0.23	2.34
Level III		17.57	0.66	3.76

phosphatase, and goat anti-mouse IgG polyclonal antiserum that has been covalently immobilized to 1.1-μm particles. Localization of the reagents in the cassette and the assay format were described above. Assay precision data are shown in Table 2. Within-run assay precision was determined by assaying 14 replicates of three levels of control material; between-run precision was assessed by assaying four replicates of three levels of control material over 4 days. Recovery (Table 3) was determined by spiking blank serum with nine levels of TSH. Dilution recovery studies (Table 4) yielded values of 98–108%.

The effect of potentially interfering endogenous substances as presented in Table 5 was determined by spiking TSH into commercially prepared control materials containing elevated levels of hemoglobin, bilirubin, and triglycerides. Protein concentrations up to 12 g/dl do not effect the assay. No significant cross-reactivity was noted for luteinizing hormone (LH; <1200 μIU/ml), follicle-stimulating hormone (FSH; <1200 μIU/ml), or human chorionic gonadotropin (hCG; <107,000 μIU/ml).

Table 3 TSH Immunoassay Spike Recovery

Sample	Initial TSH (μIU/ml)	TSH added (μIU/ml)	Theoretical yield (μIU/ml)	Actual yield (μIU/ml)	Recovery (%)
1	0	0.02	0.02	0.01	50
2	0	0.04	0.04	0.02	50
3	0	0.075	0.075	0.07	93
4	0	0.125	0.125	0.10	80
5	0	0.25	0.25	0.25	100
6	0	0.56	0.56	0.47	84
7	0	1.2	1.2	0.99	83
8	0	12.50	12.50	12.74	102
9	0	25.00	25.00	26.14	104

Table 4 TSH Immunoassay Dilutional Recovery

Dilution	Expected value (μIU/ml)	Actual value (μIU/ml)	Recovery (%)
Neat		40.76	100
1 : 2	20.38	20.02	98.2
1 : 4	10.19	11.05	108.4
1 : 8	5.09	5.53	108.6
1 : 16	2.55	2.61	102.4

A fall in the assay dose response at high TSH concentrations ("high-dose hook effect") is observed only at levels of TSH greater than 1000 μIU/ml. Specimens with high concentrations of TSH may be reassayed following dilution with the zero calibrator. By TSH dilution, the minimum detectable concentration is 0.04 μIU/ml. The assay dynamic range is from 0.04 to 50 μIU/ml. A typical assay standard curve is shown in Fig. 9. A method correlation study comparing 84 patient samples assayed by the Abbott IMx TSH (North Chicago, Illinois) and the Eclipse ICA method is shown in Fig. 10. Whole blood, plasma, or serum can be used for the TSH assay. A matched specimen correlation of 26 whole-blood, plasma, and serum samples showed no statistically significant difference, at the 99.5% confidence level using the Student *t*-test, when whole blood and serum, whole blood and plasma, or serum and plasma were compared.

B. Digoxin Assay Performance

The Eclipse digoxin immunoassay is a simultaneous competitive immunoassay wherein the antiserum (sheep anti-digoxin) is immobilized on

Table 5 TSH Immunoassay Interfering Substances

Substance	Sample	Initial TSH value (μIU/ml)	Final concentration of interference substance in sample (mg/dl)	TSH value after spike (μIU/ml)	Recovery (%)
Hemoglobin	1	5.26	750	5.76	109
	2	21.12	750	19.82	94
Bilirubin	1	5.26	20	5.16	98
	2	5.26	20	5.11	98
Lipemia	1	5.26	750	5.52	105
	2	21.12	750	20.94	99

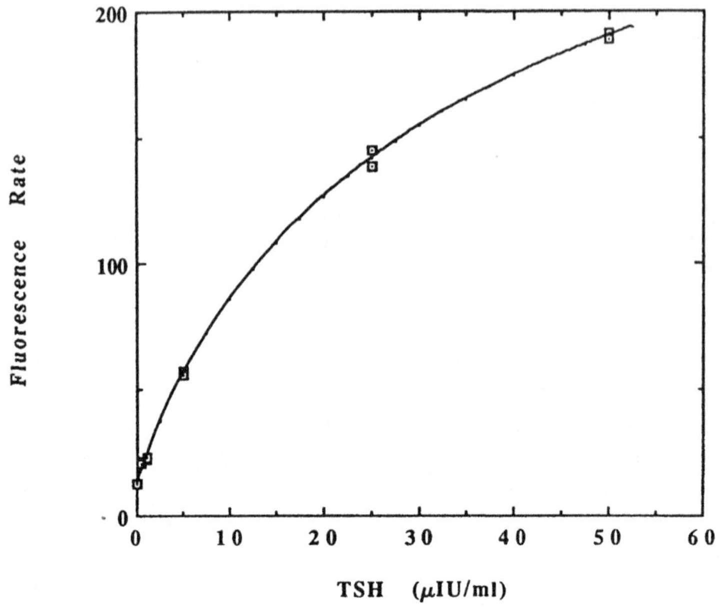

Figure 9 An Eclipse TSH standard curve. The data were fitted using a four-parameter logistic curve.

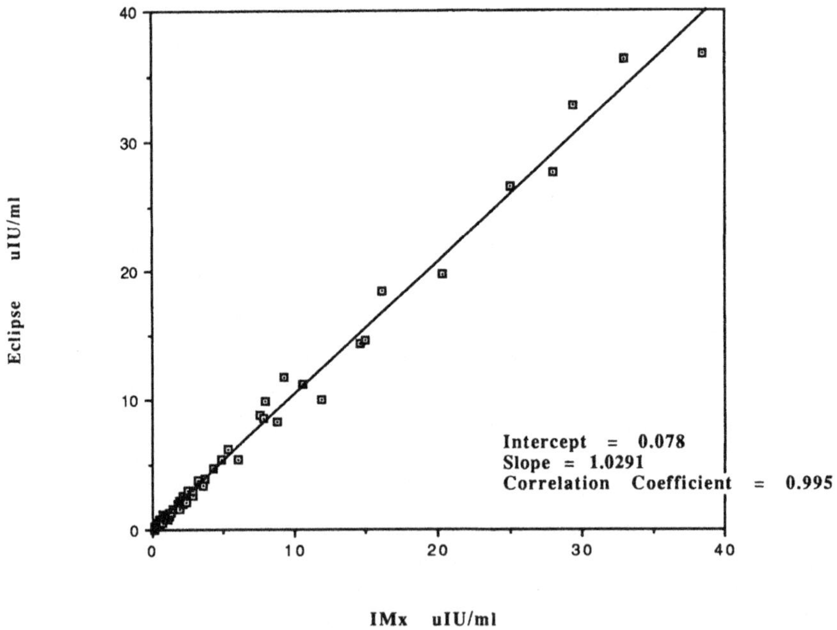

Figure 10 TSH method correlation comparing the Eclipse TSH and the Abbott IMx TSH assay.

Table 6 Digoxin Immunoassay Precision

Sample	Replicates	Mean (ng/ml)	Standard deviation (ng/ml)	Coefficient of variation (%)
Within-run				
Level I	10	0.71	0.06	8.20
Level II	9	1.97	0.11	5.34
Level III	11	3.35	0.18	5.51
Between-run				
Level I		0.89	0.05	5.33
Level II		2.12	0.05	2.41
Level III		3.45	0.11	3.13

the particles. The conjugate is synthesized by covalently linking digoxigenin-3-*O*-carboxymethyloxime to calf intestinal alkaline phosphatase. In this assay, the conjugate resides in the antibody/conjugate chamber of the cassette and the particles are in the solid-phase chamber. At the delivery of sample the upper friction valve opens simultaneously, placing all of the reactants in the solid-phase chamber. Like all of the immunoassays, the total incubation time is 10 min, with the entire incubation occurring in the solid-phase chamber. The Eclipse ICA interpolates the result from a factory-set internal four-parameter logistic curve. Assay precision data are shown in Table 6. Within-run assay precision was determined by assaying multiple replicates of three levels of control material; between-run precision was assessed by assaying four replicates of three levels of control material over four days.

Recovery of digoxin from serum samples spiked with digoxin over the concentration range of 0.3–6 ng/ml ranged from 93 to 103%. The effect of potentially interfering endogenous substances as presented in Table 7 was determined by spiking the indicated substance (hemoglobin, bilirubin,

Table 7 Digoxin Immunoassay Interfering Substances

Substance	Sample	Initial digoxin value (ng/ml)	Final concentration of interfering substance (mg/dl)	Digoxin value after spike (ng/ml)	Recovery (%)
Hemoglobin	1	1.10	500	1.21	110
	2	3.47	500	3.56	103
Bilirubin	1	1.20	20	1.09	91
	2	3.24	20	3.52	109
Lipemia	1	1.21	500	1.17	97
	2	3.57	500	3.77	106

Table 8 Digoxin Immunoassay Cross-reactivities

Substance	Cross-reactivity (%)
Digitoxin	0.051
Lanatoside C	58.0
Digoxigenin	75.1
Ouabain	0.031
Prednisolone	0.0004
Prednisone	0.0006
Spironolactone	0.0003
Canrenoate	0.00016
Progesterone	0.0005
Testosterone	0.0006
Dihydrodigoxin	0.32
Digoxigenin monodigitoxiside	128.0
Digoxigenin bisdigitoxiside	94.7

and triglycerides) into serum specimens with known concentrations of digoxin. Protein concentrations up to 16 g/dl did not effect the assay. Cross-reactivity with structurally related compounds is shown in Table 8. The cross-reactivities are expressed as the ratio of the digoxin concentra-

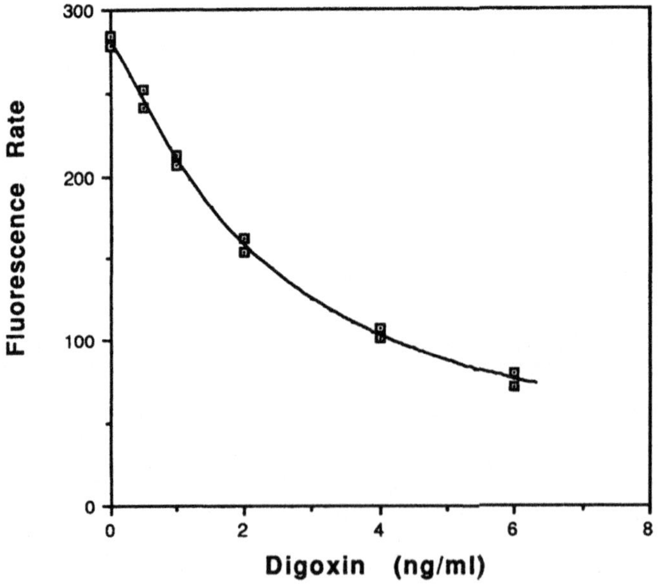

Figure 11 An Eclipse digoxin standard curve. The data were fitted using a four-parameter logistic curve.

tion to the concentration of potentially cross-reacting substances at 50% inhibition of maximum binding (ED_{50}), multipled by 100. The effect of digoxinlike immunoreactive substance (DLIS) (Graves, 1986) was assessed in samples from neonates (using cord blood; $n = 10$) and from patients with renal failure ($n = 10$). None of these patients had received digoxin. Results from assays using the Eclipse ICA were all <0.3 ng/ml.

The assay dynamic range is from 0.3 to 6 ng/ml. Specimens with concentrations of digoxin exceeding 6 ng/ml may be reassayed following dilution with the zero calibrator. The minimum detectable concentration is 0.2 ng/ml. A typical assay standard curve is shown in Fig. 11. A method correlation study comparing 82 patient samples assayed using the Kallestad (Sanofi Diagnostics, Chaska, Minnesota) Quanticoat ^{125}I digoxin radioimmunoassay (package insert 78214) and the Eclipse ICA digoxin assay is shown in Fig. 12. Either plasma or serum can be used. A matched-specimen comparison of 34 plasma and serum samples gave a regression coefficient of 0.993 with a slope of 0.97721 and an intercept of 0.053. Additionally, these samples showed no statistically significant difference, at the 99.5% confidence level, using the Student t-test.

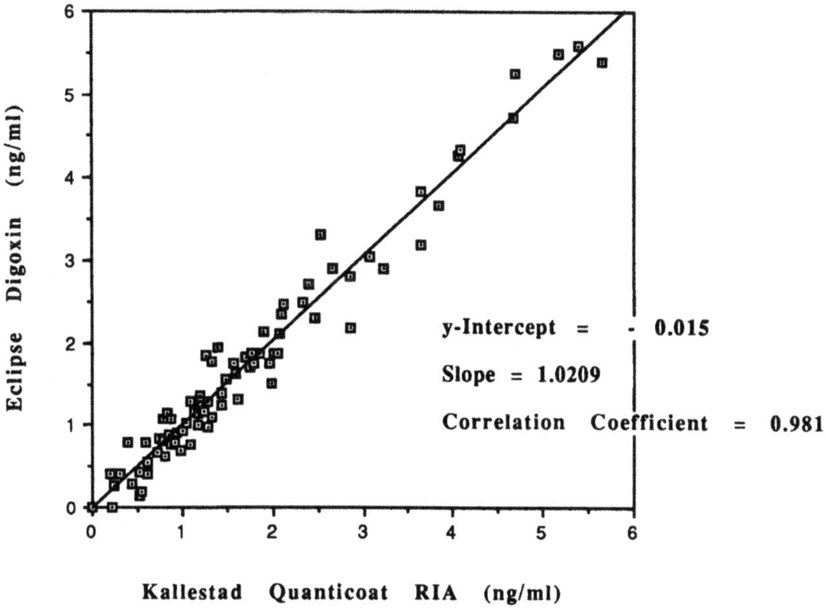

Figure 12 Digoxin method correlation comparing the Eclipse digoxin immunoassay and the Kallestad (Sanofi Diagnostics) Quanticoat RIA.

VIII. CONCLUSION

The Eclipse ICA is one of the few clinical analyzers capable of performing both immunoassays and chemistry tests. Additionally, the ease of operation allows the instrument to be used at sites (e.g., physician offices, emergency rooms, clinics) where the high level of technical expertise required in large clinical laboratories is unavailable. The versatility of the Eclipse ICA for performing a wide range of analytical procedures has been demonstrated (Table 1). Additional chemistry and immunoassay tests are under development. The assay performances of chemistry tests performed on the Eclipse ICA, although not described here, are comparable to those of standard chemistry analyzers currently in use. Analytical performance for the TSH and digoxin immunoassays described above are equivalent (as indicated in the respective manufacturer's package insert) to the comparison procedure cited. While details of the pricing for the Eclipse ICA instrument and cassettes are not available at this time, overall costs (including instrument, cassettes, and labor) will be competitive with current analyzers.

REFERENCES

Bennett, V., and Branton, D. (1977). Selective association of spectrin with the cytoplasmic surface of human erythrocyte plasma membranes. *J. Biol. Chem.* **252:** 2753–2763.

Graves, S. W. (1986). Endogenous digitalis-like factors. *CRC Crit. Rev. Clin. Lab. Sci.* **23**(3): 177–200.

CHAPTER 16

ES-300 Immunoassay System

Michael A. Sagona and William E. Collinsworth
Diagnostic Laboratory Systems,
Boehringer Mannheim Corp.,
Indianapolis, Indiana

Richard H. Gadsden, Sr.
Clinical Chemistry, Children's Hospital,
Medical University of South Carolina,
Charleston, South Carolina

I. INTRODUCTION

During the early 1970s, Boehringer Mannheim Corporation began its involvement with immunodiagnostics. Both its experience and its reputation in enzyme research, technology, and production made it a likely candidate to enter the area of immunodiagnostics.

The first immunoassay developed by Boehringer Mannheim was for digoxin in 1972, followed by insulin that same year. The first immunoassay analyzer introduced was the ES-11, a photometer that had the capability to do curve calculations. In the next few years, the ES-11 was upgraded to an ES-22, then to a semiautomated version, the ES-33. In 1986 Boehringer Mannheim introduced the ES-600, a totally automated, multichannel immunoassay instrument (Heuer, 1991). Hamilton Corporation and Boehringer Mannheim have been able to supply walk-away automation testing with flexibility and curve manipulation capabilities (Schmidt *et al.*, 1986). To date there are more than 3000 ES-22 and ES-33 analyzers, as well as more than 700 ES-600 systems, placed worldwide.

In 1990, the ES-300 immunoassay system was launched worldwide (July/United States; October/Japan; May/Europe). The ES-300 was de-

Immunoassay Automation: A Practical Guide

signed to meet the needs of the U.S. market with benchtop flexibility and walk-away capability. The new ES-300 system benefits from 5 years of field experience utilizing the same reagents and coated-tube technology as the ES-600 instrument. Boehringer Mannheim has made significant technological advancements in the manufacturing of its coated tubes. The company has developed a proprietary process that ensures lot-to-lot consistency in the tube-coating process. In addition, there is a multistep quality control program that has allowed Boehringer Mannheim to manufacture a coated tube with high degrees of assay precision (Spona, 1987; Kanst *et al.*, 1988).

II. SYSTEM DESCRIPTION

A. Instrumentation

1. Analyzer

The physical dimensions of the ES-300 analyzer are 38.5 in wide × 22 in high × 24 in deep. The weight of the instrument is 205 lb (Fig. 1). The ES-300 electrical requirements are 115 VAC, 15 A, and 60 Hz. The ES-300 is a self-contained system with distilled water, wash solution, cleaning solution, and reagents all housed on the analyzer. A waste container is attached and kept near the location of the instrument.

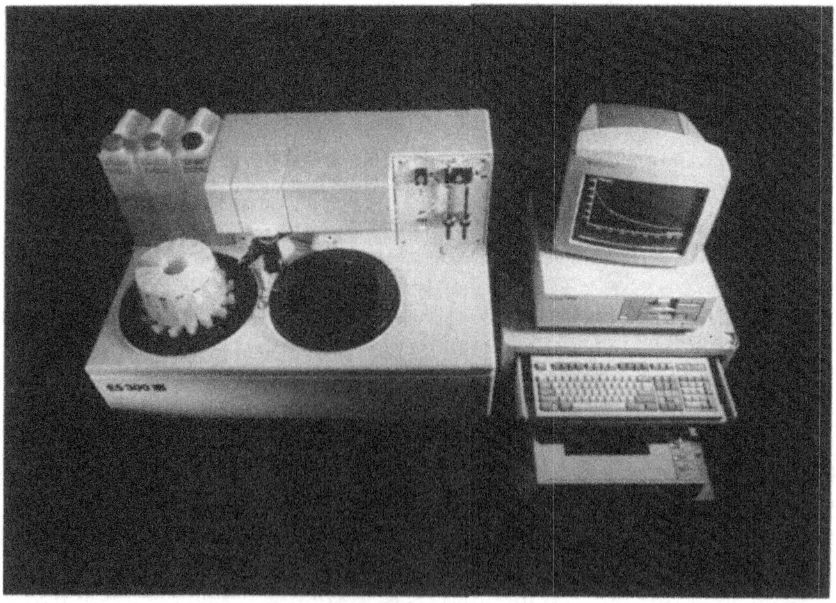

Figure 1 ES-300 system: instrument and computer.

The main components of the analyzer are:

1. The reagent rotor can accommodate 12 variable reagents as well as three designated positions: two positions for the universal substrate, and one position for the system cleaning solution.

2. The sample rotor has 150 positions for patient samples and for standards. An additional 10 positions exist for the use of universal multi-constituent controls.

3. The multifunctional arm (MFA) has four arms on which the following needle probes are located: sample/reagent needle, coated-tube wash/aspirate needle, substrate/reagent needle, and photometer/mixer needle. The arms rotate the needles 360° to pick-up and dispense sample, reagent, and substrate as well as mix, and aspirate and pick up for the reading of the sample in the cuvette. The needles provide liquid level detection to ensure accurate pipetting.

4. The dispensing system is driven by two Hamilton syringes, which have a capacity of either 250 μl or 2.5 ml. The syringe chosen depends upon the volume necessary to pipette. Better precision and accuracy will be achieved by selecting the correct volume syringe.

5. The incubator rotor has 160 positions available for coated tubes. The temperature range of the incubator rotor is 25–37°C in 0.5°C increments. The chosen temperature is maintained by six Peltier units mounted under the incubator rotor. The Peltier units have the capability of either cooling or warming the rotor to the correct temperature.

6. The photometer detects light from a halogen lamp that flows through a culminating lens, the 422-nm filter, then through a quartz flow-through cuvette (path length 3 mm), and is collected by a receiver diode. The 422-nm filter is mounted on a filter wheel with three additional filter positions, which allow for future expansion of the ES-300 test menu. There is a reference diode and feedback circuit, which regulates the lamp to maintain a constant output. The flow-through cuvette temperature is maintained at the same temperature as the incubator rotor by means of a single Peltier unit.

2. Computer and Software

The ES 300 system includes a Hewlett Packard (HP) Vectra QS/16S computer, keyboard, HP VGA high-resolution monitor, and an Epson FX-850 printer (Fig. 1). The computer has an 80-386SX microprocessor with an 80387 coprocessor, 3 MB of RAM memory, 40-MB hard disk, and an HP dual asynchronous serial interface. The computer is essential to the system in that it carrys out all the necessary operations from instrument control to evaluation of results, data storage, and quality control functions, as well as bidirectional interfacing for uploading and downloading patient information. The ES 300 analyzer is connected to the HP computer through the serial RS232C port. The Epson FX850 printer is operated through an RS232C parallel port on the computer.

The ES 300 software called TWIN is divided up into the following four blocks: (1) run—execution/evaluation of testing; (2) quality control—quality control monitoring; (3) system parameter—operational programming/mainframe interfacing/calculation mode; and (4) system functions—system testing/troubleshooting.

ES 300 operators spend the majority of the time using the RUN block mode. To initiate a run the operator first enters the patient requisition. This includes the patient's name, I.D. number, and the testing or test profile selection. The patient's demographics may also be entered at this point, or after the run has been started. Several operator-defined functions exist to allow for rapid requisition of entries. Once the sample requests have been made, it is then possible to segregate the tests for a run by back-ordering either specific samples or specific tests.

In addition to the flexibility in sample handling, options are also available for the standard curve as well as the controls that are used. The standards are recommended to be run in duplicate, with patients run singly. The operator may select to perform a full calibration curve, a one- or two-point recalibration curve, and finally no standards run and simply using the stored curve function. As many as three different controls can be run per test. Also, the operator can select controls to be run at the beginning of the run at the end of a run, and/or after a specified number of patient samples.

Other functions within the RUN block include:

1. Loading status. This provides a printed summary of the requested run with the rotor position number, patient I.D., and tests ordered for that patient. It also generates an easy-to-follow load list for the necessary reagents, samples, cleaning solution, substrate, sample tubes, and coated-uncoated tubes; it determines the volumes that are necessary for the run and indicates the appropriate positions for all constituents on the reagent, sample, and incubator rotors.

2. Run optimization by overlapping sequences (ROBOS). This is a function of the software, which determines the appropriate pipetting sequences to allow the assays of a specific run to be performed during the shortest possible time period and thus optimize the work-load management (Fig. 2). Tests are overlapped so that the incubation period of previous assays can be used to perform other functions such as wash, aspirate, dispense, and read other tests. If the operators wish they can change the order sequence set by the software by simply assigning priorities to specific tests.

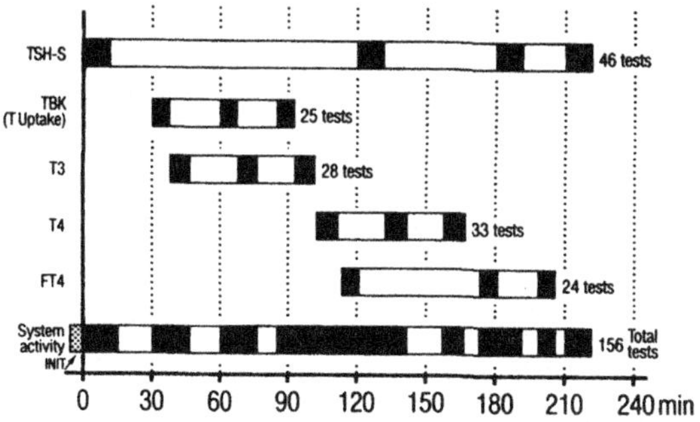

Figure 2 Diagram of run optimization by overlapping sequences (ROBOS).

3. Run status. This module provides the operator at any time during the run the ability to determine the system's progress. It also allows one to see the procedural steps for each of the assays in progress. It indicates pipetting, incubation, and photometric schemes, as well as their individual starting and finishing times.

4. Documentation module. From this module one can generate four different types of reports, and it also provides the ability to review and edit the standard curve.

5. Data conclusion/archive. This allows the operator the choice of whether to accept the standard curve and quality control values as well as the ability to release patient results. The archiving function allows one to store patient data and system programming.

6. System cleaning is performed on a monthly basis. Each month the operator requests via the computer the system cleaning procedure. The system initiates a complete system cleaning with minimal technologist involvement to assure consistency in pipetting and patient results.

B. Reagent

The methodology behind the chemistry on the ES-300 is the enzyme-linked immunosorbent assay (ELISA). The ELISA methodology on the ES-300 is a heterogeneous system, as opposed to a homogeneous system. Heterogeneous assays are able to measure both high- and low-molecular-weight compounds in very low concentrations and thus are capable of measuring a wide range of analytes. Currently, most assays are configured on the ES-300 using antibody-coated tubes. Horseradish peroxidase (POD) is the enzyme of choice, tagged to either the antibody or antigen. In addition, a patented universal substrate, ABTS, is used. The assay formats are either competitive, one- and two-step sandwich, or modified competitive. Each assay has five to seven standards for a full curve calibration. The calibration curve stability lasts for 2 weeks. In between the 2-week full curve calibrations, it is recommended to perform a one-point recalibration with each run using one of the designated standards.

The standard curve is calculated from the absorbances of the standards and is dependent upon the chosen evaluation and calibration mode.

The Rodbard calculation is used for most chemistries to generate the standard curve:

$$y = \frac{\text{P1} - \text{P4}}{1 + (x/\text{P2})^{\text{P3}}} + \text{P4}$$

where y is the absorbance of sample, x the concentration of sample, and P1–P4 the curve parameters.

Hyberbola, linear regression, cutoff, pos/neg, and absorbance readings are the optional calculation methods that are available for standard curve calculation, dependent upon the operator's selection.

Future assays will be formatted around a universal streptavidin tube. The tube walls will be coated with the tetrameric protein, streptavidin. The advantage of this technology lies in the unusual strength of the avidin/biotin bond. The free energy of the association is 21 kcal/mol with an association constant of $10^{15}\ M^{-1}$. Each avidin molecule binds four molecules of biotin, resulting in an excess of binding sites, which will allow for any minute imprecision in the tube molding process, thus contributing a smaller amount of the overall imprecision of the assay and allowing sensitive assays of those analytes in extremely low concentration such as progesterone and estradiol.

III. PERFORMANCE

A. Technical Evaluation

1. Precision

With the incorporation of the heterogeneous enzyme immunoassay chemistry on the ES-300 the performance is equivalent to the precision, sensitivity, and accuracy of current radioimmunoassays (RIAs). Within-run coefficients of variation (CVs) of all assays are between 3 and 10%, and between-run CVs are 8–12%. Table 1 demonstrates the within-run precision using a control in the normal range and a control in the abnormal range. The next table (Table 2) reveals the precision on all assays performed in duplicate over a given concentration range (range of samples) and analyzed by linear regression statistics with the means and standard deviations of the two populations.

Table 1 Precision of Enzymun Methods on ES 300
Within-Run Precision

Analyte	Control material[a]	Concentration	CV%
Cortisol	PNIM	12 ng/ml	<4
	PPIM	50 ng/ml	<3
Digoxin	PNIM	1 ng/ml	<4
	PPIM	3 ng/ml	<3
Ferritin	PNIM	70 ng/ml	<4
	PPIM	40 ng/ml	<3
FSH	PNIM	10 mU/ml	<6
	PPIM	30 mU/ml	<5
hCG	PNIM	6 mIU/ml	<12
	PPIM	30 mIU/ml	<4
IgE	PNIM	100 U/ml	<4
	PPIM	160 U/ml	<4
Insulin	PNIM	10 mU/ml	<8
	PPIM	60 mU/ml	<4
Prolactin	PNIM	15 ng/ml	<5
	PPIM	40 ng/ml	<3
T3	PNIM	1.5 ng/ml	<5
	PPIM	3.0 ng/ml	<3
T4	PNIM	7 μg/ml	<4
	PPIM	20 μg/ml	<3
fT4	PNIM	0.9 ng/ml	<7
	PPIM	4.0 ng/ml	<3
TBG	PNIM	8.2 μg/ml	<3
	PPIM	16 μg/ml	<5
TBK	PNIM	0.7 TBI	<7
	PPIM	1.25 TBI	<3
TSH-s	PNIM	7 μU/ml	<5
	PPIM	4 μU/ml	<4
Progesterone	PNIM	10 ng/ml	<4
	PPIM	30 ng/ml	<3
AFP	PNIM	12 ng/ml	<4
	PPIM	50 ng/ml	<3
Estradiol	PNIM	150 pg/ml	<7
	PPIM	600 pg/ml	<8

[a] PNIM, precinorm control; PPIM, precipath control.

2. Accuracy/Sensitivity

The analytical sensitivity of each analyte is revealed in Table 3, along with the method used for standardizing each test to give maximum accuracy.

Table 2 Precision of Enzymun Methods on the ES-300

Method	N	Regression equation	Correlation	Mean X	SD X	Mean Y	SD Y	Range of samples
Thyroid assessment								
Enzymun T_4	62	$Y = 0.998X + 0.1$	0.996	8.50	3.47	8.51	3.44	2.0–16 μg/dl
Enzymun T_3	62	$Y = 0.986X + 0.62$	0.998	1.07	0.58	1.06	0.58	0.4–3.6 ng/dl
Enzymun FT4	50	$Y = 1.002X + 0.001$	0.999	1.46	0.92	1.47	0.93	0.5–5.0 ng/dl
Enzymun TSH-S	46	$Y = 1.001X - 0.004$	0.998	2.84	3.33	2.84	3.32	0.01–16.8 μU/ml
Enzymun TBK[a]	58	$Y = 1.008X + 0.001$	0.998	1.00	0.27	1.01	0.27	0.2–2.0 TBI
Fertility assessment								
Enzymun FSH	50	$Y = 0.993X - 0.025$	0.997	16.54	14.00	16.40	13.94	6.0–60 mIU/ml
Enzymun LH	50	$Y = 1.002X - 0.10$	0.999	5.91	6.99	5.82	7.00	4.0–40 mIU/ml
Enzymun prolactin	50	$Y = 0.983X + 0.004$	0.996	33.83	42.10	33.26	41.55	10.0–150 ng/ml
Enzymun hCG	54	$Y = 0.997X + 0.25$	0.999	67.21	64.86	67.77	64.54	10.0–300 mIU/ml
Tumor markers								
Enzymun AFP	66	$Y = 0.987X + 0.68$	0.998	46.10	24.3	46.17	24.0	20.0–140 ng/ml
Enzymun CEA	69	$Y = 0.997X + 0.21$	0.999	49.8	117.7	49.9	117.4	1.0–800 ng/ml
Other assays								
Enzymun ferritin	62	$Y = 0.884X + 2.5$	0.987	229.3	449	219.6	384.3	150.0–800 ng/ml
Enzymun IgE	42	$Y = 0.986X + 0.52$	0.999	176.6	181.2	174.7	178.9	30.0–300 IU/ml
Enzymun digoxin	54	$Y = 0.998X - 0.008$	0.999	1.43	0.8	1.42	0.8	0.4–3.3 ng/ml
Enzymun cortisol	62	$Y = 1.023X - 0.33$	0.998	17.08	11.8	17.15	12.1	2.0–45 μg/dl
Enzymun insulin	62	$Y = 0.991X - 0.15$	0.999	20.04	31.66	19.71	31.43	2.0–80 μU/ml

[a] T_4 uptake (TBI units).

Table 3 Sensitivity and Accuracy of Enzymun on ES-300 Sensitivity/Accuracy

Assay	Sensitivity	Standardization
T_3	0.25 ng/ml	N/A
T_4	0.5 μg/dl	GC-MS
fT4	0.2 ng/dl	Equilibrium dialysis
TSH-S	0.07 μU/ml	2nd IRP (80/558)
TBK	0.2 TBI	N/A
TBG	2.0 μg/dl	N/A
hCG	1.5 mIU/ml	1st IRP (75/537)
LH	0.7 mIU/ml	1st IRP (68/40)
FSH	0.7 mIU/ml	2nd IRP (78/549)
Prolactin	2.0 ng/ml	WHO Std. (75/504)
IgE	1.5 IU/ml	2nd IRP (75/502)
Insulin	3.5 μU/ml	N/A
Digoxin	0.3 ng/ml	N/A
Cortisol	1.0 μg/dl	ID-MS
Ferritin	5.0 ng/ml	NIBSC (80/602)
Ferritin-S	2.0 ng/ml	NIBSC (80/602)
AFP	1.8 ng/ml	CDC Biological Std.
Progesterone	0.4 ng/ml	ID-MS
Estradiol	10 pg/ml	ID-MS

3. Interferences

Bilirubin (<60 mg/dl) and lipemia (<1000 mg/dl triglycerides) provide no interferences with any of the existing Enzymun-Test reagent menu. Hemolysis (<1 g/l) has no effect on any of the assays, except insulin, where a negative interference is caused by the release of insulin-degrading enzymes from the ruptured erythrocytes (Figs. 3–5).

B. External Evaluation

Tunn *et al.* (1990) demonstrated in a multicenter evaluation the precision of the Enzymun one-step cortisol assay. The within-run imprecision was less than 8% and the between-run imprecision was less than 12%. The detection limit was discovered to be 30 nmol/l (11 μg/l). There was excellent agreement between the Enzymun cortisol and the reference method, ID-MS, $r = 0.98$ and $y = 1.02x - 0.45$.

Hintze *et al.* (1990) have shown, using the Enzymun fT4 assay, a within-run imprecision of between 0.8 and 9.8%, depending on the reference material used. The between-run imprecision had a CV of between 1.0 and 13.2%, once again depending on the reference material used. When the new fT4 assay was compared to the calculation for a free throxine index

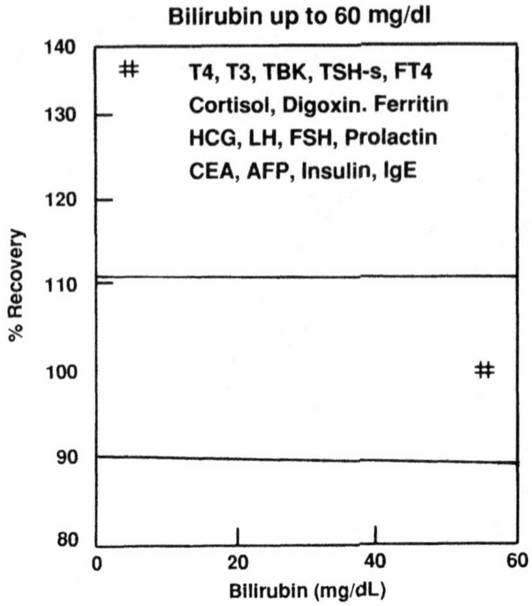

Figure 3 Interferograph for bilirubin with Enzymun test reagents on the ES-300.

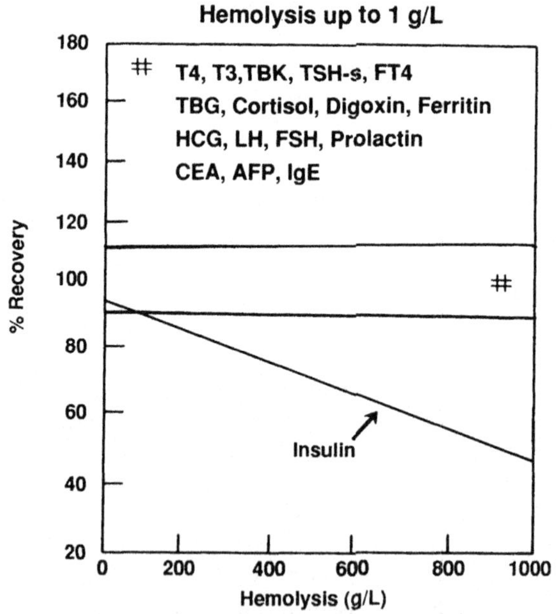

Figure 4 Interferograph for hemolysis with Enzymun test reagents on the ES-300.

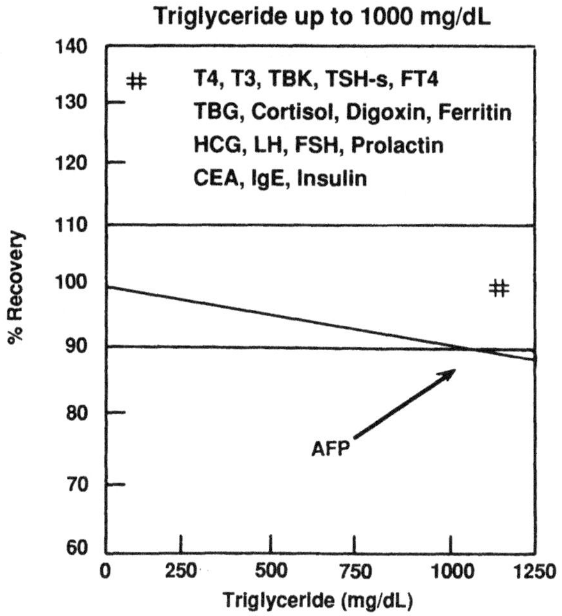

Figure 5 Interferograph for lipemia/triglycerides with Enzymun reagents on the ES-300.

with a number of samples in the hypothyroid, euthyroid, and hyperthyroid condition, a good correlation was obtained.

Spona (1987), in a multicenter evaluation of Enzymun CEA, demonstrated that the intraassay CV was between 1.3% at 23.0 μg/l of CEA and 13.9% at 1.3 μg/l of CEA. Interassay precision ranged from 3.6 to 19.2%. The sensitivity for the CEA assay proved to be 0.5 μg/l of CEA. A good correlation was found between the Enzymun CEA assay and six other CEA enzyme immunoassay (EIA) and RIA methods. The correlation coefficients ranged from 0.933 to 0.998. The slope and intercepts ranged from 0.842 to 1.222 and from −1.176 to 0.693, respectively. A recovery experiment in spiked human sera used equal amounts of a solution of purified CEA and human sera containing 0–5.47 μg/l, mixed. The percent recovery ranged from 88 to 106% of CEA.

IV. CONCLUSION

The ES-300 has walk-away capability with 18 fully automated heterogeneous enzyme immunoassays ranging from FT4 to the streptavidin progesterone assay. The ES-300 heterogeneous enzyme-linked immunosorbent assay is equivalent to current RIA methodology based upon its high degree of sensitivity, precision, and accuracy. It has fully automated the difficult process of the heterogeneous assay.

There are a number of test concepts that have been incorporated into the system: the competitive assay, one- and two-step sandwich assays, and modified competitive as well as enzyme-labeled antigen and enzyme-labeled antibody test formats. From the technical data presented, the ES-300 ensures both excellent precision and accuracy, as well as the needed sensitivity to give clinically reliable results.

The future universal tube assays will incorporate the uniqueness of the streptavidin/biotin bond to give even greater precision and sensitivity, as well as shortening the incubation/turnaround time of the assays. This, along with the true walk-away capability due to the fully automated features on the ES-300, will create greater efficiencies for the immunoassay laboratory and has put the ES 300 in a new generation of immunoassay analyzers.

REFERENCES

Heuer, M. (1991). A pioneer in advanced research. *J. Clin. Immunoassay* **13**(4),

Hintze, G., Briehl, E., Jaworek, D., Kunst, A., and Kobberling, J. (1990). Evaluation of a new enzyme immunoassay system for free thyroxine (Enzymun-Test FT4). *J. Clin. Chem. Biochem.* **28**(6), 427–433.

Kunst, A., Seidenschwarz, E., Burk, H., Schauer, S., Haug, M., Lehmann, P., and Ehrhardt, V. (1988). New one-step enzyme immunoassay for free thyroxin. *Clin. Chem.* **34,** 1830–1833.

Schmidt, H., and Heuer, M. (1986). ES 600. *Lab. Clin. Pract.* **4,** 83–87.

Spona, J. (1987). Multi-center study of a new CEA enzyme immunoassay using monoclonal antibodies. *J. Clin. Chem. Biochem.* **25**(1), 53–59.

Tunn, S., Pappert, G., Willnow, P., and Kreig, M. (1990). Multicenter evaluation of an enzyme-immunoassay for cortisol determination. *J. Clin. Chem. Biochem.* **28**(12), 929–935.

CHAPTER 17

IMx SYSTEM

Peter P. Chou
American Medical Laboratories, Inc., Fairfax, Virginia

I. INTRODUCTION

Increased demand for tests from the clinical laboratories as well as development of automated instruments to perform these tests occurred at about the same time during the 1950s. Automation allowed laboratories to process a much larger workload without a comparable increase in the number of staff (Maclin and Young, 1986). However, most of the automated instruments are available in the areas of clinical chemistry, hematology, and microbiology. There are still a few areas, such as immunoassay, that remain constrained by manual testing procedures (Fiore *et al.*, 1988). But the light is on the horizon, and all systems described in this book are developed in order to improve and/or automate various immunoassays.

Conventional radioimmunoassay and enzyme immunoassay are manual techniques, characterized by long incubation time, laborious wash and transfer steps, and poor reproducibility. Attempts to automate these technologies have frequently resulted in large, costly instruments aimed at high-volume analytes and are not optimal for the majority of clinical laboratories. Therefore, Abbott Laboratories has developed a fully automated, benchtop instrument, the IMx. This system is capable of processing a batch of 20 or 24 samples in 20–50 min with no operator intervention. Its operation is based on two analytical approaches to processing immunoassays: a novel technology known as microparticle capture enzyme immunoassay (MEIA) for high-molecular-mass/low-concentration analytes, and fluorescence polarization immunoassay (FPIA) for low-molecular-mass analytes (Jolley, 1981a,1981b; Popelka *et al.*, 1981).

FPIA is the technique used in the Abbott TDx instrument that has been applied to the determination of many low-molecular-mass analytes, such as therapeutic drugs and some hormones. Please refer to the chapter on TDx analyzer (Chapter 9) for a detailed description of this part of the operation. The combination of these two technologies into a single instrument has made this system capable of performing a wide range of immunoassay tests.

II. SYSTEM DESCRIPTION

A. Instrumentation

The IMx analyzer weighs 43.2 kg. Its dimensions are 62 × 70 × 36 cm (d × w × h). The system is designed to operate within an ambient temperature range of 15°–30°C and a relative humidity range of 15–85%. The complete system consists of a benchtop analyzer; MEIA reagent packs and reaction cells; FPIA reagent packs, sample cartridges and cuvettes; and calibrators and controls. The analyzer (Fig. 1) consists of the following

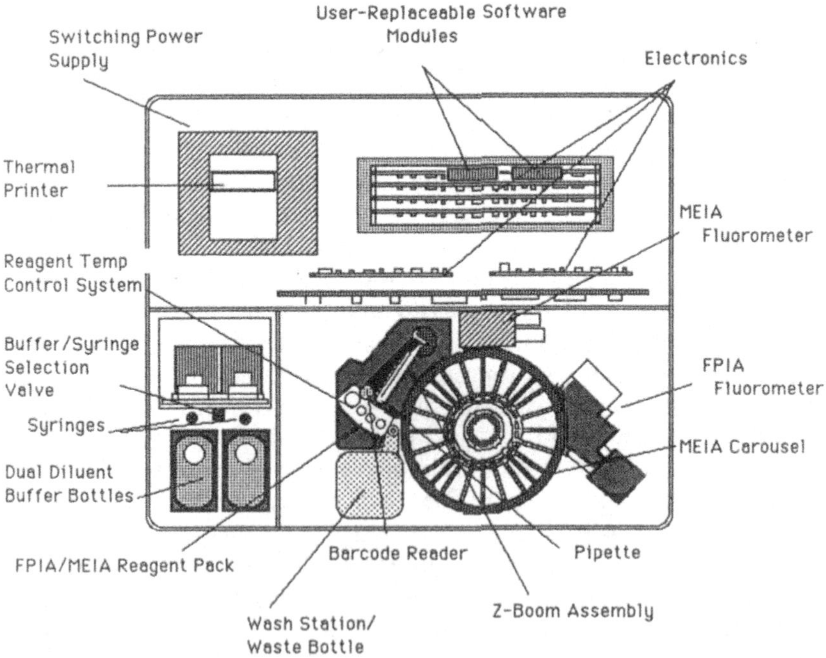

Figure 1 Major components of the IMx analyzer.

major components: MEIA carousel containing 24 MEIA reaction cells or FPIA carousel containing 20 sample cups and cuvettes; MEIA front-surface fluorometer; FPIA optics system; reagent heater block; air heater system; diluent heater system; robotic (two degrees of freedom) pipetting system, which includes the reagent bar-code reader system; fluid delivery system; pipette wash/waste-container system; optics interface circuitry; memory and computer circuit boards; user-changeable memory modules (system and assay); MEIA lamp power-supply system; printer; operator interface; and dual RS-232 interfaces.

The specific features of various components will be discussed in Section IIC in detail except for the FPIA portions of the instrument, which are similar to the TDx analyzer and are described in Chapter 9 of this book.

FPIAs are performed in 20-test batches with a 30-min assay time, and MEIAs are performed in 24-test batches in 30–50 min, with serum samples requiring no pretreatment. However, the instrument can predilute samples automatically. There are 100 assays per reagent pack, and calibration curves are stable at least 2 weeks.

B. Principle and Method

MEIA technology is based on two key features: increased kinetics through the use of very small particles (0.47 μm in diameter) as the solid phase, and efficient separation of bound from unbound material by capture of the microparticles in a glass-fiber matrix.

A suspension of microparticles provides far greater effective surface area than a conventional polystyrene-bead or coated-tube solid phase. The area available for reaction with the bead is 1.27 cm^2, whereas the total surface area of the particles used in a typical MEIA assay approaches 6.11 cm^2 (Bangs, 1985). This fivefold increase in reactive surface area increases reaction kinetics and reduces incubation times so that assays are completed within 30–50 min. An additional benefit of using suspensions of microparticles is that they are easily manipulated by instrument robotics, for relatively simple automation of assay protocols.

The particles are separated from the reaction mixture via "microparticle capture" onto a glass-fiber matrix, a process that relies on the high affinity of glass fibers for the protein-coated microparticles. The microparticles adhere to the surface of the fibers irreversibly, whereas nonspecifically bound material can be effectively removed by washing the matrix. The matrix also provides a precisely located mechanical support for the microparticles during the optical measurement phase of the assay protocol. Finally, because capture takes place on the surface of the glass fibers, one can use fiber matrices with large pore sizes, which are less susceptible to clogging by viscous samples.

MEIA can be used in either a "sandwich" or a competitive ligand format. In the sandwich format, the latex microparticles are covalently coated with capture antibody. When incubated with the unknown sample, they form the capture complex. An enzyme-labeled antibody conjugate is then incubated with the particles to form the second half of the sandwich complex (Brown, 1987; King *et al.*, 1987). In the competitive format, antibody-coated microparticles are incubated with sample containing the analyte and an enzyme-labeled analyte (conjugate). Removal of unbound conjugate after equilibrium is accomplished with the glass-fiber surface. Substrate is then added and the resulting fluorescence signal is measured. The enzyme/substrate system used in both MEIA assay formats is alkaline phosphatase (EC 3.1.3.1)/4-methylumbelliferyl phosphate (4-MUP).

C. Specific Features

1. MEIA Reaction Cell

The MEIA reaction cell (Fig. 2a) comprises in a single unit a sample well, dilution well, incubation well, and capture matrix with blotter. It is not assay specific and can be used with all MEIA assays.

2. MEIA Carousel

Different carousels are used to process FPIA and MEIA assays. The MEIA carousel (Fig. 2b) holds 24 MEIA reaction cells. It incorporates a locking feature that ensures that the reaction cells are held firmly under the front-surface fluorometer to give a high degree of positional repeatability. The reaction cells are loaded into the appropriate location in the carousel and firmly locked into place by twisting the locking ring. Before each run, an indicator on the locking ring is optically scanned by a detector in the instrument to verify that the carousel is locked. This indicator also allows the instrument to identify which type of carousel, MEIA or FPIA, has been loaded. At the end of each run, the reaction cells are disposed of by twisting the locking ring in the opposite direction and inverting the carousel over a waste container.

3. Pipette System and Fluid Delivery System

The pipette system involves a two-degrees-of-freedom robotic arm that holds the pipette/probe assembly and allows it to be positioned over the reagent bottles, the reaction cells, and the wash station. Stepper motors move the pipette system up and down (Z direction) as well as radially (R direction).

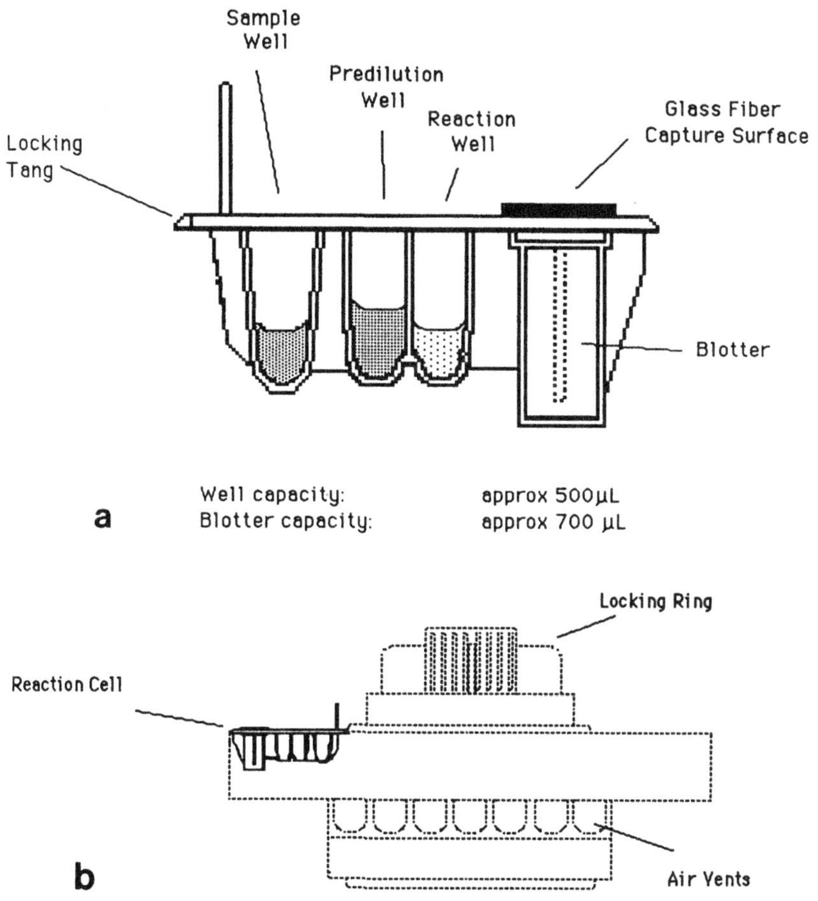

Figure 2 (a) MEIA reaction cell; (b) MEIA carousel.

The pipette/fluid delivery system transfers reagents from reagent bottles to reaction cells and from well to well within a reaction cell. The pipette itself is a drawn stainless-steel tube, Teflon coated to minimize carryover. Fluid levels are sensed by measuring electrical conductivity between the pipette/probe tip and an external electrode.

The pipette system also incorporates a bar-code reader assembly that is automatically moved over the reagent pack before a run to identify the test specified.

The fluid-delivery system consists of two syringes: a 250-μl sample syringe and a 2500-μl diluent syringe, both driven by stepper motors. A stepper-motor-driven valve allows both syringes to be connected to either of the two buffer bottles (MEIA or FPIA). These 1-liter bottles of diluent buffer stay in the instrument at all times and their levels are monitored by the computer. Switching between diluent buffers is completed automatically by means of the valve, and an assay run cannot be initiated unless sufficient buffer is in the appropriate bottle. The valve also allows the syringes to be connected to the pipette to allow for aspiration and delivery of fluids from the reagent bottles and the wells of the reaction cells.

Carryover between samples and reagents is minimized by washing the pipette/probe over a specially designed wash station. The inside as well as the outside of the pipette is washed with about 1.2–2.5 ml of diluent buffer.

4. Temperature-Control System

Enzyme immunoassays require precise temperature control to achieve repeatable performance. Temperature must be accurately controlled during all incubation steps of the assay protocols. The effect of temperature on the activity of alkaline phosphatase-mediated conversion of substrate is about 3–5% per °C (McComb *et al.*, 1979).

The instrument relies on three separate systems to control the temperature: the reagent temperature is controlled in reagent vials by a closed-loop heating block; assay diluent buffer temperature is controlled by a flow-through heater block; and reaction-cell temperature is controlled by a forced-air heating system.

Before a run, reagent vials are placed into a heating block in the instrument; a cast aluminum assembly holds the vials precisely to permit access to the reagents by the pipette system. The block is heated by integral electric heater rods, and the temperature of the block is sensed by an embedded thermistor that is in contact with the walls of the two central reagent vials. An analog feedback circuit compares the thermistor sensor output with a setpoint temperature set by the computer and maintains the block at 35.0° ± 0.5°C. Diluent buffer is precisely heated (35.0° ± 0.5°C) so that the pipette is warmed before the aspiration and dispensing of reagents and sample. Before additions of temperature-sensitive reagents, heated diluent buffer may be cycled through the pipette and into the wash station. Any sample dilutions are also performed with this heated diluent buffer.

MEIA reaction cells are heated in their perspective carousels by forced air from below the carousel. Ambient air is drawn in by a fan and forced over a heating element, past a thermistor, and up toward the carousel where it warms the reaction cells. An analog circuit compares the thermistor temperature against a setpoint determined in the software. In this way, the computer can control the air temperature of the output from the heater system to minimize warmup time at the beginning of a run and can maintain air temperature in the vicinity of the reaction cells such that the temperatures of the reaction-cell wells stay constant during changing ambient conditions.

During a run, temperature control is accomplished by reading an additional "remote" thermistor placed in the air flow in the immediate vicinity of the reaction cells. Figure 3 shows the relative locations of the carousel, air flow, and remote thermistor, as well as a schematic represen-

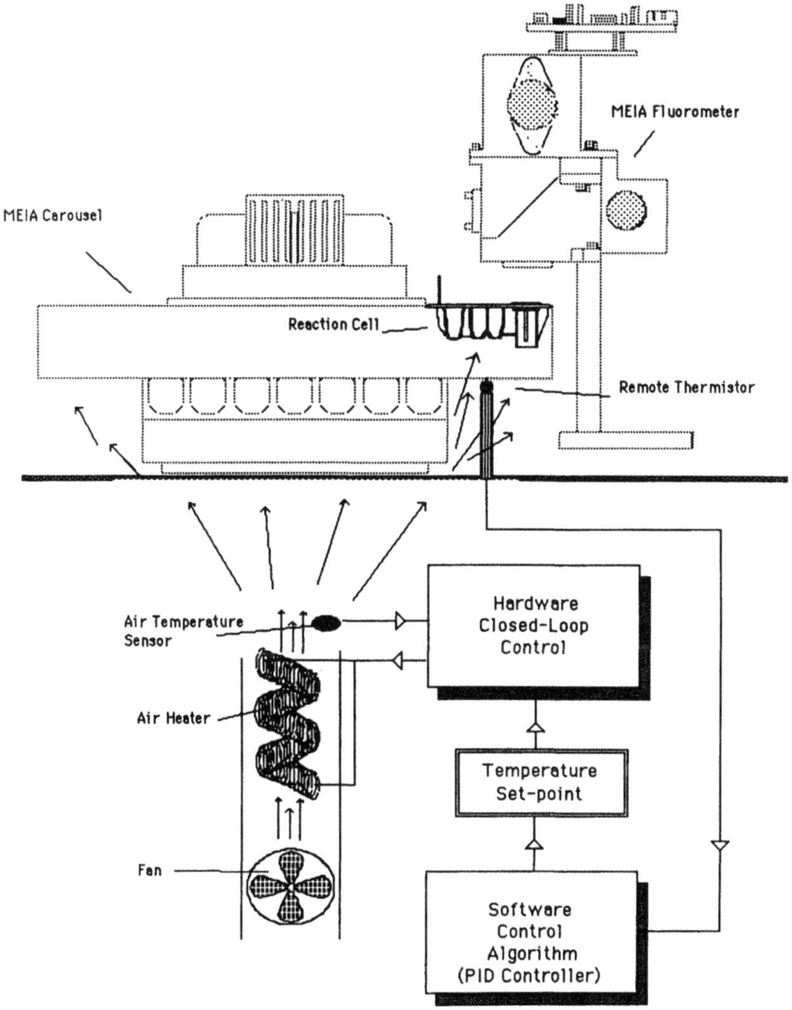

Figure 3 Schematic representation of reaction-cell temperature-control scheme.

tation of the control strategy. A single-point calibration is performed that relates a manual measurement of the temperature of an aliquot of diluent buffer in a well of the reaction cell (at equilibrium) to the temperature measured at this remote thermistor. During a run, the computer controls the air-heater control circuit, in response to readings on the remote thermistor to implement closed-loop control at the remote thermistor location. The equilibrium temperature at this location has been related to the liquid temperature of the reaction cell during a prior calibration, so that closed-loop control of the reaction mixture in the reaction cell is achieved. The reaction well temperature is maintained at 34.0° ± 0.7°C, even though the ambient operating temperature of the laboratory may range from 15° to 30°C. Temperature calibration of the instrument is stable for at least 1 week. Precision of the reaction-cell temperature during a run is ± 0.5°C. The algorithm used to control reaction-cell temperature is based on a proportional integral differential controller (Dorf, 1980).

5. Front-Surface Fluorometer (MEIA)

MEIA results are determined by quantifying the rate of fluorescence development when substrate is converted by the action of an enzyme-labeled conjugate. The substrate (4-MUP; Abbott Labs.) is dephosphorylated to 4-methylumbelliferone (4-MU; Abbott Labs.) by alkaline phosphatase. Abbott Laboratories has developed a front-surface fluorometer that selectively excites and quantifies emission from 4-MU in the presence of 4-MUP. The fluorometer (Fig. 4) consists of a low-pressure mercury lamp, an excitation bandpass filter and dichroic beamsplitter, focusing/collection lens, photodiode, photodiode filter, emission longpass filter, emission bandpass filter, photomultiplier tube, and signal-processing electronics. Excitation energy derived from the low-pressure mercury arc lamp is enhanced by an integral phosphor coating that converts light from the predominant mercury line (254 nm) to 365 nm. This energy is then filtered by the excitation bandpass filter to produce energy predominantly at 365 nm to excite 4-MU molecules. The bandpass characteristic of this filter is customized to limit transmission below 345 nm to <0.01%, minimizing excitation of 4-MUP. Light transmitted through the excitation bandpass filter then strikes the dichroic beamsplitter, which is reflective at 365 nm and transmissive at 448 nm.

A portion of this 365-nm energy passes through the dichroic beamsplitter, passes through the ultraviolet filter glass, and strikes a photodiode. The signal developed at the photodiode is representative of the 365-nm energy sent to the reaction matrix and is used to normalize the fluorescence rate data. This signal is also proportional to the lamp output and is used to generate a control signal that is used by the lamp power supply to control lamp current; this maintains the intensity of the 365-nm

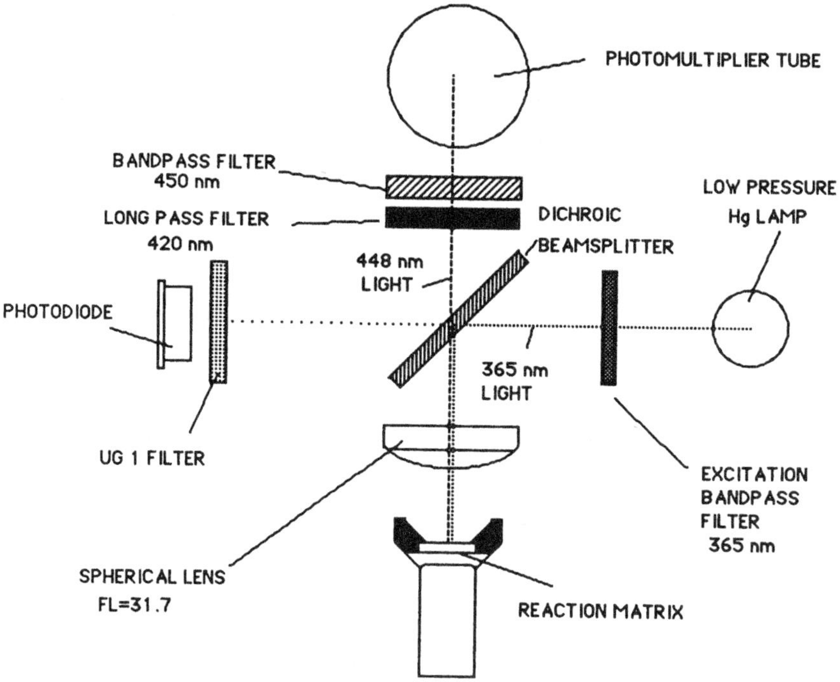

Figure 4 Optical schematic of front-surface fluorometer.

energy measured at the photodiode within 5% over the useful life of the lamp. The 365-nm light reflected from the front face of the dichroic beamsplitter is focussed through a lens (focal length, 31.7 mm) onto the reaction matrix. The lens also serves as the collector for 448-nm light that is generated on the matrix during a fluorescence measurement. The 448-nm energy passes through the dichroic filter and additional longpass and bandpass filters. The longpass (GG 420) filter keeps out wavelengths <400 nm and the bandpass filter's characteristic is centered on the maximum emission energy band of 4-MU. In this way the effects of stray 365-nm excitation energy and any 387-nm (noise) emitted from 4-MUP will be minimum. Figure 5 shows the transmission characteristics of the major filters superimposed on the 4-MU/4-MUP excitation and emission spectra.

Thin-film dielectric interference coatings on the dichroic beamsplitter and the excitation bandpass filters are designed to minimize environmental effects that could contribute to optical drift (Brunsting *et al.*, 1986). The entire fluorometer system resides inside the thermally controlled environment of the analyzer so that thermal drift is also minimized.

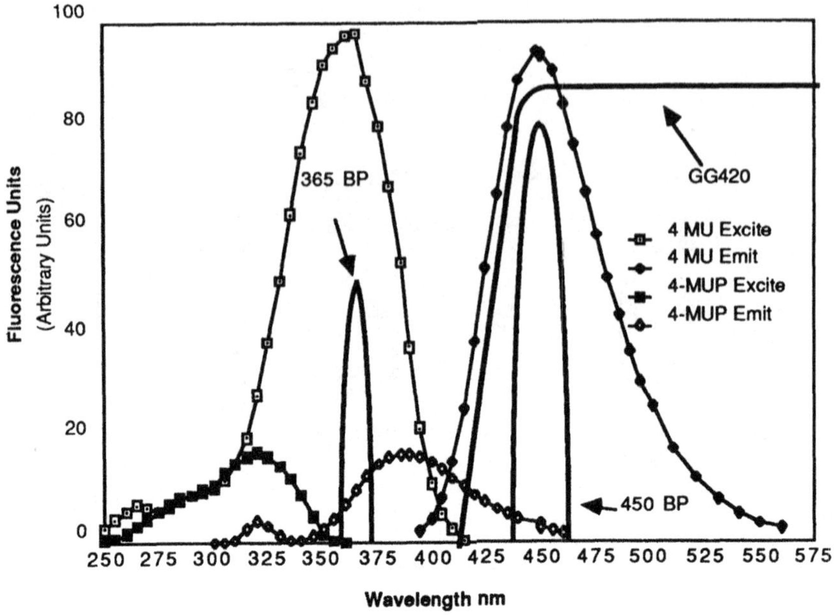

Figure 5 Relative excitation and emission spectra of 4-MUP and 4-MU, 1.5 nmol/l each, in a standard reaction mixture at pH 10.3.

A set of six specially constructed reaction cells loaded with discs containing specific amounts of an inorganic europium phosphor in a durable ceramic matrix is used to check the calibration of the fluorometer system. The discs are formulated to give three intensities of fluorescence to cover the entire dynamic range of fluorescence signal possible in an assay.

Photomultiplier tube gain is varied to set the signal of the middle fluorescent standard to nominal calibrated value. A linear check is then performed to verify that the photomultiplier tube is still operating in the linear region over the entire range of assay fluorescence values at the new gain setting. Because lamp intensity is controlled and the stability of the rest of optical components is held to a tight tolerance, large changes in gain of the photomultiplier tube are not necessary to maintain system calibration.

III. PERFORMANCE

A. Data Reduction and Assay Calibration

The IMx postprocessor uses linear regression analysis to convert the fluorescent measurement data to rates, which are proportional to analyte concentration. All rate calculations are based on eight fluorescent measurements of 500 ms each, with 0–1000 ms pause intervals between each measurement, depending on specific assay requirements. The y-intercept from this analysis (at t = time of the first fluorescent measurement) provides an indication of substrate contamination. If the maximum limit placed on this variable is exceeded, indicating that a substantial amount of 4-MUP has been converted to 4-MU, the corresponding rate will be invalid and no results for that sample will be generated. Additional checks performed on the rate to determine its validity include evaluation of the correlation coefficient and the normalized root mean square error (NRMSE), an indication of scatter about the regression line, calculated as follows:

$$\text{NRMSE} = \frac{\sqrt{\dfrac{\Sigma(y_i - \hat{y})}{n - 2}}}{\text{Rate}}$$

where y_i is the actual counts per second for each reading, $\hat{y}$ the predicted counts per second from curve, $y_i - \hat{y}$ the residual, and n = the number of readings (8; i.e., $n - 2 = 6$). A maximum limit is set on this parameter and a minimum limit is set on the correlation coefficient. All evaluation criteria must be met for the rate to be valid. Once this has been established, the analyte concentration in the sample is then calculated from a stored standard curve.

Three calibration modes are available for IMx assays: CAL, a full calibration that is stored; Mode 1, a one-point adjustment of the stored calibration; and Mode 2, no adjustment to the stored calibration. The user selects the appropriate mode from the front panel before pressing RUN. MEIA and FPIA assays are initially calibrated by preparing a carousel with six concentrations of calibrators in duplicate. Samples and controls may be optionally added, in singlet. After loading the carousel and reagent pack into the analyzer, the user simply closes the door, selects CAL mode, and presses RUN. The appropriate protocol is loaded from the assay memory module and the carousel is processed automatically. A postprocessing routine analyzes the obtained data and, if results are considered valid, generates a calibration curve by using one of the following data-reduction methods: point-to-point, linear regression, or four-parameter logistic curve fit. Control and sample concentrations are then determined from the calibration curve and a hard-copy report is printed. The calibration curve is stored in memory and remains stable for a minimum of 2 weeks.

For maximum precision of results between full calibration runs, some MEIA assays require one calibrator (designated as Mode 1 calibrator) to be run in singlet with every carousel. The rate obtained for the Mode 1 calibrator is divided by the corresponding rate from the fitted curve to yield the Mode 1 factor, which is then used to adjust the stored calibration curve. Control and sample concentrations run in Mode 1 are determined from the adjusted curve. All FPIA and some MEIA assays can be run in Mode 2. The user inserts a carousel of samples and controls into the analyzer, closes the door, selects Mode 2, and press RUN. Concentrations are derived from a stored calibration curve for that assay.

B. Operational Performance

Operation of the instrument is straightforward. All interaction with the instrument is completed through a keypad and front panel display. The display is arranged as 40 alphanumeric characters on two lines, with the top line used to give prompting and status messages and the bottom line used to label five "command keys," software-configured multiuse controls that enable the user to operate the instrument. Numeric data are input with an adjacent numeric keypad. The command key approach eliminates complex control panels with many dedicated keys and also enhances user friendliness by presenting only control functions that are appropriate for the particular operation being performed. By coupling the presentation of control functions with prompting and status messages, error-free operation is enhanced and user training is minimized. Assay results and other vital data are presented on a 40-column printout and can also be accessed via an RS-232 port for automatic data collection by a host computer. An additional RS-232 port is available for service testing.

Present software design allows all results to be printed only at the end of the assay. However, instantaneous printout of results as they become available would be nice.

Servicing the instrument is simplified by use of a one-piece removable enclosure that provides access to all subsystems. The instrument remains operational with the enclosure unit removed. Diluent buffer bottles and the interior of the instrument are accessed through hinged doors to facilitate loading of reagents and carousel, changing of lamps, and other routine maintenance procedures. A waste container located in the instrument holds the washing and the instrument will prompt users to empty the container.

During the evaluation, it was noticed that for assays that require excessive washing of the sample probe, this waste container needed to be emptied frequently. The capacity of this waste container should be larger to allow more assays to be completed, or it could simply be connected to a drain line.

C. Assay Performance

An example of a typical sandwich-type protocol is the IMx assay for alpha-fetoprotein (AFP). In the first step of this assay, the sample is incubated with a suspension of alpha-fetoprotein-specific antibody-coated microparticles. After the binding of the analyte in the sample to the capture antibody is complete, an aliquot of the mixture is transferred to a glass-fiber matrix. As the mixture flows through the matrix, the microparticles adsorb to the glass fibers. A second antibody, labeled with the alkaline phosphatase, is added and incubated on the matrix. After incubation, the matrix is washed with on-line diluent to remove excess sample and unbound conjugate. Separation is both rapid (<3 s) and efficient (requiring <200 μl of wash solution). The 4-MUP substrate is then added to the matrix for detection and measurement. The concentration of analyte is directly proportional to the rate of fluorescence emitted from the surface of the matrix. The rate of fluorescence is measured and compared with a calibration curve stored in the instrument to obtain AFP concentration.

The integrity of the glass-fiber matrix is critical to the performance of the assay. In other words, users must inspect all reaction cells to make sure that there are no defective cells. Several defective cells (pieced matrix material, not well-seated matrix material) have been noticed during the evaluation, and erroneous results were obtained from those defective reaction cells.

Temperature control of the environment appears to be very important to the proper performance of the IMx system. It was noticed that certain assays such as thyroxine demonstrated extreme sensitivity to heat. In addition, this instrument generates heat continuously; therefore, proper ventilation is also required.

The lifespan of the mercury lamp is not consistent. It varies from 1 to 6 months in our laboratories.

D. Clinical Performance

Analytes evaluated in this study include thyroxine (T_4), T_3 uptake (T-up), human thyroid-stimulating hormone (hTSH), triiodothyronine (T_3), human chorionic gonadotropin (hCG), ferritin, creatine kinase-MB (CK-MB), luteinizing hormone (LH), and follicle-stimulating hormone (FSH). Each analyte was evaluated for precision and sensitivity. One reference method was selected and used for the correlation study. Carryover study was performed for ferritin and hCG.

1. Interassay Precision Study

Analyte	Mean	SD	CV	*N*
T_4 (μg/dl)	4.4	0.36	8.2	87
	7.6	0.46	6.0	89
	14.8	0.53	3.6	88
T-uptake (unit)	0.51	0.02	3.8	100
	0.99	0.02	2.1	100
	1.49	0.02	1.5	100
hTSH (μIU/ml)	0.25	0.02	8.5	32
	6.6	0.28	4.3	33
	51.9	2.43	4.7	35
T_3 (ng/ml)	0.64	0.05	7.7	30
	1.40	0.11	8.0	30
	3.52	0.15	4.3	30
hCG (mIU/ml)	24.2	2.18	9.0	44
	141.8	9.24	6.5	40
	313.2	24.76	7.9	40
Ferritin (ng/ml)	8.33	0.66	7.9	42
	20.53	0.94	4.6	41
	158.94	7.48	4.7	39
	412.12	15.31	3.7	45
CK-MB (ng/ml)	5.1	0.29	5.7	48
	20.3	1.02	5.0	48
	111.9	7.38	6.6	48
LH (mIU/ml)	5.37	0.47	8.7	48
	43.2	2.8	6.4	48
	82.5	5.1	6.2	48
FSH (mIU/ml)	5.0	0.4	8.0	48
	24.9	2.2	8.9	48
	70.3	8.2	11.7	48

2. Sensitivity Study

Sensitivity was calculated by determining the mean and standard deviation of the rates of the zero calibrator through repetitive analyses of the zero calibrator within the same run. The rate at 2 SD above the mean of the zero calibrator, calculated from the original calibration curve, yielded the calculated sensitivity. This value represents the lowest measurable concentration of an analyte that can be distinguished from zero.

Analyte	*N*	Calculated sensitivity
T_4	14	1.03 μg/dl
hTSH	10	0.05 μIU/ml
T_3	10	0.16 ng/ml
hCG	10	0.26 mIU/ml
Ferritin	12	1.16 ng/ml

(continues)

Analyte	*N*	Calculated sensitivity
CK-MB	10	0.19 ng/ml
LH	10	0.5 mIU/ml
FSH	10	0.2 mIU/ml

Alternatively, one can calculate the minimum detection limit by serially diluting a low control or patient specimen, analyzing all specimens, and observing the diminishing of the signal. The value before the diminished signal is referred to as the minimum detection limit or observed sensitivity. However, this study was not performed in this evaluation.

3. Carryover Study

Sample carryover must be held to a minimum to reduce the likelihood of contaminating a negative sample and reporting a false-positive result. Carryover for the hCG assay was evaluated by assaying three samples with high hCG concentrations (10,000; 100,000; and 1,000,000 mIU/ml). Each sample was immediately followed by two replicates of the hCG zero calibrator. No detectable carryover within the claimed sensitivity limits (2.0 mIU/ml) of the assay was observed. In addition no high-dose hook effect was noted at values up to a concentration of 1,000,000 mIU/ml.

Carryover for the ferritin assay was evaluated by assaying a specimen containing 22,000 ng ferritin/ml. The zero calibrator placed immediately after this elevated ferritin sample showed no detectable ferritin.

4. Correlation Study

Analyte	Reference method	Slope	*y*-Intercept	*r*	*N*
T_4	Abbott TDx T_4 PLUS	1.03	−0.79	0.992	264
T-uptake	Abbott TDx T-uptake	0.99	−0.01	0.977	263
hTSH	Abbott hTSH-EIA	0.83	−0.20	0.997	138
T_3	Amersham Amerlex-T_3	0.97	0.20	0.955	143
hCG	Hybritech Tandem-E	0.87	0.70	0.972	185
Ferritin	Abbott Ferrizyme	1.09	8.5	0.976	453
CK-MB	Ciba-Corning Magic-Lite	0.83	−2.16	0.988	200
LH	DPC Double Ab	0.90	1.8	0.966	647
FSH	Serono MAIACLONE	0.81	1.3	0.987	697

IV. CONCLUSIONS

Traditionally, all immunoassays are performed either in duplicate or triplicate in order to minimize imprecision. However, the precision on IMx appears to be excellent for all assays evaluated. Therefore, it is possible to perform these assays in singlet, which will improve the productivity for immunoassays.

During this evaluation study, it appeared that the calibration curves were valid for much longer than the 2-week stability that the manufacturer is claiming. We noticed that several calibration curves were stable for as long as 6 weeks. This extended stability of the calibration curves should also improve productivity.

Space is a premium in most clinical laboratories. Therefore, the relatively small size of this instrument plus the fact that it is a bench-top unit will enhance the marketability of this instrument. However, there is still a need to redesign the plastic MEIA kit boxes for two reasons: (1) the boxes are larger than needed, which causes problems in storage in refrigerators, and (2) the enclosure will not stay shut and the lid pops open. During the evaluation, many kits were received open as a result of this design flaw. This is particularly a problem with the standards, where many vials are included and jar loose during shipment.

This system is designed to be used by medium-size hospital laboratories. High-volume users will find the throughput of this system to be too low. The carousel approach limits the throughput for this system. In addition, the IMx system is not a random access instrument, and it becomes very ineffective for profile analyses. Finally, there is no positive specimen identification system for this instrument.

Despite the deficiencies mentioned earlier, the IMx system provides a very attractive alternative for immunoassays. It uses no isotopic labels. It is easy to operate and maintain. It can provide stat analyses around the clock. It is a true walk-away system and thus reduces hands-on time and improves productivity. The combination of MEIA and FPIA technologies has greatly enhanced the capability and versatility of this instrument.

REFERENCES

Bangs, L. B. (1985). "Uniform latex particles." Seragen Diagnostics Inc., Boston.

Brown, W. E. (1987). Microparticle-capture membranes: Application to TestPack hCG-urine. *Clin. Chem.* **33,** 1567–1568.

Brunsting, A., Kheiri, M. A., Simonaitis, D. F., and Dosman, A. J. (1986). Environmental effects on all-dielectric bandpass filters. *Appl. Optics.* **25**(18), 3235–3241.

Dorf, C. D. (1980). "Modern control systems." 3rd ed. pp. 380–383. Addison-Wesley, Reading, Massachusetts.

Fiore, M., Mitchell, J., Doan, T., Nelson, R., Winter, G., Grandone, C., Zeng, K., Haraden, R., Smith, J., Harris, K., Leszczynski, J., Berry, D., Safford, S., Barnes, G., Scholnick, A., and Ludington, K. (1988). The Abbott IMx automated benchtop immunochemistry analyzer system. *Clin. Chem.* **34**(9), 1726–1732.

Jolley, M. E., Strope, S. D., Wang, C-H. J., Panas, H. N., Keegan, C. L., Schmidt, R. L., and Schwenzer, K. S. (1981a). Fluorescence polarization immunoassay I. Monitoring aminoglycoside antibiotics in serum and plasma. *Clin. Chem.* **27**(7), 1190–1197.

Jolley, M. E., Strope, S. D., Schwenzer, K. S., Wang, C. J., Lu-Steffes, M., Hill, H. D., Popelka, S. R., Holen, J. T., and Kelso, D. M. (1981b). Fluorescence polarization immunoassay. III. An automated system for therapeutic drug determination. *Clin. Chem.* **27**(9), 1575–1579.

King, W. J., Brown, W. E., George, S. *et al.* (1987). An automated, microparticle-based fluorometric enzyme immunoassay for the measurement of carcinoembryonic antigen in human serum and plasma [Abstract]. *Clin. Chem.* **33**(6), 920.

Maclin, E., and Young, D. S. (1986). Automation in clinical laboratory. In "Textbook of Clinical Chemistry" (N. W. Tietz, ed.), p. 236. W. B. Saunders, Philadelphia.

McComb, R. B., Bowers, G. N., and Posen, S. (1979). "Alkaline phosphatase." Plenum Press, New York.

Popelka, S. R., Miller, D. M., Holen, J. T., and Kelso, D. M. Fluorescence polarization immunoassay II. Analyzer for rapid, precise measurement of fluorescence polarization with use of disposable cuvettes. (1981). *Clin. Chem.* **27**(7), 1198–1201.

CHAPTER 18

THE MAGIC LITE SYSTEM AND ACRIDINIUM ESTER-BASED IMMUNOASSAYS

John F. O'Brien, George G. Klee, and C. L. Shellum
Department of Laboratory Medicine and Pathology, Mayo Clinic, Rochester, Minnesota 55905

I. INTRODUCTION

Laboratories engaged in immunoassays have an ever-increasing array of improved test methodologies and automation hardware available to them. One of the fastest-growing methodologies is the use of chemiluminescence detection. This chapter will discuss one particular chemiluminescence-based format, the Magic Lite system developed by Ciba-Corning Diagnostics. It makes use of acridinium ester as the chemiluminescent label. Chemiluminescence, in general, has emerged as a practical and very sensitive signal method in immunoassay. Chemiluminescent labels have been reported with detection limits in the sub-attomole range (1,2), and the techniques have shown excellent speed, simplicity, and dynamic range as well as applicability to a diverse array of analytes. Since the first chemiluminescence immunoassays were reported in the late 1970s with luminol as the chemiluminophore (3–5), a variety of other chemistries including acridinium esters (1) have been developed and applied to immunoassay. The last few years have been particularly exciting, with the development of two innovative classes of enzyme substrates for chemiluminescence and bioluminescence (2,6,7). The subject of chemiluminescence immunoassay has

Immunoassay Automation: A Practical Guide

been well reviewed (8–15) and is a major topic in several recently published books (15–17). Only a brief overview will be given here.

II. THE PRINCIPLE OF CHEMILUMINESCENCE

In general terms, chemiluminescence (CL) is the emission of light accompanying selected chemical reactions. These particular reactions share the principle of having one of the products promoted to its excited state, which can potentially emit light upon relaxation to the ground state. This is direct chemiluminescence. Alternatively, the excited reaction product can transfer some of its excess energy to another substance, which can in turn emit light (indirect CL). Most chemiluminescing species can undergo some form of indirect CL if an appropriate energy acceptor is available. This mechanism is often used to enchance CL sensitivity by use of an efficient fluorophore as the energy acceptor. Bioluminescence (BL) can also be applied to immunoassay (7). Both CL and BL are identical in their conversion of chemical energy to light, but BL reactions require specific enzyme mediated biological systems (15–17).

For immunoassay the CL label can be either the light-emitting species (i.e., acridinium ester or luminol) or an enzyme that catalyzes the CL reaction (horseradish peroxidase, alkaline phosphatase, and others). Many examples of both label types have been described. Competitive or two-site chemiluminescence-based immunoassays are carried out like those using any other label. In the final step, the reagent(s) necessary for the CL reaction are added to the system and the ensuing light emission is measured. If the reaction is very fast, such as the case for acridinium esters ($t_{\frac{1}{2}}$ = 0.9 s) (1), the reagents must be forcefully injected into the sample while the sample is in the luminometer, directly in front of the photomultiplier detector. Slower reactions can be initiated on a bench top if desired and the light measurement made at some appropriate later time, usually at the time of maximum emission intensity.

Instrumentation for CL and BL detection is inherently simple. The instruments (luminometers) need only inject appropriate reagents into the sample and collect the light from the reaction. As noted above, slow CL reactions do not necessarily require the reagent injection feature and can be initiated outside of the luminometer. In either case, CL detection is much simpler from an instrument point of view than is fluorescence, absorbance, electrochemical, or other detection systems where the instrument must both probe and measure the resulting signal. The simplicity of CL detection can lead to the fabrication of very small instruments, such as the 8-cm-long photodiode-based detector made by Dynatech Laboratories or numerous compact camera luminometers that are commercially available (18). Camera luminometers are useful for measuring CL from microtiter plates, membrane blots, and other techniques using flat geometry. Except in specially designed equipment, photographic detection is used for the slower types of chemiluminescent labels only, where the reaction is initiated before insertion into the camera enclosure.

Chemiluminescent detection is very sensitive for a couple of reasons. First, the detection of light with photomultipliers (or photographic film) is in itself extremely sensitive, and second, the noise level is inherently low. The sample is in a dark, sealed compartment, and unless there is some type of background emission, the detector receives no signal until the CL reaction is initiated. The only noise is instrumental electronic noise, which is very low. For nonchemiluminescent detection methods, the act of probing and detecting simultaneously always leads to some type of noise. In fluorescence detection, for example, the fluorescence emission is induced by an excitation light source and this leads to background, scattered light hitting the detector. There is also the possibility of interference by extraneous fluorescing molecules. Time-resolved detection using lanthanide elements as fluorophores, as also discussed in this book, can minimize this problem and significantly improve sensitivities over more standard fluorescent immunoassays.

Although many chemiluminescent and bioluminescent systems have been adapted for immunoassay detection, very few of them are commercially available. Immunoassays using luminol or isoluminol as a label have been commercially available the longest. These are the basis of the Amerlite system (Amersham) discussed in Chapter 11 and are also used by Henning-Berlin (Lumitest) and Byk-Sangtec (LIA test). Acridinium compounds are used commercially by several companies including Ciba Corning, London Diagnostics, and Hoescht-Bering for immunoassay and Gene Probe for DNA/RNA probe assays. A third interesting and commercially available class of compounds is the dioxetane enzyme substrates (2,6). These are CL compounds whose light emission can be enzymatically triggered. Enzymatic cleavage of a specific group (phosphate, beta-galactose, etc.) on the dioxetane leads to the production of a molecule capable of either direct or indirect CL. For indirect CL, energy is transferred to a fluorophore such as fluorescein, which emits at its characteristic wavelength. These substrates are interesting because they can be used directly to improve the sensitivity of ELISAs by simply substituting a CL end point for the colorimetric end point.

As noted above, acridinium ester (AE) is the label employed in the Magic Lite system. The chemiluminescence of AE in the presence of dilute alkaline hydrogen peroxide was first reported by McCapra in 1976 (19). This work led to the synthesis of an AE derivative for use as a labeling reagent for chemiluminescent immunoassays (1). This is commercially available and quite straightforward to use for in-house labeling of proteins. It couples via lysine residues under mild conditions (pH 8), and the CL efficiency is not adversely affected by the coupling process. For labeled antibodies, the above reference reported labeling to an incorporation ratio of 3 mol label per mole of antibody without an adverse affect on the ability of the antibody to bind antigen. Our laboratory has found incorporation ratios of up to 5 mol of label per mole of antibody to work well, but the optimal amount varies from antibody to antibody.

Other acridinium derivatives with improved properties have been synthesized and applied to immunoassay. Dimethyl acridinium ester is utilized in Magic Lite assays and has stability superior to the original derivative (20). A new class of acridinium derivatives (*N*-sulfonylcarboxamides) has been recently synthesized by Hoechst AG (21). The company has reported both superior stability and a 2- to 5-fold increase in CL efficiency over the original compound. Other compounds have also been reported or are in developmental stages (10).

The general reaction leading to AE chemiluminescence is shown in Fig. 1, where R is the labeled protein. An oxidation reaction is triggered by alkaline hydrogen peroxide solution. A dioxetanone intermediate is formed, which decomposes to form the emitting species, *N*-methyl acri-

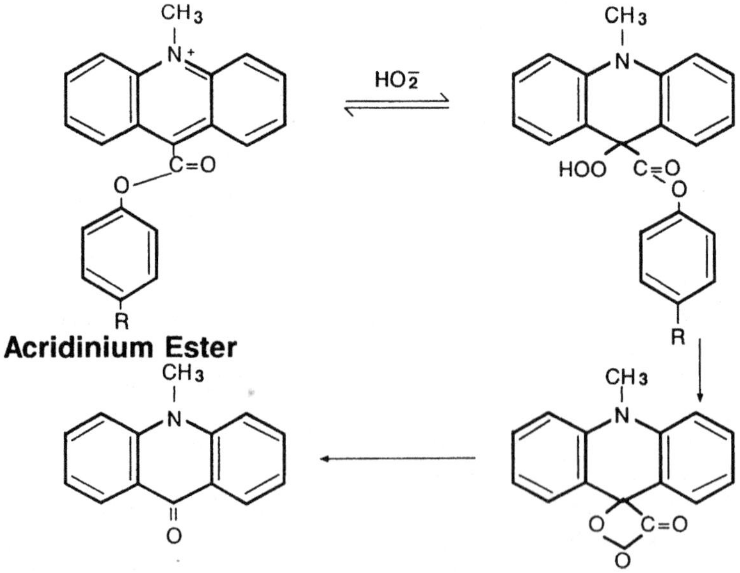

Figure 1 The chemiluminescent reaction of acridinium esters.

done (1). The light emission is at 430 nm, and the reaction is very fast with complete emission within 2 s (Fig. 2). Note that the emitting species is dissociated from the protein. Thus, no loss in emission efficiency occurs as a result of coupling the label to a protein. In practice (Magic Lite system) the actual reaction is triggered by two injections. The first is hydrogen peroxide in nitric acid. The function of the acid is to lower the pH to convert all the AE to its acid form. An equilibrium between acid and pseudo-base forms exists, and the latter form does not emit light (1). Immediately following this injection is an injection of a mixture of sodium hydroxide, to initiate the reaction, and a surfactant to enhance the CL yield (22).

In general, the use of acridinium ester is simple and leads to rapid and sensitive detection. Besides its commercial application to immunoassays, our laboratories have found the acridium esters very useful for research and developmental work. The labeling reaction requires only 30 min, followed by gel filtration and dialysis to remove uncoupled label. We have used acridinium esters for labeling a variety of peptides, antibodies, and antigens ranging in molecular weight from 2000 to 660,000. At a molecular weight of 469, the coupled acridinium ester is less likely than an enzyme label to modify binding and behavior.

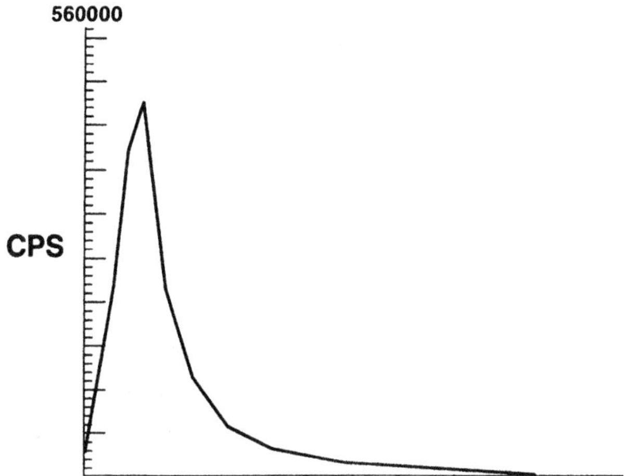

Figure 2 Kinetics of acridinium ester light emission expressed in terms of photon counts per second (cps) over the duration of the reaction (seconds).

III. DESCRIPTION OF THE MAGIC LITE SYSTEM

The Magic Lite system, as with its radioisotope-based predecessor, the Magic RIA system, makes use of micrometer-size derivatized paramagnetic particles to facilitate magnetic separation of bound from unbound label. The particles are used for both competitive and sandwich-type (Fig. 3) immunoassay formats. The acridinium ester label is amenable to either format and has been used as a label in assays spanning the size range from thyroxine (T_4) (competitive) to ferritin (antibody excess). The assays are conducted in a semiautomated format, or, as recently introduced, with a fully automated random access instrument, the ACS 180. Both will be described. The assays available in each format are listed in Table 1.

A. Semiautomated Format

The format and order of reagent addition differ from assay to assay but the general idea can be illustrated by the Magic Lite T_4 assay. The assay for T_4 uses a competitive binding format where the sample is incubated with acridinium ester-labeled T_4 conjugate and anti-T_4 coupled to paramagnetic particles. After the incubation, the particles are magnetically separated

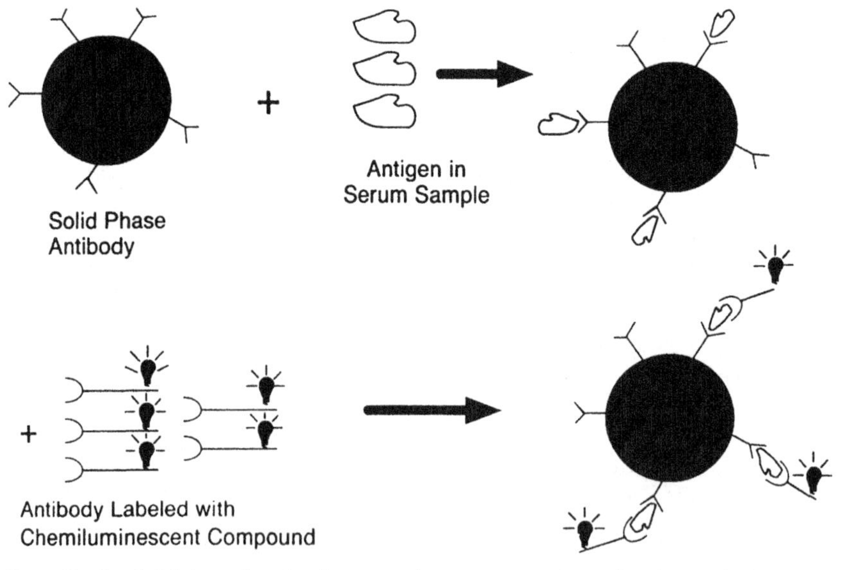

Figure 3 Sandwich-type chemiluminescence immunoassay using antibody-coupled paramagnetic particles as the solid phase.

Table 1 Magic Lite Assays Currently Available (A) or in Development (D)

	Analyte	ACS:180 analyzer	Original format
Thyroid	Thyroxin (T_4)	A	A
	Triiodothyronine (T_3)	A	A
	T_3 uptake	A	A
	Thyrotropin	A	A
	Free T_4	A	A
	Free T_3	D	D
Fertility	Choriogonadotropin	A	D
	Prolactin	A	D
	Estradiol	D	—
	Lutropin	D	D
	Follitropin	D	D
	Progesterone	D	D
	Testosterone	—	D
Anemia	B12	A	A
	Folate	A	A
	Ferritin	A	A
Cancer	Carcinoembryonic antigen	D	D
	α-Fetoprotein	A	D
	Prostate-specific antigen	D	—
Therapeutic drug monitoring	Digoxin	A	D
	Theophylline	A	—
Miscellaneous	Parathyrin	D	A
	IgE	D	D
	Cortisol	A	D
	β_2-Microglobulin	D	—
	Creatinine kinase MB	A	A
	Chlamydia	—	A

and the supernatant is decanted. For separation, racks holding up to 60 tubes are placed over a magnetic base and all samples are pelleted and decanted simultaneously. Figure 4 illustrates the pelleting using magnetic separation. After a wash and second separation/decantation step, the chemiluminescence from the bound label is measured in the luminometer (Bertholdt), which automatically injects the hydrogen peroxide and base necessary to initiate the light reaction. Samples are processed in the luminometer at a rate of 1 sample per 6 s. The photon output (inversely proportional to T_4 concentration) is measured and the data reduction is done by the luminometer.

These assay formats require manual manipulations but can be automated to a degree (Enhanced Magic Lite System). The initial addition of

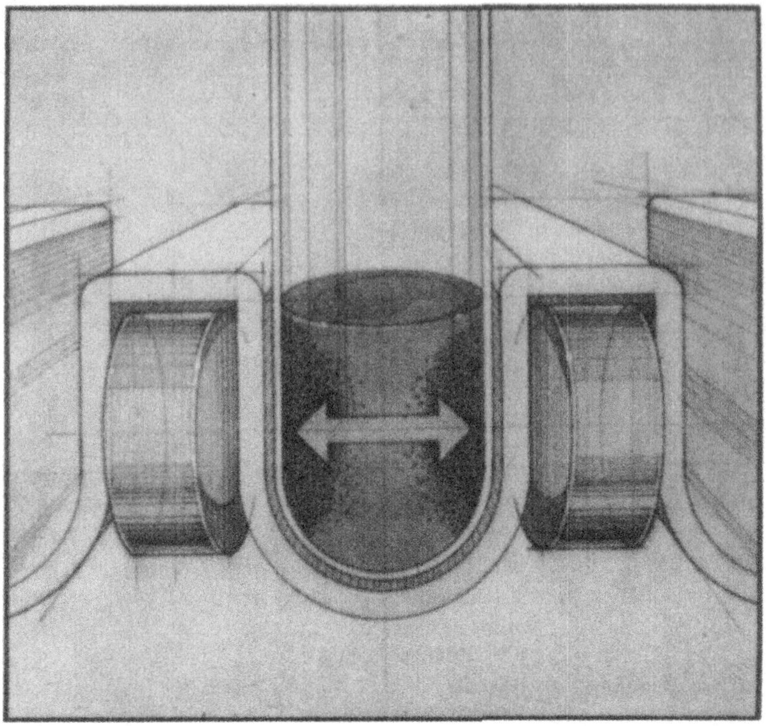

Figure 4 Contents of an assay tube after separation using the Corning magnetic separation unit.

samples and reagents, including the paramagnetic particles, can be done by a liquid handling system. The separation and decanting is done 60 tubes at a time by hand using the magnetic rack system. For signal measurement, the tubes must be manually loaded into the luminometer, where they are then measured automatically.

B. Fully Automated Random Access Instrument

Recently, a fully automated random access instrument (ACS:180) has been introduced (23). Although the instrument is quite distinct from the original methodology, it still makes use of the paramagnetic particle solid phase and acridinium ester label (Fig. 5).

Basically, the samples, reagents, and antibody- or antigen-coupled magnetic particles are automatically placed in a cuvette, which is carried along through a 37°C incubation chamber to an automated magnetic sepa-

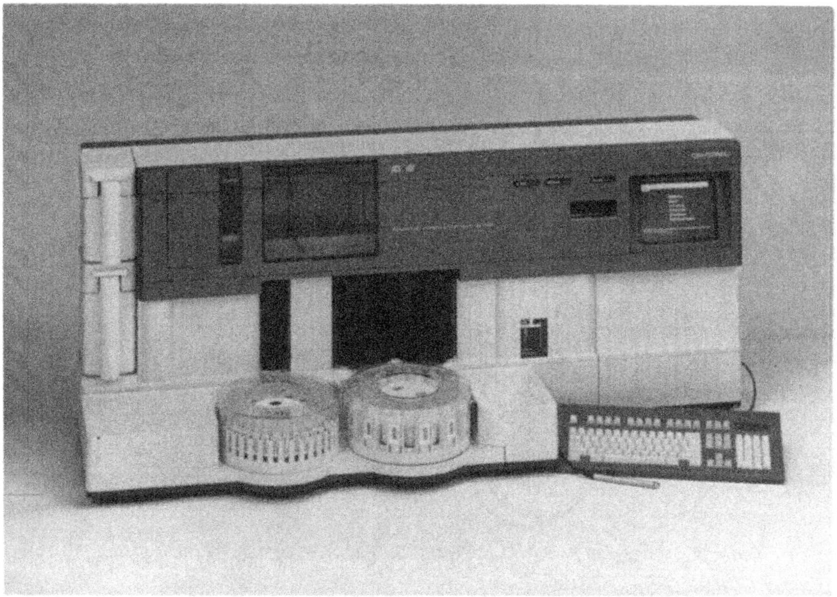

Figure 5 The ACS:180 Analyzer.

ration/wash station. After separation of unbound label, the cuvette continues to the detection station, where light initiation reagents are injected (Fig. 6).

The ACS:180 can do up to 180 samples per hour, with the first result in 15 min and following results every 20 s. Other features include the choice of 13 on-board assays chosen from those in Table 1, a bar-code reader in conjunction with the sample tray, a bidirectional computer interface with the ability to automatically transfer results to the laboratory information system (LIS), and stat (random access) assay capabilities. The success of this instrument must, at this point, be qualified until clinical studies evaluate all tests in the proposed menu.

In designing a rapid, heterogeneous immunoassay system, the kinetic limitations of diffusion and binding must be addressed if adequate sensitivity is to be achieved. The combination of a micrometer-size particulate solid phase and elevated reaction temperature (37°C) helps to offset the reduced binding times (23). In the assay for creatine kinase MB (CK-MB), for example, the 37°C incubation approximately triples the amount of captured label antibody compared to the binding at 22°C. The sensitivity and rapid reaction rate of the acridinium ester label also aid in producing a rapid assay.

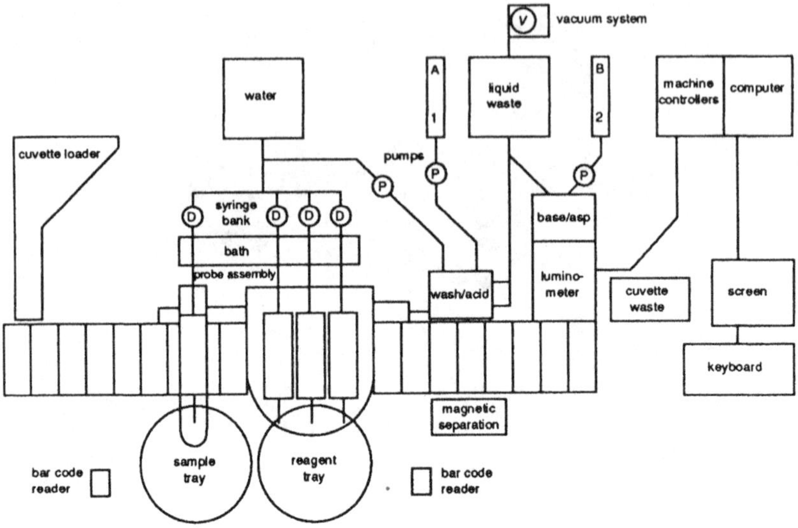

Figure 6 Components of the ACS:180 Analyzer: D, diluter; P, pump; A1, acid pump; B2, base pump; V, vacuum source.

IV. PERFORMANCE OF THE MAGIC LITE SYSTEM AS EXEMPLIFIED BY THE CK-MB AND TSH ASSAYS

A. CK-MB Analysis

1. Importance of CK-MB Measurement and Current Methods

Creatine kinase isoenzyme MB (CK-MB) is the enzyme test requiring the most frequent consultation in the clinical laboratory. This is understandable because a positive CK-MB and/or lactic acid dehydrogenase isoenzyme (LD-1) is one of the World Health Organization's (WHO) three criteria for a myocardial infarction (MI) (24). The sensitivity and specificity of CK-MB can be greater than 90%, and they are uniformly better than LD-1. Galen and Gambino (25) have presented data that suggest that CK-MB outperforms all other criteria for MI.

Because of the clinical utility of CK-MB determinations, optimizing the assay has occupied laboratorians for some time. For many years, the most popular methodology for estimating CK-MB has been electrophoresis. The reason for the persistence of electrophoretic technique is largely that the method allows the electrophoretic equipment to be used for both serum protein separation and separation of other isoenzymes. Further automation of the electrophoretic method has reduced the time required to do the assay. The current interest in the resolution of isoforms of CK-MM, and more recently of CK-MB, has further encouraged continued use of electrophoresis. The generality that an electrophoretic picture is worth a thousand numbers has some validity when comparing the newer immune methods with electrophoresis. One claim that has been frequently used in substantiating the use of electrophoresis, particularly when compared with immunoinhibition methods, is that atypical forms of the enzymes can be distinguished from the usual three isoenzymes. However, the occurrence of a macroenzyme whose electrophoretic migration is identical to MB has been established (26). Moreover, because the newer two-site assays will not detect unusual forms of CK-BB, their use could eliminate confusion and actually be considered desirable. These factors would seem to eliminate the advantages of electrophoresis. To clarify confusion on samples having elevated CK activity not attributable to MB by immunemethods, they might reasonably be run on electrophoresis to see if unusual migrating forms of CK are present.

The heterodimeric structure of CK-MB make it ideal for constructing a two-site immune assay. Hybridoma technology has facilitated the selection of monoclonal antibodies that react with the heterodimeric MB exclusively (27,28). Given monospecific antibodies, sandwich-type assays using antibody to M, B, or MB to immobilize CK followed by an antibody with specificity to an alternative epitope can be used.

2. Magic Lite CK-MB Assay

In the Magic Lite assay the antibodies used are bead-bound anti-B to immobilize MB, and acridinium ester–labeled anti-MB as the signal-antibody. The anti-B ferromagnetic particles, patient serum, and labeled anti-MB are incubated simultaneously for 30 min at room temperature. After the incubation, the supernatant is decanted with the aid of the magnetic separation and washed twice before resuspension in 100 μl H_2O and chemiluminescence analysis in the luminometer.

The novelty of the Magic Lite assay as first described by Piran *et al.* (28) is not so much in the specificity imparted by production of MB-specific antibody, inasmuch as any "sandwich" approach would result in equivalent specificity, but rather in the sensitivity achieved by use of the chemiluminescent technology. It allows for detection of CK-MB down to 1 ng/ml. This should allow the measurement of changes in CK-MB over time well within those suggested by Helena in the 4- to 8-h postinfarct period (29). Furthermore, with a large prospective menu of chemiluminescent tests, commonality of detection instrumentation becomes possible.

3. Performance of Magic Lite Relative to Electrophoresis

A number of publications have addressed the performance of CK-MB Magic Lite relative to the electrophoretic (30,31) and other immunological (32–34) methods. Because CK-MB Magic Lite will very frequently be instituted in laboratories using electrophoresis, correlation data from this laboratory is included below (Fig. 7). Our data suggest that for patients representative of the majority to be assessed for acute cardiac ischemia (i.e., hospitalized patients who have not undergone surgery), the Magic Lite MB method has a sensitivity and specificity slightly better than that of electrophoresis. The best cut off, which imparts the highest specificity even at some loss of sensitivity, was chosen by the cardiologists at the Mayo Clinic. This range of 1.7–9.6 ng/ml allows for nearly 100% specificity with an approximate 78% sensitivity. This method was used to collect the data in Figs. 7 and 8 and Table 2 and is inferred in any reference to U/L or RI in the text (Table 2 and Fig. 8).

Two generalities could be stated for any mass-based measurement of CK-MB when compared to electrophoresis. First, it has been recognized that even with extensive chart review to categorize patients without use of CK-MB data, because of the current reliance on such data, one is never sure that it was not used in the diagnosis. Given this possibility, the CK-MB can greatly influence the diagnosis and therefore the ROC curve. However, were CK-MB used in the diagnosis, the new method, if it is to be better than the existing one, must presumably have a compensatory higher

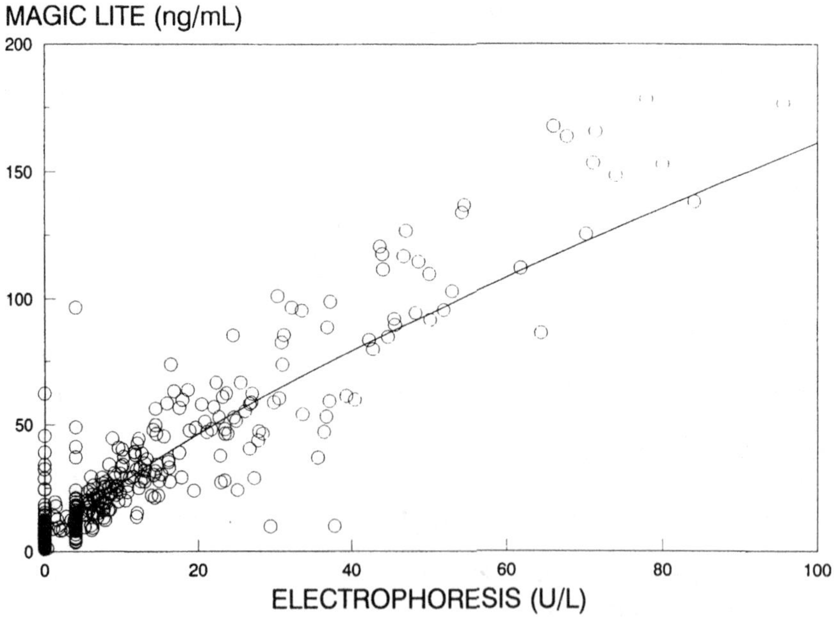

Figure 7 Correlation between CK-MB concentration measured by the Magic Lite system and electrophoresis.

Table 2 Comparison of Magic-Lite CK-MB Results in Two Patient Populations

	Hospitalized without surgery	Myocardial infarction
Number of patients	28	134
Lowest observation	2.97 ng/ml	2.06 ng/ml
Highest observation	9.33 ng/ml	550.6 ng/ml
−2SD	1.74	−112.9
+2SD	9.72	251.5
Median	5.12	27.8
Skewness	Not significant	N/A

sensitivity and specificity not only to be judged better but even to be equal in efficiency to the current method.

Second, in specifically addressing the comparison with electrophoresis, it is clear that undetectable MB levels occur in patients who have grossly elevated total CK activities. This is because for MM quantitation to be accurate, a dilution or smaller-than-usual application volume must be

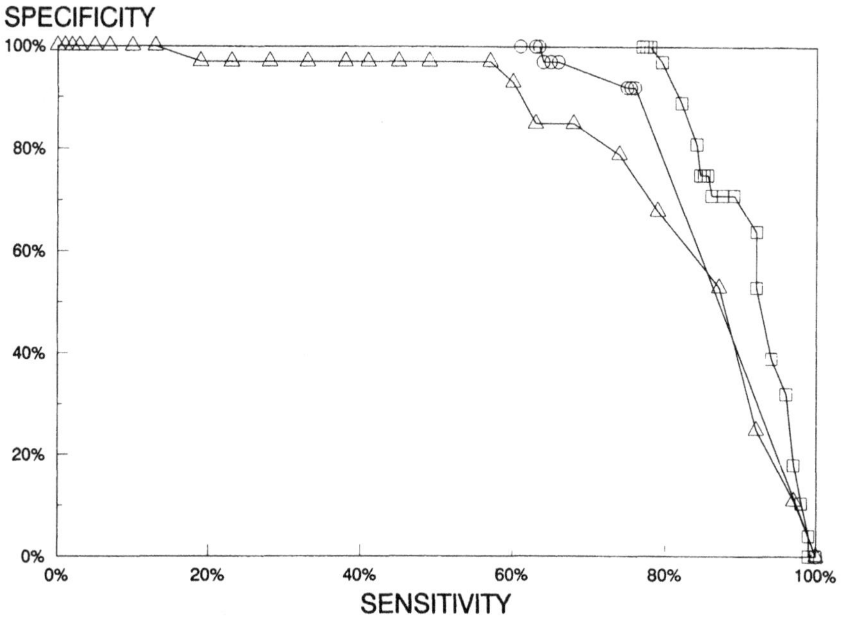

Figure 8 Comparison of Magic Lite (□), electrophoresis (○), and relative index (△) [Magic Lite (ng/ml)/CK-total (μ/l)] in a population of hospitalized nonsurgical patients. Two test values are included on each line for reference.

used. If, in such cases, the CK-MB value falls below 5 U/l (99 URL for males) applied to the electrophoresis medium, the patients are often considered to have none or at most a trace of MB. However, in the same sample using a mass technique, the CK-MB may be over the limit set for normals. This results in more positive patients by Magic Lite and a diagnostic quandary for clinicians because of noncardiac sources of MB, and tends to give a negative impression to cardiologists whose current modus operandi is to emphasize specificity in CK-MB testing. For this reason, normal ranges should be established in more relevant normals, that is, hospitalized, history-read, noncardiac patients. Finally, the accuracy for electrophoretic data below 5 U/l is of real question. The calculation of these levels is made necessary for comparison of the data but is usually reported as trace in practice.

[For reference, the electrophoretic data in U/l was calculated by multiplying percent MB times the total CK activity. At the time of the study, our method gave relatively low activity owing to the nonoptimized activator and the temperature (30°C) at which the assay was run. The method used resulted in an upper reference limit (URL) of 97 u/l for males.]

In patients in whom CK-total is substantially elevated, a separate normal range for the Magic Lite assay (ng/ml) would perhaps best address the nonspecificity brought about by the small but significant amount of CK-MB presumably evolving from skeletal muscle. Alternatively, we suggest that the relative index (RI) (i.e., ng/ml CK-MB + total CK activity U/l) be used. More recently we would further amend the use of RI to include any patient whose skeletal muscle enzyme represents the major source of any CK. Thus, one would be led to use RI not only in the case of trauma or surgery, but also when cardiac enzyme is a significant percentage of the total CK, which remains in the normal range as would be expected in myocardial infarctions involving a relatively small mass of the heart.

It is important to recognize the relative index cutoffs chosen are specific not only to the mass measurement method but also the method for quantitation of CK-total in activity units. We have recently changed our method for CK-total activity (NAC activation at 37°C) so that the URL for males is 336. Under these circumstances, the most sensitive and specific RI is 3.6, which is very similar to that recommended by Latner *et al.* (30).

4. Magic Lite versus the Stratus

For the most part, laboratorians will compare the Magic Lite CK-MB to the Stratus CK-MB (Baxter), a method addressed in Chapter 22. Both have advantages, and final proof of the best assay is still being sought. The sensitivity comparison between the Stratus and Magic Lite would suggest there is little advantage of one method's sensitivity over another (32,33). The anomalous 68% response of the Stratus versus the Magic Lite method suggests that the matrix may affect the assays in different ways. Specificity has been a problem in a small percentage of patients when the radial-wash method (Stratus) is used (34,35). Further formulation of substrate-wash reagents, which include a new liver alkaline phosphatase (ALP) inhibitor, have apparently resolved this specificity problem for a majority of samples (36).

From a practical standpoint, it could be argued that the Stratus methodology is best owing to its speed (8 min) and the method's automation. As currently configured, the Stratus is most compatible with the expertise of technologists covering the laboratory around the clock and for use with single (nonbatch) samples.

5. Modification for Shorter Analysis Time

It has been suggested that stat CK-MB will allow assignment of critical care patients more efficiently. However, due to the nature of the temporal rise and fall of CK-MB, a negative test may merely mean that the test must be repeated on a later sample to rule out the possibility that the CK-MB has not yet risen to a level consistent with MI, no matter the sensitivity of the method. Triaging patients who have received thrombolytic therapy, to either group those who have been successfully reperfused or to group those requiring angioplastic disruption of the infarction, could require a more sensitive, rapid test (23). In order to make the Magic Lite method (in the semiautomated mode) more adaptable to stat assays, we have evaluated the possibility of a 10-min incubation assay. The results indicate that a 10-min incubation time should be sufficient since the RLU value for 5 ng/ml is still over 10-fold the background. Its comparability to the 30-min assay is shown in Fig. 9. This is also apparent from the results with the ACS-180, which has only a 7-min incubation time. If the incubation is shortened to 10 min, the timing of reagent addition must be done very carefully to avoid within-run differences in exposure to tracer and sequestration antibody. Using the shorter incubation times, the Magic Lite method can be completed in 25–30 min. Use of the ACS 180 will result in a 15-min assay in the random access mode.

B. High-Sensitivity TSH Measurement

1. Clinical Impact

The recent introduction of high-sensitivity TSH assays that can measure subnormal concentrations has greatly expanded the clinical role of this analyte. Traditionally, TSH measurements have been the cornerstone for the diagnosis of primary hypothyroidism, with elevated TSH in a

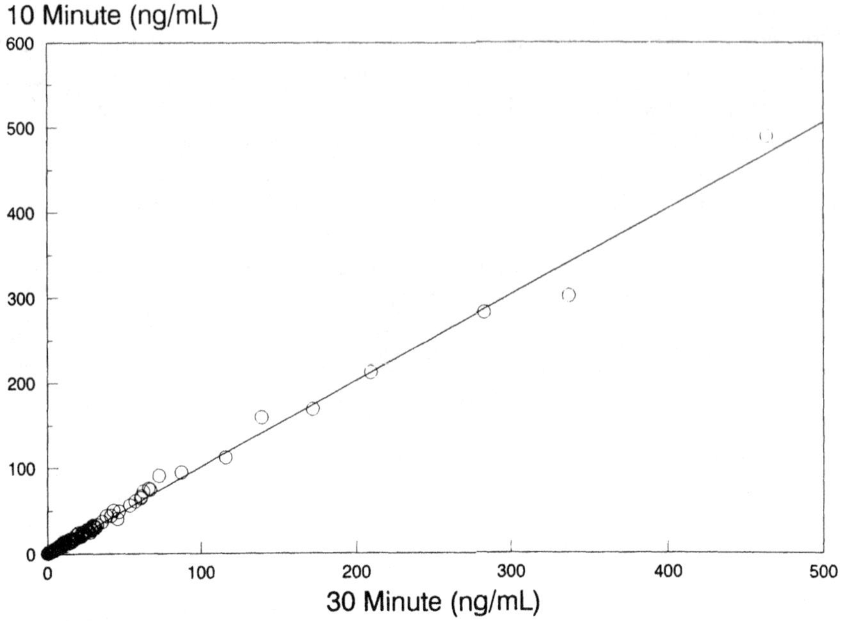

Figure 9 Comparison of results of Magic Lite assays done using 30 min (standard assay time) versus 10 min.

patient with clinical symptoms being "sine qua non" for the diagnosis. Confirmation of primary hyperthyroidism, however, depended on performance of stimulation tests in which the injection of thyrotropin-releasing hormone (TRH) failed to produce a rise in serum concentration of TSH. Currently, basal TSH measurements are used for the diagnosis of both primary hypothyroidism and primary hyperthyroidism. Through negative feedback the high thyroxine concentration of hyperthyroidism suppresses the basal concentration of TSH. With sensitive assays these basal concentrations can be measured and have been shown to correlate with the results of TRH testing. In this expanded role, TSH has become the single most useful marker of metabolic thyroid disease, and many physicians are using this for the initial assessment of thyroid disease. The two key assay characteristics that have led to this expanded role of TSH are increased analytic sensitivity and faster measurement time. Although other assay systems are available for sensitive TSH measurements, CL methods are particularly well suited for the requirements of sensitivity and speed and are sufficiently robust so they perform well in routine practice.

2. Evolving Sensitivity and Specificity Requirements

The performance requirements for sensitive TSH assay have been the subject of many discussions, and specific characteristics are not uniformly agreed upon. The American Thyroid Association (ATA) recently developed recommendations that state that sensitive TSH assays should have (37):

1. Accuracy within ±5% of the stated WHO or MRC standard.
2. Interassay precision stated with a goal of CV < 20% at 0.1 mU/l.
3. Recovery of standard material within ±10% over entire range of assay.
4. Linearity of diluted patient specimens within ±10% of standard curve.
5. Thyrotoxic sera reading within ±5% of signal for zero calibrator.
6. No significant interference from heterophile antibodies and cross-reactivities <0.1% with other glycoprotein hormones—LH, FSH, and hCG.
7. No "hook" effect with flattening or down turning of standard curve up to 300 mU/l.
8. Clear separation of hyperthyroid and euthyroid patients with a goal of <5% overlap of these groups.

In addition, Dr. Spencer and colleagues have preliminary data that even more sensitive assays may provide further information in the assessment of the degree of hyperthyroidism (38). For this expanded role, they advocate that assays should be capable of measuring concentrations as low as 0.005 mU/l with an interassay coefficient of variation of <40%. As illustrated in Fig. 10, most "sensitive assays" currently measure down to a concentration of approximately 0.1 mU/l, with interassay variation increasing substantially below that level. This lower detection level of 0.005 is well within the capability of CL but is not routinely achieved by most assays.

3. Magic Lite TSH Assay—The Procedure and Its Performance

The Ciba Corning Magic Lite TSH procedure is a two-site chemiluminometric assay. The signal system (acridinium ester) is covalently attached to an antibody recognizing the β-subunit of TSH. The separation system (paramagnetic particles) is covalently bound to a second antibody. Duplicate aliquots of 100 μl of the signal antibody are incubated for 2 h ± 5 min at room temperature. Then 500 μl of the paramagnetic particle-coupled antibody is added and incubated for an additional 30 ± 5

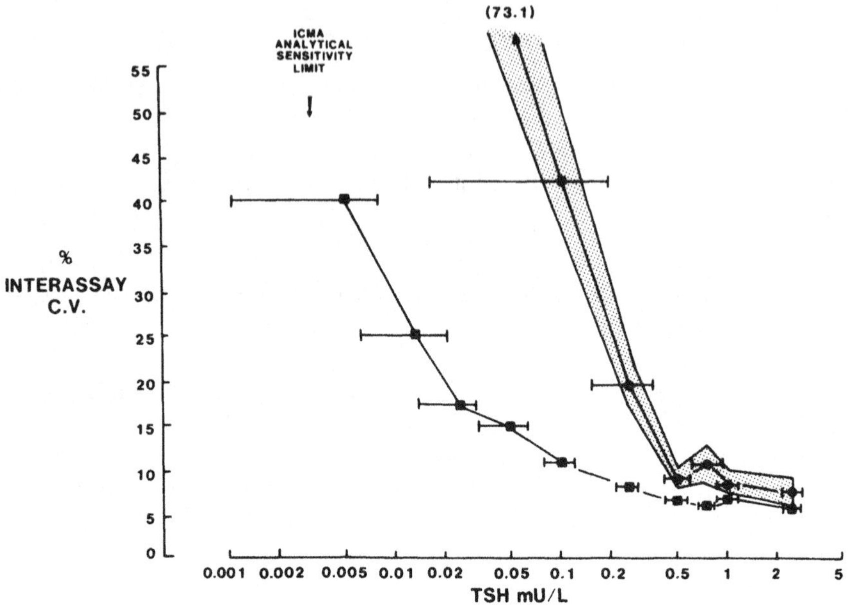

Figure 10 TSH ICMA interassay precision profile (■) contrasted with 10 other TSH immunometric assays (●) previously studied. Mean SE is shown by shading. The horizontal bars represent the 95% confidence limits of measurement. Reprinted from ref. 51, with permission.

min. The "acridinium ester antibody I TSH antibody II-bead" sandwich complex is then separated from the unreacted reagent and washed with deionized water using magnetic separator racks. The final step is to resuspend the pellet of magnetic particles and measure the CL signal using an automated MLA-II luminometer. Normally, duplicate zero and high-range calibrators and three levels of controls are analyzed with each batch of patient specimens. The full standard curve consists of 10 points ranging from concentrations of 0 to 100 mIU/l, with RLU (relative light units) ranging from approximately 2500 to 1,000,000. These points define the master curve that is supplied with each lot of reagents. The software in the luminometer uses third-degree polynomials to fit a spline curve to these data. The position of this master curve is adjusted mathematically for each run using the values of the two calibrators.

The Magic Lite TSH assay is standardized with the WHO 80/558 standard. Between the concentrations of 1.8 to 83.8 mIU/l, stated recoveries range from 80 to 123% with a mean of 103%. Interassay precision is less than 6.2% for concentrations ≥1.0 mIU/l and 10.4% at 0.59 mIU/l. The stated sensitivity of the assay is 0.02 mIU/l (39). In our laboratory the assay has a detection limit of 0.06 mIU/l and has interassay precision (based on mean of duplicate determinations) decreasing from 18% at 0.11 mIU/l to 5% at 0.41 IU/l using the WHO-IRP 68/38 standard. The cross-reactivity with LH, FSH, and HCG are all less than 0.1%. We have found the system to dilute linearly within ±7% over the range of 90 mIU/l to 3 mIU/l to 100 mIU/l with no interference caused by anti-mouse antibodies. We found recovery of added WHO standard to be within ±8% over the range of 2–33 mIU/l. We have encountered no "hook effect" up to 250 mIU/l. There was 4% overlap between values found in patients with untreated Graves disease and euthyroid subjects (40).

The current Magic Lite TSH assay is a robust procedure that works well for diagnosing and monitoring both hypothyroid and hyperthyroid patients. Suppressed values frequently are found in patients on thyroid hormone replacement, but this often is related to the dose of medication, and TSH values generally return to the normal range when the thyroxine replacement dose is reduced. Very sick hospitalized patients also may have suppressed values, especially if they are receiving glucocorticoids (41). This assay is not sensitive enough to distinguish degree of hyperthyroidism, and currently this is accomplished by additional measurements of free or total T_4 and/or T_3 .

The Ciba Corning company recently developed a TSH procedure for use on their ACS:180 automated analyzer. This procedure uses a polyclonal antibody attached to paramagnetic particles and an acridinium ester–conjugated monoclonal antibody as the tracer. The assay uses 200 μl of serum and has a working range of 0.05–100 mIU/l calibrated with the WHO 2nd IRP 80/558 reference material. No high-dose "hook" effect is reported for up to 2000 mIU/l (42). The mean detection limit based on differentiation from the zero standard with $p < .05$ confidence is reported at 0.046 mIU/l. The linearity of three diluted specimens was within 94–113% of the standard with an average of 105%. Recovery of additions of TSH ranging from 3.3 to 52.8 mIU/l was within the range 91.6–101.8%, with an average of 96.5%. Cross-reactivity with LH of 200 IU/l, FSH of 200 IU/l, and hCG of 200,000 IU/l was insignificant and less than 0.1%. Intraassay precision ranged from 4.7% at 2.1 mIU/l to 9.1% at 9.6 mIU/l. Low-range precision data and the performance of this assay with thyrotoxic sera or the operation of hyperthyroid and euthryoid patients were not presented.

The CL technology should provide greater analytic sensitivity than currently available in the Magic Lite TSH reagents. Ultrasensitive CL assays require high-affinity antisera, low background noise, and tight manufacturing tolerances. The results reported by Spencer *et al.* (41) provide an intriguing target for TSH testing, but only time and further studies will prove if this goal can be routinely achieved in clinical practice. In the meantime, the guidelines developed by the ATA provide useful benchmarks for evaluating current TSH assays. The Ciba Corning Magic Lite TSH procedure meets most of these recommendations with the exception of low-end precision and the accuracy of some of the recovery experiments. Future refinements will undoubtedly continue to improve these performance characteristics.

V. NEW APPLICATIONS OF ACRIDINIUM ESTERS

A. Flow Injection Immunoassays

Two fully automatable immunoassays using acridinium esters in flowing systems have been reported (43,44). In the first, the entire assay, including detection, takes place in a transparent 20-μl immunoreactor (immunoaffinity column). A two-site immunoassay is accomplished by the consecutive injection of the sample, acridinium ester–labeled antibody, and alkaline hydrogen peroxide to initiate chemiluminescence. The light emission is collected directly from the transparent immunoreactor, which is then regenerated in preparation for the next sample injection. The time required per sample is approximately 10 min and depends on the buffer flow rate that is chosen. Mouse immunoglobulin G (IgG), the test analyte for this system, has a detection limit of 200 amol IgG when run at a rate of 10 min per sample. A system such as this is inherently easy to automate, requiring only an automatic sample injector and control over the pump and buffer selection valve.

The second flow system reported (44) also uses a small immunoreactor. The sample and labeled antibody are injected as in the above system but the detection process is different. For detection, the buffer is changed to the elution buffer and the sample and labeled antibody are eluted from the immunoreactor. This stream merges with a stream of alkaline hydrogen peroxide immediatedly before flowing into the detector cell, where the light from the ensuing reaction is collected. The analysis of PTH was demonstrated with a detection limit of 50 amol and a rate of 6 min per sample.

B. Liposome-Enhanced Immunoassays

Many groups are exploring the use of liposomes for signal amplification in immunoassay (44,45,20). The specific antigen or antibody is coupled to the surface of the liposome and the liposome encapsulates a solution of the detection molecule, which can be electrochemically active, fluorescent, colored, chemiluminescent, etc. The immunoassay is done in a standard manner, and as a final step, the liposome is lysed and the detection molecule is released and detected. Because of the possibility of encapsulating 10^5 or more molecules per liposome, the theoretical sensitivity enhancement is enormous. The performance of these systems depends on many factors but perhaps most significantly on the stability of the liposomes. Significant leakage of the liposome's contents can cancel the potential advantages.

Ciba-Corning has synthesized a rather hydrophilic acridinium ester derivative for use in liposome encapsulation (20). Their standard dimethyl-acridinium ester derivative is too hydrophobic and the rate of leakage from the liposome is quite high. The new derivative has a leakage rate of 1.3% in 7 days at 4°C. It has been applied to TSH analysis and has resulted in a dose-response curve in a 5-min assay that is comparable in sensitivity to the standard Magic Lite assay with 2.5 h of incubation time.

C. Homogeneous Immunoassays

Homogeneous (nonseparation) immunoassays using CL have been demonstrated (46–49) but have not resulted in sensitivity comparable to heterogeneous assays. One interesting method makes use of the phenomenon of chemiluminescence energy transfer in an immunoassay for cyclic AMP (38). The method is based on the transfer of energy from the excited state of cAMP-labeled isoluminol to fluorescein-labeled anti-cAMP antibody. The fluorescent compound undergoing indirect CL is termed the energy acceptor. The unbound isoluminol-labeled antigen emits light at 460 nm and the antigen–antibody complex emits at 525 nm, fluorescein luminescence. A standard curve can be set up with antigen concentration on the *x* axis and the ratio of emission at 460/525 nm on the *y* axis. The slope of the dose-response curve is positive.

Although homogeneous immunoassays have not as yet been demonstrated with acridinium esters, a potentially appropriate derivative has been synthesized (10) and work is underway to evaluate its feasibility. This has been termed an N-functionalized acridinium ester. These derivatives differ from the other acridinium labels in that they are coupled to protein through a functional group on the nitrogen of the acridinium. Upon reaction with H_2O_2, the emitting acridone will remain attached to the protein rather than diffusing away as is the case for the other acridinium labels. The goal is for it to function in a homogeneous energy-transfer assay analogous to the isoluminol-based assay discussed above. A problem with both of these methods, however, is the effect of elevated pH on the antigen-antibody binding. The energy transfer must occur before the two species have uncoupled and diffused away from one another. The future may likely bring more research in this area.

REFERENCES

1. Weeks, I., Beheshti, I., McCapra, F., Campbell, A. K., and Woodhead, J. (1983). Acridinium Esters as High-Specific-Activity Labels in Immunoassay. *Clin. Chem.* **29,** 1474–1479.
2. Schaap, A. P., Akhavan, H., and Romano, L. J. (1989). Chemiluminescent substrates for alkaline phosphatase: Application to ultrasensitive enzyme-linked immunoassays and DNA probes. *Clin. Chem.* **35,** 1863–1864.
3. Arakawa, H., Maeda, M., and Tsuji, A. (1977). Enzyme immunoassay of cortisol by chemiluminescence reaction of luminol-peroxidase. *Bunseki Kagaku* **26,** 322–326.
4. Schroeder, H. R., Boguslaski, R. C., Carrico, R. J., and Buckler, R. T. (1978). *Methods Enzymol.* **57,** 424–459.
5. Hersch, L. S., Vann, W. P., and Wilhelm, S. A. (1979). A Luminol-assisted competitive-binding immunoassay of human immunoglobulin G. *Anal. Biochem.* **93,** 267–271.
6. Bronstein, I., Edwards, B., and Voyta, J. C. (1989). 1,2-Dioxetanes: Novel chemiluminescent enzyme substrates. Applications to immunoassays. *J. Biolum. Chemilum.* **4,** 99–111.
7. Miska, W., and Geiger, R. (1989). Luciferin derivatives in bioluminescence-enhanced enzyme immunoassays. *J. Biolum. Chemilum.* **4,** 119–128.
8. McCapra, F., Watmore, D., Sumun, F., Patel, A., Beheshti, I., Ramakrishnan, K., and Branson, J. (1989). Luminescent labels for immunoassay—From concept to practice. *J. Biolum. Chemilum.* **4,** 51–58.
9. Wood, W. G. (1989). Routine luminescence immunoassays—Dream or reality. *J. Biolum. Chemilum.* **4,** 79–87.
10. Zomer, G., and Stavenuitter, J. F. C. (1989). Chemiluminogenic labels, old and new. *Anal. Chim. Acta* **227,** 11–19.
11. Kricka, L. J., and Whitehead, T. P. (1987). Chemiluminescent and bioluminescent immunoassays. *J. Pharm. Biomed. Anal.* **5,** 829–833.
12. Grayeski, M. L. Chemiluminescence analysis. *Anal. Chem.* **59,** 1243–1256A.
13. Weeks, I., Sturgess, M. L., and Woodhead, J. S. (1986). Chemiluminescence immunoassay: An overview. *Clin. Sci.* **70,** 403–408.
14. Seitz, R. W. (1984). Immunoassay labels based on chemiluminescence and bioluminescence. *Clin. Biochem.* **17,** 120–125.
15. Campbell, A. K. (1988). "Chemiluminescence: Principles and Applications in Biology and Medicine." Ellis Horwood Ltd., Chichester, U.K.
16. Van Dyke, K. (ed.) (1990). "Luminescence Immunoassay and Molecular Applications." CRC Press, Boca Raton, Florida.
17. Scholmerich, J., Andreesen, R., Kapp, A., Ernst, M., and Woods, W. G. (eds.) (1987). "Bioluminescence and Chemiluminescence: New Perspectives." John Wiley, Chichester, U.K.
18. Bronstein, I., and Kricka, L. J. (1990). Instrumentation for luminescent assays. *Am. Clin. Lab.* **Jan/Feb,** 33–37.
19. McCapra, F. (1976). Chemical mechanisms in bioluminescence. *Acc. Chem. Res.* **9,** 201–208.
20. Law, S., Miller, T., Piran, U., Klukas, C., Chang, S., and Unger, J. (1989). Novel poly-substituted aryl acridinium esters and their use in immunoassay. *J. Biolum. Chemilum.* **4,** 88–98.

21. Kinkel, T., Lübbers, H., Schmidt, E., Molz, P., and Skrzipczyk, H. J. (1989). Synthesis and properties of new luminescent acridinium-9-carboxylic acid derivatives and their application in luminescence immunoassays. *J. Biolum. Chemilum.* **4,** 136–139.
22. Bagazgoitia, F. J., Garcia, J. L., Diéquez, C., Weeks, I., and Woodhead, J. S. (1989). Effect of surfactants on the intensity of chemiluminescence emission from acridinium ester labelled proteins. *J. Biolum. Chemilum.* **4,** 121–128.
23. Boland, J., Garey, G., Drodel, E.,and Kwiatkowski, M. (1990). The Ciba Corning ACS:180 benchtop immunoassay analyzer. *Clin. Chem.* **36,** 1598–1602.
24. Report of the Joint International Society and Federation of Cardiology/World Health Organization Task Force on Standardization of Clinical Nomenclature. (1979). Nomenclature and Criteria for Diagnosis of Ischemic Heart Disease. *Circulation* **59,** 607–609.
25. Galen, R. S., and Gambino, S. R. (1975). "Beyond Normality: The Predictive Value and Efficiency of Medical Diagnoses." John Wiley and Sons, New York.
26. Venta, R., *et al.* (1989). IgA-CK-BB complex with CK-MB electrophoretic mobility can lead to erroneous diagnosis of acute myocardial infarction. *Clin. Chem.* **35,** 2003–2008.
27. Vaidya, H. C. *et al.* (1986). Direct measurement of creatine kinase-MB activity in serum after extraction with a monoclonal antibody specific to the MB isoenzyme. *Clin. Chem.* **32,** 657–663.
28. Piran, U. *et al.* (1987). Immunochemiluminometric assay of creatine kinase MB with a monoclonal antibody to the MB isoenzyme. *Clin. Chem.* **33,** 1517–1520.
29. Helena Laboratories Educational Bulletin. (1988). CK Isoforms in AMI and Thrombolytic Therapy.
30. Latner, B. P., Skale, J. S., and Burns, W. (1989). Measuring creatine kinase MB isoenzyme in a maintenance hemodialysis population: Chemiluminometric compared. *Clin. Chem.* **35,** 1965–1968.
31. Murthy, V. V. (1990). Creatine kinase-MB immunoassay using chemiluminescence labelled MB-specific antibody. *Diag. Clin. Test.* **28,** 45–48.
32. Wu, A. H. B., *et al.* (1989). Role of rapid immunoassays for urgent ("stat") determination of creatine kinase isoenzyme MB. *Clin. Chem.* **35,** 1752–1756.
33. Wu, A. H. B., and Schwartz, J. G. (1989). Update on creatine kinase isoenzyme assays. *Diag. Clin. Test.* **27,** 16–19.
34. Apple, F., Heiler, G., and Preese, L. (1990). Falsely increased CK-MB results obtained with the new reformulated CK-MB wash IV solution in the Stratus analyzer. *Clin. Chem.* **36,** 405–406.
35. Bachem, M. G., and Greisner, A. M. (1988). Evaluation of a chemiluminescence immunoassay for determination of the mass concentration of serum creatine kinase MB isoenzyme. *J. Clin. Biochem.* **26,** 736.
36. Eisenberg, P. R., *et al.* (1989). Concordance of creatine kinase-MB activity and mass. *Clin. Chem.* **35,** 440–443.
37. Hay, I. D., Bayer, M. K., Kaplan, M. M., Klee, G. G., Larsen, P. R., and Spencer, C. A. (1992). American Thyroid Association assessment of current free thyroid hormone and thyrotropin measurements and guidelines for future clinical assays. Accepted for publication, *Clin. Chem.*
38. Spencer, C. A., LoPresti, J. S., Patel, A., Guttler, R. B., Eigen, A., Shen, A., Gray, D., and Nicoloff, J. T. (1990). Applications of a new chemiluminometric thyrotropin assay to subnormal measurement. *Clin. Endocrinol. Metab.* **70,** 453–460.
39. Klee, G. G., and Hay, I. D. (1988). Sensitive thyrotropin assays: Analytic and clinical performance criteria. *Mayo Clin. Proc.* **63,** 1123–1132.
40. Package insert for "TSH Magic Lite," Ciba Corning Diagnostics Corp., 63 North Street, Medfield, Massachusetts 02052.
41. Spencer, C., Eigen, A., Shen, D., Duda, M., Qualls, S., Weiss, S., and Nicoloff, J. (1987). Specificity of sensitive assays of thyrotropin (TSH) used to screen for thyroid disease in hospitalized patients. *Clin. Chem.* **33,** 1391–1396.

42. Kwiatkowski, M., Long, L., Seery, J., Blake, D., *et al.* (1990). An automated chemiluminescence immunoassay for thyroid stimulating hormone (TSH). Presented at the 1990 AACC meeting in San Francisco, California.
43. Shellum, C. L., and Gübitz, G. (1989). Flow injection immunoassays with acridinium ester-based chemiluminescence detection. *Anal. Chim. Acta* **227,** 97–107.
44. Hage, D. S., and Kao, P. C. (1991). Automated PTH assay by HPLC with chemiluminescence detection. *Anal. Chem.* **63,** 586–595.
45. Plant, A. L., Brizgys, M. V., Locasio-Brown, L., and Durst, R. A. (1989). Generic liposome reagent for immunoassays. *Anal. Biochem.* **176,** 420–426.
46. Plant, A. L., Locascio-Brown, L., Brizgys, M. V., and Durst, R. A. (1988). Liposome-enhanced flow injection immunoanalysis. *Bio/Technology* **6,** 266–269.
47. Kohen, F., Kim, J. B., Barnard, G. J., and Lindner, H. (1980). An Assay for urinary estriol-16α-glucuronide based on antibody-enhanced chemiluminesence. *Steroids* **36,** 405–408.
48. Patel, A., Davies, C. J., Campbell, A. K., and McCapra, F. (1983). Chemiluminescence energy transfer: A new technique applicable to the study of ligand-ligand interactions in living systems. *Anal. Biochem.* **129,** 162–169.
49. Campbell, A. K., and Patel, A. (1983). A homogeneous immunoassay for cyclic nucleotides based on chemiluminescence energy transfer. *Biochem. J.* **216,** 185–189.

CHAPTER 19

The OPUS System

Michael Lehrer
Division of Biochemistry, Long Island Jewish Medical Center, New Hyde Park, New York, and Department of Laboratory Medicine, Albert Einstein College of Medicine, Bronx, New York

Laurel Miller and Joanne Natale
PB Diagnostic Systems, Inc., Westwood, Massachusetts

I. INTRODUCTION

The OPUS Immunoassay System is a bench-top, continuous-access immunoassay analyzer that operates in random-access and stat modes with the additional options of preset panel and batch operation (Fig. 1). Analyzer operation is totally dry; there are no liquid reagents or tubings to change. There is no sample or reagent carryover, since disposable pipette tips are used for each pipetting step.

OPUS performs quantitative, *in vitro* testing for therapeutic drugs (Grenner *et al.*, 1989; Inbar *et al.*, 1990; Ackermann *et al.*, 1990; Blackwood *et al.*, 1990; D'Eon *et al.*, 1990; Bahar *et al.*, 1990), fertility hormones (Havelick *et al.*, 1990), thyroid function (Grenner *et al.*, 1989), tumor markers (Pothier *et al.*, 1990), and other analytes, and performs qualitative and quantitative testing for infectious diseases (Freeley *et al.*, 1990).

The analyzer is best suited to be used in small- and medium-sized hospitals and physicians' office laboratories for a wide range of immunoassays. OPUS also provides stat capabilities in higher-volume settings. It requires only short setup times and little maintenance. This combination of random access and automatic operation means that the operator has long

Immunoassay Automation: A Practical Guide

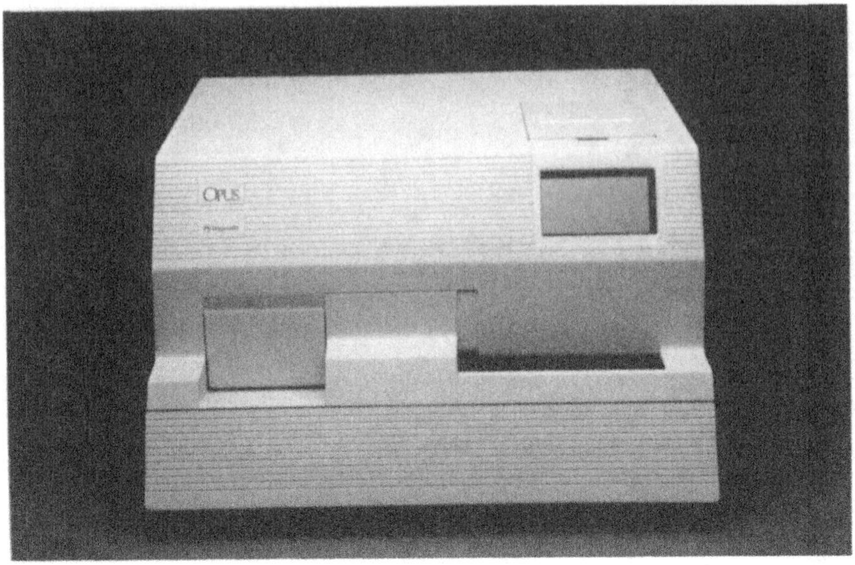

Figure 1 The OPUS Immunoassay Analyzer.

walk-away intervals during which time he can operate a second, complimentary analyzer or perform other duties (Lauer *et al.*, 1990).

OPUS employs a unit module concept to allow true random-access capability. Each test module contains all reagents needed for that test. Sample pretreatment is unnecessary [except for total triiodothyronine (T_3), where a single dilution step is required]. Hands-on time is limited to touchscreen data entry, loading of test modules, filling sample cups, loading sample and pipette tip trays, and emptying the waste drawer when prompted.

This capability for true random access increases the flexibility of automated immunoassay. No longer is it necessary to schedule batch runs for low-volume testing. Turnaround times are shortened and effective throughput is increased.

OPUS runs any combination of tests simultaneously. The operator has access to analyzer operation at virtually all times. OPUS offers stat capability continuously. For example, during a typical random-access run of several anticonvulsants, digoxin, and theophylline, a stat human chorionic gonadotropin (hCG) request arrives in the laboratory. The operator can select stat mode and have a reportable result for the hCG within a half hour.

II. SYSTEM DESCRIPTION

OPUS is a complete immunoassay system that performs sample handling, test incubation at constant temperature, signal detection, and conversion of signal into a test result. It consists of assay-specific test modules and a continuous-access analyzer.

A. Test Modules

Each module is ready for insertion into the analyzer and contains all reagents needed for a specific assay. There are two types of test modules: a multilayer film test module and a fluorogenic ELISA test module.

1. The Multilayer Film Test Module

The multilayer film test module (Fig. 2) is a 1 ½-in plastic module that contains dry reagents coated on a film chip; it is used in the analysis of

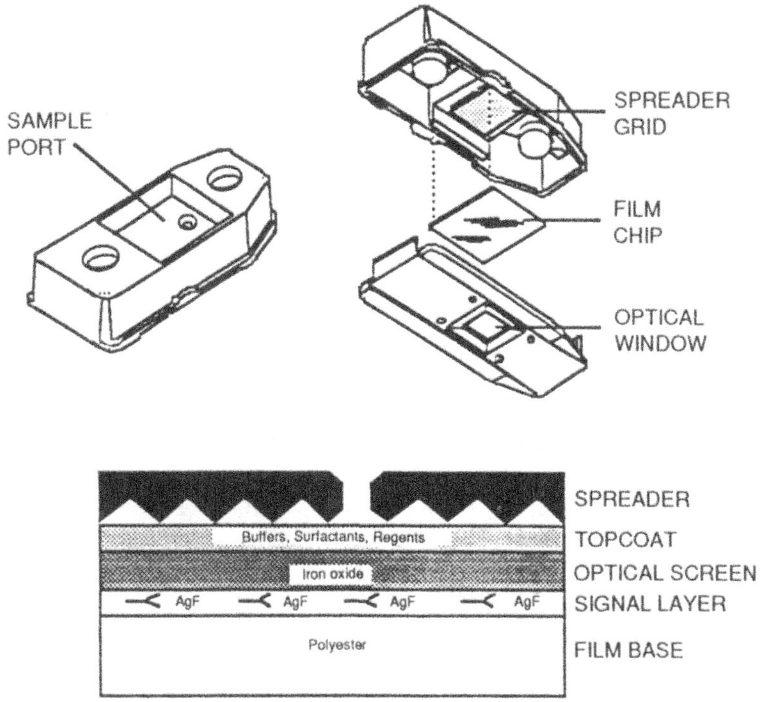

Figure 2 Multilayer film test module.

low-molecular-weight analytes and some thyroid function assays. This module consists of a clear polyester base coated with an agarose matrix containing an immobilized immune complex (an antibody bound to fluorescent-labeled analyte). Above this "signal" layer is a second layer of agarose containing iron oxide, which blocks the passage of light to the upper layers. The top layer contains additional reagents, surfactants, buffers, etc. This layer blocks the passage of high-molecular-weight molecules and allows only the smaller analyte molecules to pass.

The top layer is in contact with a molded, grooved surface to accomplish uniform spreading and metering of sample. The fluorescent signal is read from below through an opening in the base of the plastic module.

2. The Multilayer Film Assay

Sample introduced into the test module spreads uniformly across the top surface of the film chip. The serum sample penetrates and rehydrates the layers of agarose. The analyte passes rapidly through the iron oxide screen layer and comes into contact with the immune complex in the signal layer. The analyte then competes with fluorescent-labeled analyte for a limited number of antibody binding sites. The displaced fluorescent-labeled analyte can only diffuse into the layers and volume above, where it is not detected by the optical system. Since the signal layer is only 1–2% of the total film thickness, most of the free fluorescent conjugate diffuses above the optical screen. The fluorescent signal is generated from the remaining bound fluorescent-labeled analyte. The measured fluorescence is inversely related to the level of analyte in the patient sample. This multilayer immunoassay technique has been described previously (Grenner *et al.*, 1989; Inbar *et al.*, 1990).

3. The Fluorogenic ELISA Test Module

Employing variations of the enzyme-linked immunosorbent assay (ELISA) technique, the fluorogenic ELISA assays are based on the capture of antigens or antibodies from a solution to an insoluble solid phase. These assays are used to determine concentrations of higher-molecular-weight analytes, to indicate the presence of antibodies, or for analysis of some haptens.

The fluorogenic ELISA test module (Fig. 3) is a 1½-in plastic module with individual foil-covered wells containing the reagents. The reaction zone contains antibody immobilized on a fibrous glass matrix. At one side of the sample port is an enzyme conjugate well. A substrate well and a wash port are located on the opposite side of the sample port. The wash port is used as the dispensing port for the substrate wash.

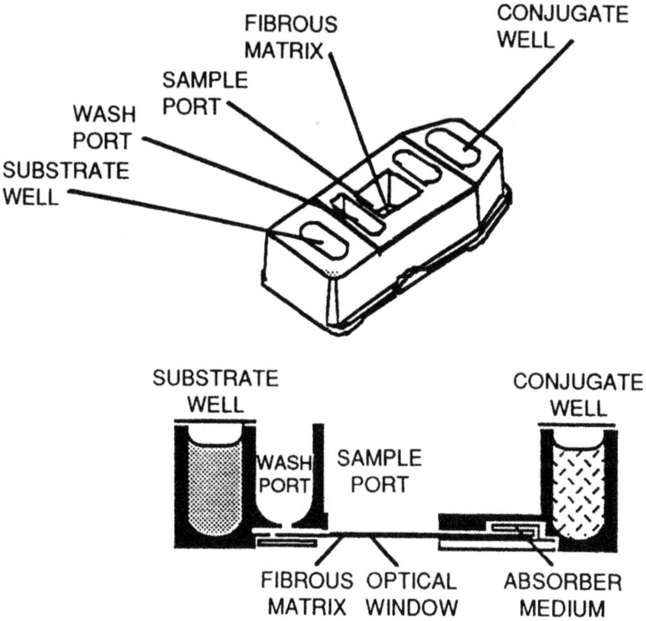

Figure 3 Fluorogenic ELISA test module.

4. Fluorogenic ELISA Assay

The specimen is pipetted onto the fibrous matrix and allowed to incubate for a few minutes to allow analyte to bind with antibody in reaction zone. OPUS then pipettes an enzyme conjugate onto the reaction zone and the incubation is continued. A sandwich immune complex is formed. Substrate is dispensed into the wash port and migrates by capillary action through the reaction zone. The immobilized enzyme conjugate converts the substrate into a fluorescent product; the substrate simultaneously washes unbound conjugate from the reaction zone. The resulting fluorescence is measured and the amount of fluorescence detected may be either directly or inversely related to the concentration of analyte in the patient sample, depending on the ELISA methodology used. Variations in the use of the different ports and wells allow these test modules to be utilized for different types of ELISA reactions. The use of the ports and wells as described below is specific for a sandwich-type ELISA reaction.

B. The OPUS Analyzer

1. Analyzer Components

OPUS's operator interface consists of a touchscreen display and a thermal printer. All functions are initiated using the interactive touchscreen, the RS-232C bidirectional interface, or with an optional bar-code wand. When prompted, the operator inserts an assay-specific test module into the loading port of the instrument.

A bar-code reader, located inside the loading port, verifies that each test module corresponds to the test module prompt on the display screen. OPUS uses a positive ID bar-code system to identify its test modules. Each module is coded with the assay type and test module lot numbers. An optional bar-code wand is located inside the instrument's front panel. This wand can be used to enter alphanumeric patient information directly from the sample tube and assay information from a bar-coded label located inside the instrument's front panel.

Figure 4 presents an internal view of the analyzer. The loader/ejector moves test modules into the rotor and, ultimately, ejects them into the waste drawer. The tray assembly holds a single tray of patient samples and two trays of pipette tips.

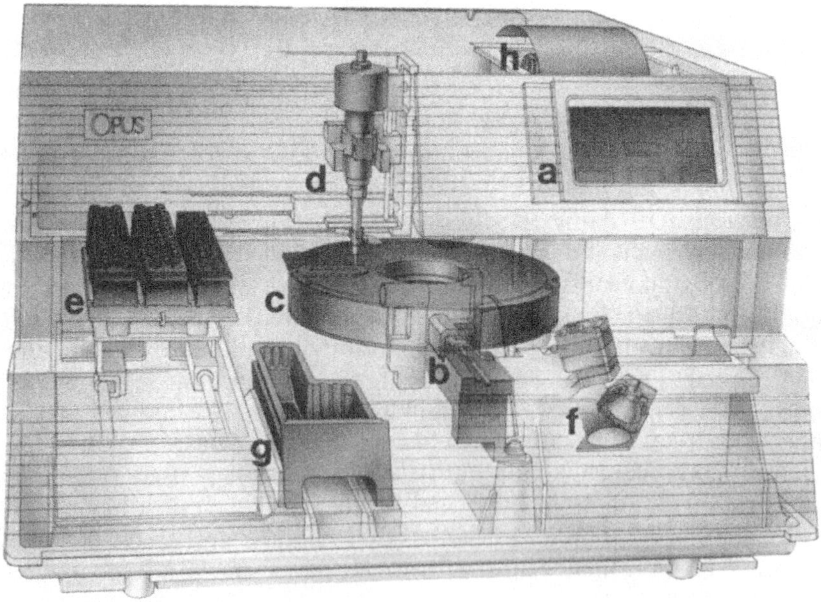

Figure 4 Internal view of the OPUS Analyzer.

An automatic pipettor, located between the tray assembly and the incubator, pipettes specimen from the sample cup to the sample port of the test module; each pipette tip is used once and discarded.

Test modules are incubated at a constant 37°C. A thermistor, mounted directly above the reading position of the incubator monitors the incubator temperature. The rotor transports test modules within the incubator.

OPUS uses an 80286 microprocessor for timing and monitoring events, controlling mechanical actions, digitizing the optical signal, controlling the temperature, and reducing data. Software performs operational checks, enables flexible user interaction, and provides HELP and ERROR messages. The software interface is easily mastered. Battery-protected nonvolatile random access memory (NOVRAM) permanently stores assay calibration data, standard curve parameters, test module lot numbers, reference ranges for assays, and the 100 most recent assay/control results. A flexible assay protocol (FAP) circuit board stores the specific assay protocols. It is designed to be easily replaced when assays are added or updated.

The fluorimeter consists of a tungsten–halogen light source, excitation and emission filters, and two photodiodes. Figure 5 presents a diagram of this optics module. Output from the lamp is directed to a three-position filter wheel that contains two pairs of matched excitation/emission narrow

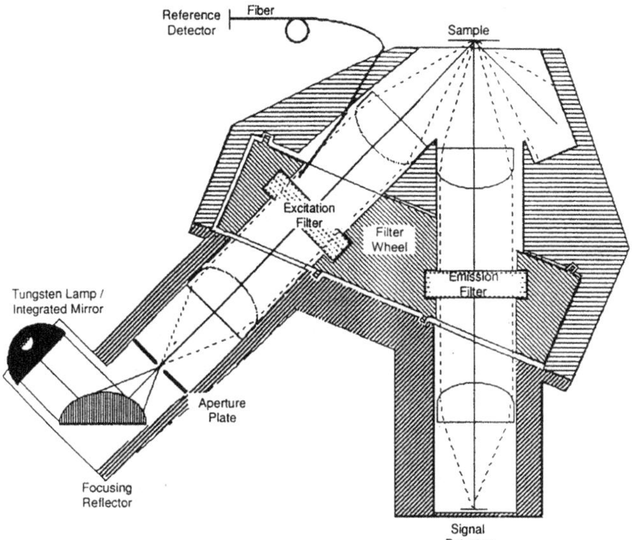

Figure 5 Fluorimeter/optics module.

band filters and one signal-blocking position. When an excitation filter is moved into the light path, the corresponding emission filter is moved into the detection arm of the optics module. The excitation/emission wavelengths of the filter pairs for ELISA-based assays are 360/45 nm; they are 550 and 580 nm for multilayer film assays.

Light from the fluorimeter is focused onto the test module, and fluorophore molecules are excited to fluoresce. The emitted light is passed through the appropriate emission filter and focused onto the active surface of a silicon photodiode. The photodiode produces a current that is proportional to the intensity of the incident light. A second photodiode converts light from the excitation filter to provide a reference reading.

Offset in the signal processing electronics is removed by measuring the output of the two photodiodes with the filter wheel in the blocking position. Signals from the detectors are measured for each test module with the filter wheel in both the pass and block positions. Excitation and emission signals are converted to digital values for data reduction, storage, and printout. For multilayer assays, two fluorometric readings contribute to the determination of analyte concentration. Multiple readings are taken for ELISA-based assays. The change in these readings over time is used in the determination of analyte concentration.

2. Analyzer Operation

OPUS should be left on 24 h/day. A laboratory may run controls according to their own quality control schedule.

To operate OPUS in random-access mode, the operator selects Random Access on the touchscreen. He assigns a patient identification number (up to 12 digits) to the sample cup; the instrument can autoassign this number, if desired. He then selects tests for that sample; as many as three tests can be selected for each sample cup.

When each of the patient samples and tests has been entered, OPUS is ready to accept test modules. The Load Screen is displayed and both the LOAD LIST and LOAD keys flash. This prompts the operator to touch the LOAD LIST key, which, in turn, prints the Load List (Fig. 6). Using the Load List as a guide, the operator pipettes sample into the proper sample cups. A maximum of 20 samples can be loaded into each tray. Up to 60 tests may be performed on these samples. Sample volumes aspirated vary between 10 and 40 μl, depending on the test. It is recommended that a sample cup be filled with 130 μl of sample for a single test and with 250 μl for up to three tests.

The Load List also indicates the numbers of each test module needed for the run. The Load Screen prompts the operator to load test modules. They are inserted, one at a time, into the instrument loading port. OPUS accepts 20 modules in approximately 2 min.

LOAD LIST
16 Jan 1991 12:02:59
TRAY: 1

CUP	PID	TEST
1	A965	Theophylline

SUPPLY	TEST
1	Theophylline

Required Tips	Tips Available
1	76

Random Access Load List

ASSAY CALIBRATION
09 Jan 1991 16:02:09
Theophylline x2
TRAY: 1

CUP	CALIBRATOR
1	0.0 ug/mL
2	2.5 ug/mL
3	5.0 ug/mL
4	10.0 ug/mL
5	20.0 ug/mL
6	40.0 ug/mL

SUPPLY	TEST
12	Theophylline

Required Tips	Tips Available
12	76

Assay Calibration Load List

Figure 6 Load List printout.

Random-access processing begins automatically after the filled sample tray and two pipette tip trays are inserted into the tray assembly. The test modules are equilibrated to 37°C. OPUS picks up a new pipette tip, aspirates sample, and dispenses sample into the proper test module.

The operator can now walk away; he needs to return only to retrieve results, request additional tests, add sample and pipette tip trays, or load more test modules. The operator can enter up to 99 test requests and access reports while the assays are in progress. A new sample tray can be loaded when pipetting from the previous tray is completed.

There is an internal counting system for pipette tips, waste drawer capacity, and assay-specific test modules. The internal counter compares the number of pipette tips used against the number required from inspection of the Load List. OPUS notifies the operator when to add pipette tips. The operator also has the option of beginning any run with two full trays of pipette tips, avoiding the need to return to the instrument to replenish the supply for that run. A second counter keeps track of the number of used test modules and pipette tips in the waste drawer; it prompts the operator to empty the waste drawer when a new sample tray is introduced. OPUS also tracks the number and type of test module needed when new tests are requested.

After further incubation, the rotor transports the test module to the "read" position and the fluorimeter measures its fluorescence. The rotor then moves the used test module to the loader/ejector, which discards it into the waste tray. The assay result is calculated by backfitting fluorescence intensity data to the calibration curve.

The first result is obtained within 6–23 min, depending on the test or panel. Additional results may be obtained in 20 seconds to 1 min to several minutes, depending on the type and volume of tests involved. Table 1 gives pertinent information on specific tests. Test modules are stored at 2°–8°C. Shelf life is at least 6 months; ongoing stability studies suggest that a considerably longer shelf life is likely.

Approximately 20–75 test results can be obtained per hour. The actual throughput depends on the specific tests and volume of tests being performed.

OPUS also allows testing of preset panels of tests. A panel is an operator-determined set of two or three assays that are chosen as one selection. The analyzer can store up to six panels, which may be reconfigured by the operator at any time.

Batch testing involves the selection of Batch on the Main Menu screen, selection of the test or panel desired, and assignment of a patient ID number to each sample. For example, an operator may choose to process 10 samples and select theophylline to be assayed. An alternative way to process in batch mode is to process 10 samples and select a panel of thyroxine, T-uptake, and TSH to be assayed.

Selection of a test in the Stat mode interrupts the processing of samples to run a single, higher-priority, patient sample. If a pipetting sequence is in progress for a particular assay, the request for a stat sample tray will not occur immediately. Upon completion of all pipetting steps, OPUS prompts the loading of the stat tray. Once stat testing is completed and the results are printed, tests that had been deferred are now allowed to continue.

3. Assay Calibration

Control samples should be run daily according to laboratory practices to validate the stability of each calibration curve. The calibration curve is stable for at least 2 weeks for fluorogenic ELISA testing and a minimum of 6 weeks for multilayer assays. It is anticipated that calibration stability will be extended to 12 weeks for many of the multilayer film assays. If test modules having a different lot number are to be used, calibration must be reestablished.

The manufacturer recommends calibration in duplicate, although the OPUS System will allow one to three calibration point replicates. Table 2 describes OPUS calibrators and calibration curve stability. Calibrators are stored at 2–8°C. OPUS's calibrators are single-assay specific.

Figure 7 presents a printout of a calibration curve for phenytoin. It includes raw data, fitted values, and data derived from curve-fitting.

Table 1 OPUS Assay Specifications

Analyte	OPUS abbreviation	Module format[a]	Reference range[b]	Assay range	Minimum detectable dose[c]	Assay time (min)	Sample accepted[d]
Theophylline	THE	MTM	10–20 μg/ml	0.36–40	0.36 μg/ml	6	Serum, plasma
Carbamazepine	CAR	MTM	8–12 μg/ml	1.01–20	1.01 μg/ml	6	Serum, plasma
Phenytoin	PHN	MTM	10–20 μg/ml	0.56–40	0.56 μg/ml	6	Serum only
Phenobarbital	PHB	MTM	15–40 μg/ml	1.49–80	1.49 μg/ml	6	Serum, plasma
Valproic acid	VPA	MTM	50–100 μg/ml	3.85–150	3.85 μg/ml	6	Serum, plasma
hCG	HCG	ETM	N/A	1.3–500	1.30 mIU/ml	16	Serum only
Total T_4	T_4	MTM	4.2–12 μg/dl	1.17–30	1.17 μg/dl	16	Serum, plasma
T Uptake	T-U	MTM	25.5–37.2%	15–55	15%	16	Serum, plasma
TSH	TSH	ETM	0.4–4.2 mIU/l	0.05–50	0.05 mIU/l	21	Serum, plasma
Digoxin	DIG	ETM	0.8–2.0 ng/ml	0.25–5.0	0.25 ng/ml	16	Serum, plasma
Gentamicin	GNT	MTM	5–10 μg/ml	0.15–14.0	0.15 μg/ml	6	Serum, plasma
FSH	FSH	ETM	N/A	0.2–200	0.2 mIU/ml	16	Serum only
CMV	CMV	ETM	N/A	N/A	N/A	15	Serum, plasma
Toxoplasma	TOX	ETM	N/A	N/A	N/A	15	Serum, plasma

[a] MTM = multilayer film test module; ETM = ELISA test module.
[b] Suggested ranges. Laboratories should establish their own ranges.
[c] Minimal detectable dose = lowest measurable level of analyte that can be distinguished from zero.
[d] Dilute HIGH dose samples with zero calibrator. For hCG, use OPUS hCG diluent.

Table 2 OPUS Calibration

Analyte	Calibrator base	Curve stability[a]	Calibrator range
Theophylline	Human serum	8 weeks	0–40 μg/ml
Carbamazepine	Human serum	8 weeks	0–20 μg/ml
Phenytoin	Human serum	8 weeks	0–40 μg/ml
Phenobarbital	Human serum	8 weeks	0–80 μg/ml
Valproic acid	Human serum	8 weeks	0–150 μg/ml
hCG	Human serum	2 weeks	0–500 mIU/ml
Total T_4	Human serum	6 weeks	0–30 μg/dl
T Uptake	Human serum	6 weeks	20–40%
TSH	Bovine serum	2 weeks	0–50 mIU/l
Digoxin	Human serum	2 weeks	0–4.0 ng/ml
Gentamicin	Human serum	8 weeks	0–14.0 μg/ml
FSH	Bovine serum	2 weeks	0–200 mIU/ml
CMV	Human serum	2 weeks	Reactive/nonreactive
Toxoplasma	Human serum	2 weeks	Reactive/nonreactive

[a] Stability studies ongoing.

The assay calibration curve is printed out only once, but the parameters are stored in NOVRAM (permanent memory) until replaced with those from a new calibration. One calibration curve is stored for each analyte assay.

C. Reports

Several reports are available continuously. These include a Load List (tests requested), Status List (tests in progress), Results List (the last 100 assay results), Assay List (a record of calibrated assays; lot numbers used, date, and time), and Patient Result reports.

D. Communications Capability

The OPUS Analyzer is provided with an RS-232C bidirectional interface and may be connected with any laboratory information system (LIS) that can use KERMIT (communications software available free of charge from Columbia University).

E. Product Availability

Shipments of the OPUS Immunoassay System commenced in the summer of 1990. The initial test menu, described in Tables 1 and 2, is avail-

PB Diagnostics
14 Jan 1991 OPUS 13:55:35
CALIBRATION
FOR
Phenytoin
LOT No.: O8 OP ID: 1

CALB.	SIGNAL	FITTED	ERROR %
0.00	19.0		
0.00	18.8		
Average	18.9	0.000	0.00
2.50	14.8		
2.50	14.8		
Average	14.8	2.55	2.15
5.00	12.8		
5.00	13.0		
Average	12.9	4.75	-5.05
10.00	10.3		
10.00	10.4		
Average	10.4	10.4	-3.50
20.00	8.20		
20.00	7.82		
Average	8.01	20.0	0.19
40.00	5.53		
40.00	5.31		
Average	5.42	39.8	-0.59

ROOT MEAN SQUARE ERROR: 2.92
CORRELATION COEFF: 0.9999

CURVE PARAMETERS:

A	-9.30805e-01
B	-9.01033e-00
C	+1.74145e+01

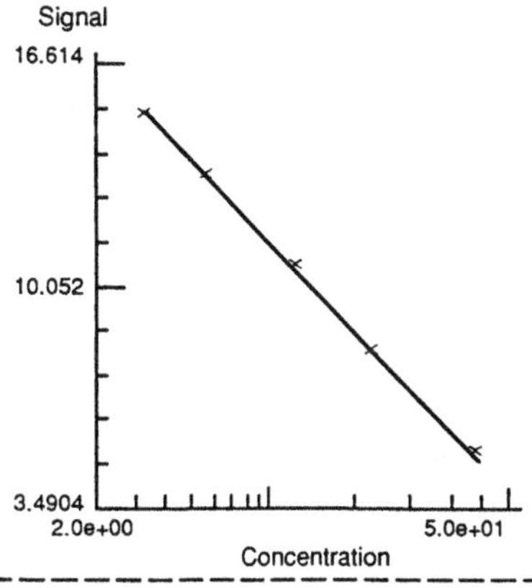

Figure 7 Calibration curve printout.

able as of the date of this publication. Tests for Tobramycin, total T3, Cytomegalovirus-IgM (CMV-M), Luteinizing Hormone (LH), Prolactin, and Ferritin are expected to be released in 1991. Further test development includes therapeutic drug monitoring tests, thyroid tests, cancer markers, cardiac tests, infectious disease, and hematology tests.

III. PERFORMANCE

The discussion that follows is based upon an investigation conducted in the Toxicology Department at the Long Island Jewish Medical Center, which served as a clinical beta site to evaluate the OPUS Immunoassay System. Various assays were investigated on the OPUS Analyzer. This section uses theophylline and digoxin as examples in relating our experience with OPUS. They serve as suitable model assays of analytes present in blood at high and low concentrations, respectively. They also serve to illustrate the two analytical techniques on the OPUS instrument: the multilayer immunoassay for theophylline and the fluorogenic ELISA for digoxin. All assays designed for the OPUS use either the multilayer or fluorogenic ELISA techniques.

Overall, the performance and lack of down time of the OPUS system is impressive. The instrument was functional within 2 h after its uncrating; during the initial 6-month evaluation period, only one service call was required. The lack of down time was a pleasant surprise, since most new, first-generation analyzers can be expected to have more than a few "bugs." Additionally, normal maintenance for OPUS is limited to monthly intervals, a welcome advancement in busy laboratories. OPUS's simple design, using very few moving parts, combined with PB Diagnostic's extensive system/reagent development and refinement, has produced a rugged and reliable instrument.

A. Multilayer Immunoassay Technique

Theophylline was selected as a model analyte to assess OPUS's competitive immunoassay performance with a compound whose blood concentrations are relatively high. The initial result is available after approximately 6 min with subsequent results generated at less than 1 min per specimen. A nominal rate of approximately 75 theophylline specimens/h is achieved. (Other low-molecular-weight compounds present at high blood levels, such as the anticonvulsants, are also assayed using the thin-film immunoassay technique.)

This throughput is achieved in spite of the fact that the assay uses an immunocomplex instead of separate layers for antibody and conjugate in the test module. The assay kinetics are fast because monoclonal antibodies with very fast dissociation rates are used. The theophylline test reaches equilibrium in less than 4 min at 37°C; the signal is stable for more than 20 min (Fig. 8). This demonstrates complete immobilization of the monoclonal antibodies in the signal layer (Grenner *et al.*, 1989).

The theophylline method showed clinically good precision at all

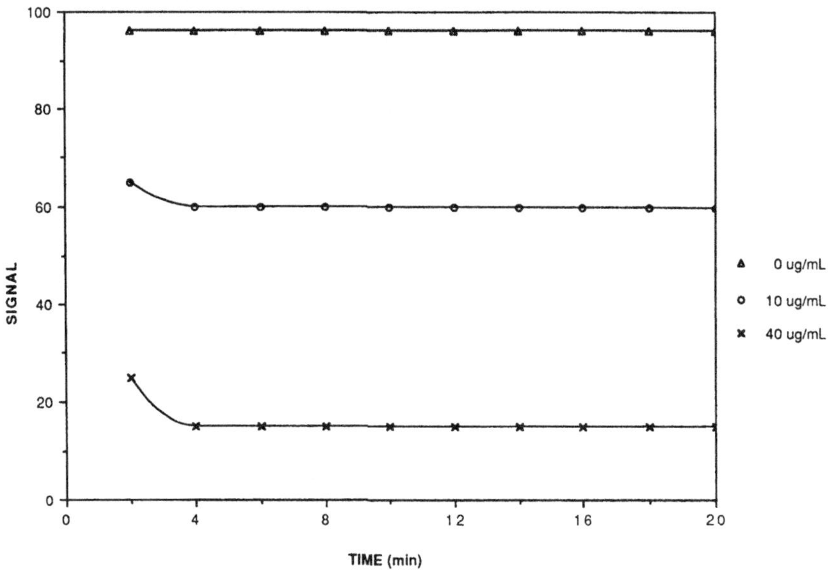

Figure 8 Theophylline assay kinetics.

levels of theophylline tested (Lehrer, 1991). A study of assay precision performed at the low, therapeutic, and toxic ranges demonstrated between-run coefficients of variation of 7.9, 2.6, and 4.7%, respectively (Table 3). Baxter's Dade controls with means of 3.8, 14.2, and 31.5 μg/ml were used. As expected, lower coefficients of variation were obtained for within-run studies (except for the mid-level control result, which was higher than its corresponding between-run level result). The standard curve for theophylline was linear in the 2.5–40 μg/ml range. Precision performance was judged to be comparable to that obtained by TDx analysis.

Table 3 Theophylline Assay Precision

	Level 1	Level 2	Level 3
Within runs (n = 20)			
Mean (μg/ml)	3.8	14.2	31.5
CV (%)	5.7	6.5	2.4
Between runs (n = 30)			
Mean (μg/ml)	4.2	14.7	31.1
CV (%)	7.9	2.6	4.7

The specificity of the assay was of particular interest. This is because the theophylline molecule falls into the xanthine class of compounds. Caffeine and theobromine are naturally occurring xanthines that are present in many foods and beverages. Their structures closely resemble theophylline (Fig. 9); the potential for cross-reactivity exists. However, none of these xanthine compounds cross-react (Table 4), attesting to the high specificity of the monoclonal antibody used in OPUS's reagents.

Furthermore, lipemic, icteric, and hemolytic samples caused no significant interference over a broad range (Table 5). At bilirubin concentrations greater than 12 mg/dl a positive interference was noted. At 20 mg/dl bilirubin levels, theophylline results appeared to be 15–20% higher than values obtained by high-performance liquid chromatography (HPLC). However, this is not a clinical problem since such high bilirubin values are rarely encountered.

A comparison of the accuracy of test results on 51 patient samples with results obtained on the TDx system showed good agreement and

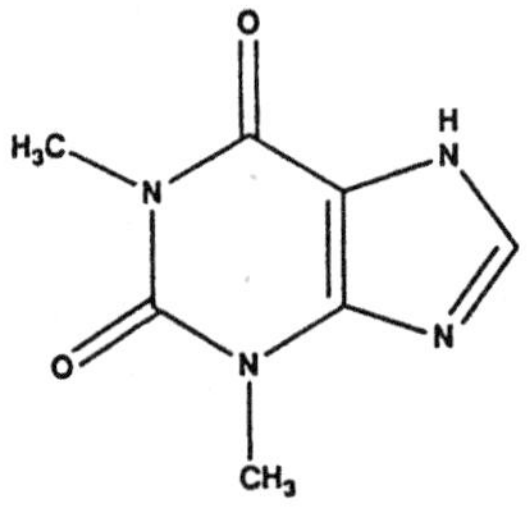

THEOPHYLLINE

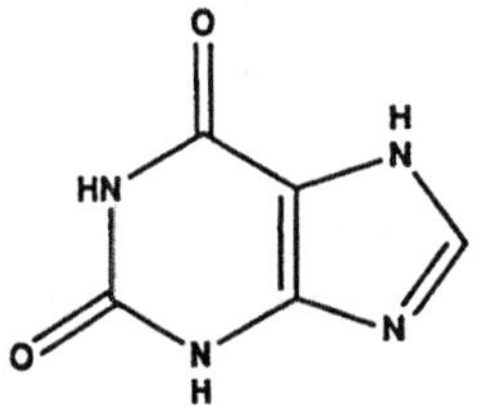

XANTHINE

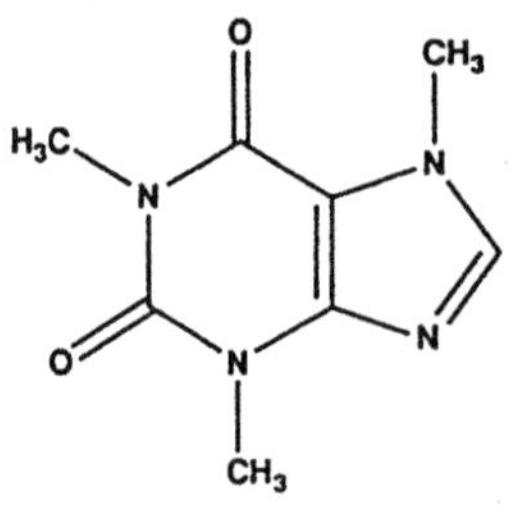

CAFFEINE

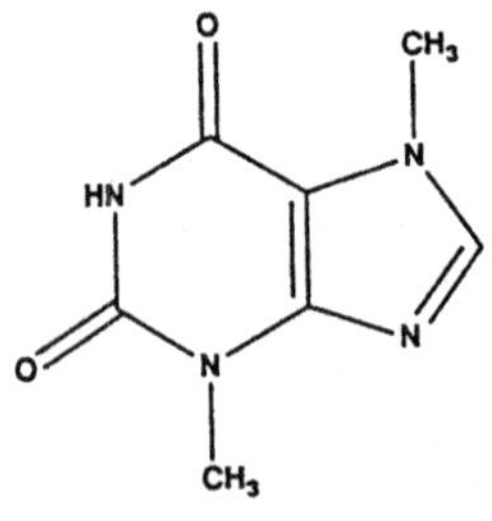

THEOBROMINE

Figure 9 Theophylline and structurally related compounds.

Table 4 Specificity of Theophylline Assay

Compound	Cross-reactivity (%)
Amobarbital	<1.0
Arterenol	<1.0
Caffeine	<1.0
8-Chlorotheophylline	3.0
1,3-Dimethyluric acid	3.8
Dyphylline	<1.0
Ephedrine	<1.0
Epinephrine	<1.0
Isoproternol	<1.0
1-Methyluric acid	<1.0
3-Methyluric acid	<1.0
Phenacetin	<1.0
Phenobarbital	<1.0
Phenylephrine	<1.0
Salicylic acid	<1.0
Theobromine	<1.0
1,3,7-Trimethyluric acid	<1.0
Uric acid	<1.0

reproducibility (Fig. 10). The resulting correlation coefficient was 0.993 with a -0.408 μg/ml *Y* intercept. During this study no samples with toxic levels of theophylline (greater than 30 μg/ml) were encountered.

B. Fluorogenic ELISA Technique

The digoxin assay is an example of a fluorogenic ELISA technique used to assay analytes present at lower concentrations (often higher-molecular-weight compounds) on OPUS. The initial digoxin result is available after

Table 5 Interference Testing[a]

Substance	Level
Hemoglobin	1000 mg/dl
Total bilirubin	12 mg/dl
Triglycerides	1100 mg/dl
Cholesterol	300 mg/dl
Total Protein	10 g/dl

[a] No interference was observed up to levels indicated.

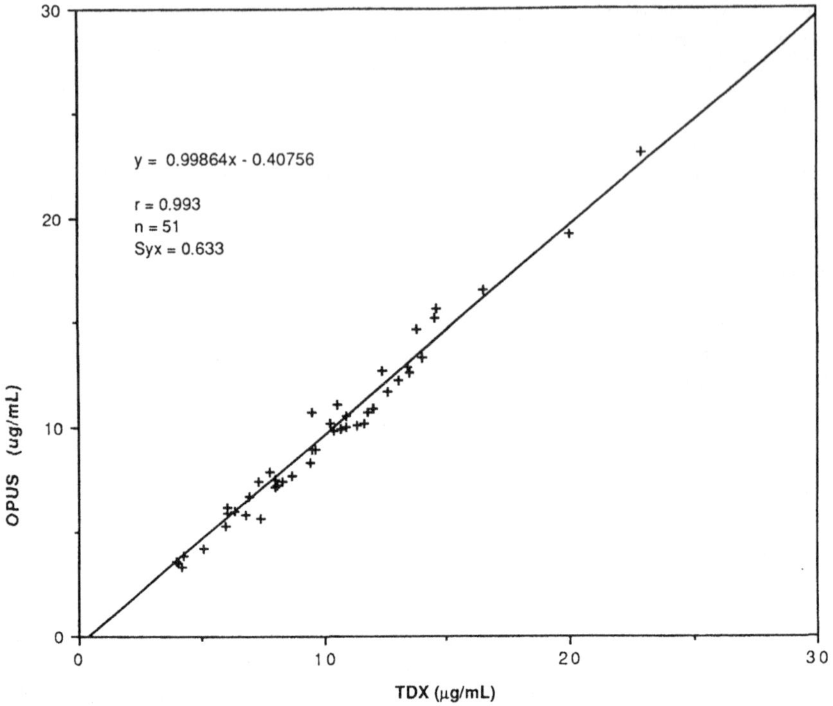

Figure 10 Theophylline correlation, OPUS versus TDx.

16 min with subsequent results generated at approximately one every 3 min. A nominal rate of approximately 20 digoxin specimens per hour is achieved. Other analytes assayed using the fluorogenic ELISA technique follow the digoxin model; only slight variations in incubation and processing times were noted.

The OPUS digoxin method demonstrated clinically good precision at all levels of digoxin tested (Meenan, 1991). The standard curve was linear in the 0.5–4.0 ng/ml range. A precision study performed at low, therapeutic, and toxic ranges showed between-run coefficients of variation of 7.9, 5.2, and 6.2%, respectively (Table 6). Similar coefficients of variation were obtained for within-run studies. Corning's CIBA controls with means of 0.84, 1.45, and 2.91 ng/ml were used. Precision performance was comparable to that obtained by TDx analysis. No significant interference was observed with lipemic, icteric, or hemolytic samples.

Comparison of results obtained with OPUS to results obtained via TDx and radioimmunoassay (RIA) (Diagnostic Products Corporation) on 46 patient samples demonstrated good agreement and reproducibility

Table 6 Digoxin Assay Precision

	Level 1	Level 2	Level 3
Within runs (n = 20)			
Mean (ng/ml)	0.84	1.45	2.91
CV (%)	7.5	5.7	5.8
Between runs [n = 30)			
Mean (ng/ml)	0.92	1.46	2.97
CV (%)	7.9	5.2	6.2

(Figs. 11 and 12). The OPUS versus TDx correlation coefficient was 0.976 with a 0.184 Y intercept; the OPUS versus RIA comparison yielded a correlation coefficient of 0.960 with a 0.256 Y intercept.

Six specimens, which originated from a single patient, were excluded from the above correlation. The results obtained on specimens from this patient demonstrated somewhat high TDx recoveries when compared to values obtained via OPUS or RIA (Table 7). It is not clear if this patient's blood contains a component that elevates the TDx results. This finding is

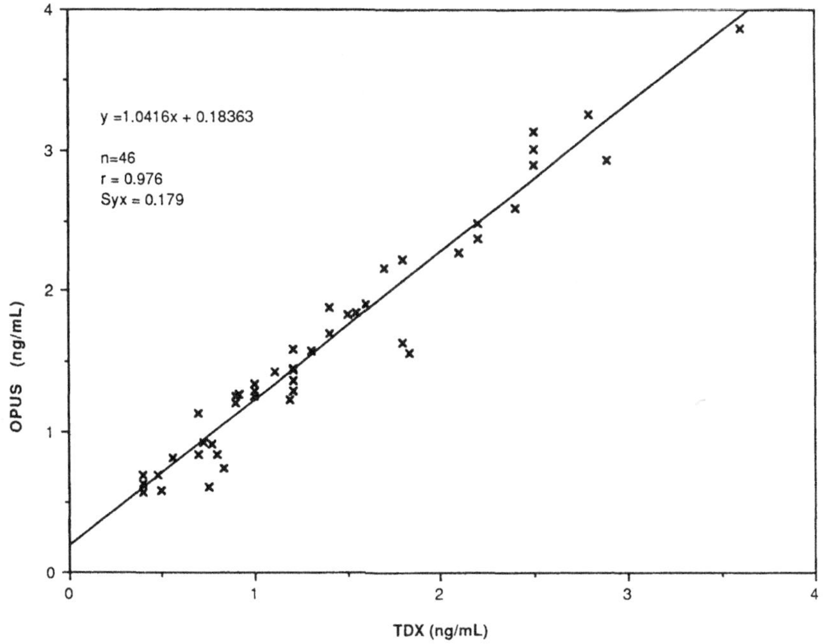

Figure 11 Digoxin correlation, OPUS versus TDx.

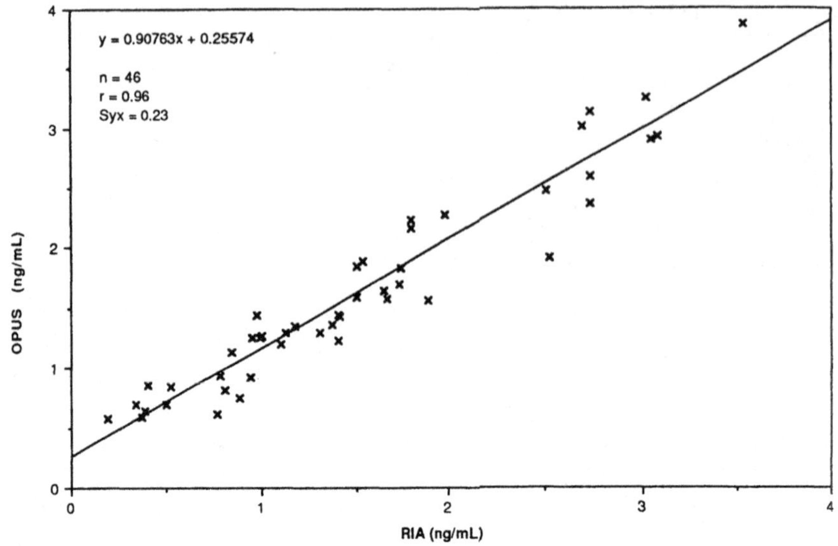

Figure 12 Digoxin correlation, OPUS versus RIA.

interesting, but more investigations are required before its significance can be assessed.

The digoxin methodology was easy to use and required no centrifugation or pretreatment of the specimen prior to an analysis. Operator hands-on time required is the same for either ELISA or multilayer immunoassays; this time ranges from approximately 1–2 min for one specimen to 10 min for a batch of 20 specimens. Following the loading of test modules, the system is totally automated and technologists can leave the instrument to perform other duties in the laboratory. Used test modules are ejected into the waste drawer and the results are printed.

Table 7 Multiple Specimens from One Patient

Specimen	OPUS	RIA	TDx
1	0.70	0.40	2.1
2	0.51	0.37	2.0
3	0.73	0.65	2.1
4	0.70	0.78	2.2
5	0.59	0.28	0.9
6	0.52	0.20	1.0

IV. CONCLUSION

The OPUS system was found to be quite versatile in our busy toxicology laboratory. The instrument can be operated in random access, batch, or stat modes. A stat request can be obtained at any time (even when the system is running in random-access or batch mode) by simply loading the sample and designating it as a stat. The OPUS will complete any pipetting steps in progress and then turn its attention to performing the stat request. When the stat determination is complete, the OPUS returns to the previous worklist and completes the remaining tests. No test is ever lost when a run is interrupted to perform a stat analysis. This is a useful feature because the stat can be any analyte of interest, regardless of which analytes are being assayed at the time. Consequently, we found OPUS useful for performing stat requests immediately upon their arrival at the laboratory. This was especially convenient because OPUS is totally random access and requires no reagent changes or sample pretreatment. The ability to order multiple tests from one sample was also advantageous. As many as three different tests can be performed from the same specimen. This is useful when multiple tests are ordered or when an analyte and its active metabolite must be measured.

Up to 20 samples can be loaded at any one time. Because everything is contained in the test modules, no external reagents or diluents arc used. It is this feature that allows the system to be totally random access. The operator functions consist of loading trays containing pipette tips and specimen cups into the analyzer, selecting the assay-specific test module(s) and removing them from their foil-sealed packages, placing module(s) on the loader, and emptying the waste drawer when prompted. The start button (stat, random access, or batch) is touched to initiate the analysis. Once the run is initiated, OPUS is totally self-sufficient and is a true "walk-away" system.

No more than 20 test modules can be loaded at any given time. Consequently, for laboratories with consistently large batches (greater than 20), the OPUS system may be less than optimal. Due to its continuous access design, additional test modules can be loaded when space on the rotor becomes available. Thus, one does not have to wait until the entire batch of 20 samples is completed before loading additional specimens. A mild disadvantage encountered with large batches results from the fact that each test module is individually sealed and that test modules must be removed from the foil-sealed package prior to loading.

Each individual test module is hermetically sealed in a foil-covered package containing a dessicant for maximum shelf life. Opened test modules are sensitive to humidity. The manufacturer recommends that test modules be removed from their package immediately before the test module is loaded into the analyzer. A minimum 15-min room-temperature equilibration of test modules is required before use. Sealed test modules can be left on the bench at room temperature for several hours; therefore, they can be immediately available for stat testing. The fluorogenic ELISA test modules are not as sensitive to humidity.

The OPUS's specimen cup has an 80-μl dead volume. Redesign of the cup to incorporate a conical shape or to incorporate a conical insert would reduce dead volume significantly. This can be advantageous with pediatric samples; it is my understanding that PB Diagnostics will try to redesign the specimen cup to reduce dead volume.

A major advantage of the OPUS is that it is ready to perform analytical tests on specimens 24 h/day. Specimens can be loaded and assays performed immediately with no warmup or calibration steps needed. There is no tubing to change, probes to wash or adjust, or pipettors to calibrate. No daily maintenance is recommended for OPUS; we found that none was needed. Monthly preventive maintenance is recommended by the manufacturer; this takes about 10 min to complete. Another advantage of inclusion of reagents and buffers in the test module is that pipetting and associated difficulties are avoided. This automation also minimizes the effects of variations in technical skill among laboratory personnel that can adversely affect precision and accuracy. Overall, the system's simplicity, ruggedness, and almost total availability to perform analytical work are impressive.

Carryover contamination of samples is not an issue with the OPUS. This is because a disposable pipette tip is used to dispense specimen into a test module and a new pipette tip is used for each pipetting step. All reagents and subsequent chemical and physical processes are confined within the test modules. This aspect of OPUS's design greatly simplifies the analytical process from the operator's perspective; it eliminates the potential for carryover contamination. Another of OPUS's advantages is that its waste products do not contain liquids. Instrument operators find this advantageous as it minimizes the cleanup process and eliminates the potential for biological waste spills.

Curve stability is good. PB Diagnostics specifies recalibration after 6 weeks for multilayer film test analytes and after 14 days for the fluorogenic ELISA analytes. These guidelines appear reasonable; we obtained the expected curve stability in our laboratory. During our beta site evaluation period, PB Diagnostics updated the system's software several times. This was done to enhance performance and to incorporate improvements resulting from feedback obtained at other beta evaluation sites. We were impressed by the flexibility of the software and by the company's ability to incorporate many enhancements so rapidly. Software updates were performed in our laboratory by PB service engineers; typically, they were completed in less than an hour.

OPUS can be purchased, leased, or obtained on a reagent rental contract. The cost of using the OPUS system is very easy to monitor. This is because there are few consumables, and those needed are generic in nature. Thus, users are not locked into the exotic rotors or other expensive disposables that seem to characterize many analyzers today. The system's design (e.g., elimination of carryover) and test-module packaging also minimize waste; there are very few situations where a test module will not yield a usable analysis. Calibration requirements are relatively infrequent and test modules have long shelf lives. The "hidden" costs are essentially nil. Consequently, effective cost management can be exercised.

Labor utilization on OPUS is extremely efficient. The system's extensive automation, minimal maintenance, infrequent calibration, and freedom from reagent preparation demands make OPUS extremely labor efficient. The importance of this factor should not be underestimated; the labor component of laboratory costs is by far the largest component.

REFERENCES

Ackermann, H., Steva, E., Blackwood, J., Inbar, S., and Metzmann, E. (1990). A dry chemistry multilayer immunoassay test for valproic acid. *Clin. Chem.* **36,** 1038.

Bahar, I., Vaupel, U., Case, A., Farrell, K., Inbar, S., and Metzmann, E. (1990). Rapid self-contained immunoassay for digoxin. *Clin. Chem.* **36,** 1028.

Blackwood, J., Cox, J., Staedter, M., Inbar, S., and Metzmann, E. (1990). A dry chemistry multilayer immunoassay test for carbamazepine. *Clin. Chem.* **36,** 1036.

D'Eon, P., Shea, M., Blackwood, J., Inbar, S., and Metzmann, E. (1990). A dry chemistry multilayer immunoassay test for gentamycin. *Clin. Chem.* **36,** 1045.

Freeley, P., Wong, P., Whitely, G., Conte, K., Dray-Lyons, K., Desplaines, K., and Metzmann, E. (1990). A human enzyme immunoassay for antibodies to human immunodeficiency virus, types 1 and 2. *Clin. Chem.* **36,** 1091.

Grenner, G., Inbar, S., Meneghini, E. W., Long, E. W., Yamartino, E. J., Jr., Bowen, M. S., Blackwood, J. J., Padilla, A. J., Maretsky, D., and Staedter, M. (1989). Multilayer fluorescent immunoassay technique. *Clin. Chem.* **34,** 1865–1868.

Havelick, J., Fure, M., Gorham, P., Doenges, P., Baker, R., Saul, R., and Metzmann, E. (1990). A rapid self-contained immunoassay for human chorionic gonadotrophin (hCG). *Clin. Chem.* **36,** 1086.

Inbar, S., Grenner, G., Blackwood, J., Long, E., Bowen, M., and Meneghini, F. (1990). Dry chemistry thin film immunoassay. *Ann. Biol. Clin.* **48,** 385–390.

Lauer, J. M., Miller, L., Monaco, S., Nipper, H. C., Cox, R. S., Jr., and McClellan, G. A. (1990). Cumputer-assisted timing of TDx and Opus. *Am. J. Clin. Pathol.* October, 1990.

Lehrer, M., and Meenan, J. (1992). Evaluation of theophylline assay via dry chemistry multilayer technique on Opus analyzer. In preparation.

Meenan, J., and Lehrer, M. (1992). Evaluation of digoxin assay by a fluorogenic ELISA technique on the Opus system. In preparation.

Pothier, S., Gentzer, W., Bessette, J., Bowser, J., Natale, J., Saul, R., and Metzmann, E. (1990). A rapid self-contained immunoassay for carcinoembryonic antigen (CEA). *Clin. Chem.* **36,** 1095.

CHAPTER 20

The Photon-ERA Immunoassay Analyzer

Roger M. Frye
Department of Laboratory Medicine,
The Johns Hopkins Hospital, Baltimore, Maryland

I. INTRODUCTION

The Photon-ERA, manufactured by Hybritech, Inc., San Diego, California, is a batch analyzer designed to automatically perform most of the operations required for the Tandem-E immunoenzymetric assays (Hybritech). Under computer control, the instrument automatically performs the pipetting, aspiration, washing, quenching, absorbance measurement, and result calculation steps. Dispensing of antibody-coated beads into assay tubes and transfer to and from off-line incubation must be performed manually.

This combination of automation with manual steps makes the Photon-ERA a transitional instrument in the evolution of immunoassay automation. It is clearly beyond the earlier automated pipetting station devices. In addition to pipetting of sample and reagents, absorbance measurement and result calculation are also provided. Computer control provides pipetting accuracy, precise timing, flexible data reduction, and the ability to use preprogrammed protocols. The assay protocol flexibility of automatic pipetting stations is not required since the Tandem enzyme immunoassays use similar standardized protocols. The next step in automation, full automation, does not require manual intervention during assay processing. The Abbott TDx and Dade Stratus are typical of this type of automation. Random access full automation, as exemplified by instru-

Immunoassay Automation: A Practical Guide

ments such as the Tosoh AIA-1200, completes the evolution to date. In general, the fully automated systems offer an additional advantage, that of modular or integral reagents requiring little or no preparation. Tandem-E reagents are packaged similarly for manual and automated operation. Bead wash solution must be diluted before use. *p*-Nitrophenyl phosphate substrate must be prepared fresh every 48 h. All other reagents are ready to use in liquid form.

II. SYSTEM DESCRIPTION

A. Instrumentation

The Photon-ERA consists of two parts: a processing unit and an IBM-PC-XT or PC clone. Communication between the two is provided by an RS232 serial interface. The only utility required is electrical power (115 V, 5 A, 50–60 Hz). Reagents (wash and quench) and waste are stored in on-board containers. The processing unit is divided into two parts. A sample processor on the left side pipettes sample and conjugate and precisely times pipetting steps. On the right side is the reaction processor, which washes beads, adds substrate and quench reagent, and measures the absorbance of the quenched assay tubes.

The computer both controls and monitors the processing unit and calculates and reports assay results. Up to 28 assay protocols can be stored, allowing for assay-specific programming of sample volume, incubation time, calibrator concentration, data for assay controls, and data reduction calculations. In processing an assay, the computer displays step-by-step prompts requiring keystroke confirmation before proceeding. These prompts are extremely helpful for the novice but may be redundant for the experienced operator. A group of electrical and mechanical sensors in the processor also allows the computer to detect and display instrument status and error messages. Also, an assay scheduling program is provided to aid in planning the day's work. Help screens are available at each level.

When not involved in controlling the Photon-ERA, the computer is a fully functional PC. A variety of IBM PC-compatible software, such as graphics and statistics programs, may be run. This is especially useful in a lower test volume laboratory where the instrument would have reasonably large blocks of idle time.

The processing unit sample and reaction processors operate independently. This, coupled with the versatility of the computer, allows for a high degree of multitasking. Different assays may be run in the sample and reaction processors simultaneously. While assays are running, assay worklists and protocols may be built or modified through the computer.

B. Reagent

The Tandem-E assays that are automated on the Photon-ERA are all solid-phase two-site immunoenzymetric assays. A sample containing the analyte is reacted with a plastic bead coated with a monoclonal antibody directed against a unique antigenic site on the analyte molecule and a second monoclonal antibody, directed against a different antigenic site, conjugated to bovine alkaline phosphatase. After the bead/analyte/enzyme–antibody sandwich is formed, the bead is washed to remove unbound labeled antibody. *Para*-nitrophenyl phosphate substrate solution is added, incubated, and the reaction stopped by addition of an alkaline quench reagent. The absorbance of liberated *para*-nitrophenol, which is directly proportional to the amount of analyte, is measured at 405 nm. The analyte is quantitated by comparison of the test absorbance to a standard curve consisting of a zero and a single non-zero calibrator. Assays are usually performed in duplicate.

The following is a list of Tandem-E assays currently available on the Photon-ERA.

Tests:	AFP	Prolactin
	CEA	PSA
	CKMB	TSH
	Ferritin	LH
	hCG	FSH
	IgE	PAP

III. INSTRUMENT PERFORMANCE

A. Technical

Initial evaluation of the Photon-ERA in our laboratory was performed beginning in December 1987 and was confined to creatine kinase MB (CK-MB), human chorionic gonadotropin (hCG), prolactin, and carcinoembryonic antigen (CEA). Discussion will be confined to CK-MB and hCG, since these assays were performed manually by the Hybritech Tandem-E method prior to the arrival of the Photon-ERA. Differences in overall assay performance reflect the impact of the Photon-ERA. The area most sensitive to automation should be precision: both overall assay precision as measured by control specimens, and agreement of sample duplicates. Each assay was assessed for within- and between-run precision and patient correlation as compared to the manual method. Tables 1 and 2 summarize precision data. Correlation data is presented in Table 3. Table 4

Table 1 Within-Run Precision: Photon-ERA

	CK-MB		hCG	
	Low	High	Low	High
N	20	18	20	17
Mean	12.9 ng/ml	49.6 ng/ml	29 mIU/ml	303 mIU/ml
SD	0.45 ng/ml	1.48 ng/ml	2.5 mIU/ml	15.6 mIU/ml
CV	3.5%	3.0%	8.7%	5.2%

Table 2 Between-Run Precision: Photon-ERA

	CK-MB manual		Photon-ERA	
	Low[a]	High[a]	Low	High
N	255	255	263	262
Mean	16.5 ng/ml	62.3 ng/ml	12.9 ng/ml	59.6 ng/ml
SD	1.03 ng/ml	4.44 ng/ml	0.84 ng/ml	3.97 ng/ml
CV	6.2%	7.1%	6.5%	6.7%

	hCG manual			Photon-ERA		
	Low[a]	Mid[a]	High[a]	Low	Mid	High
N	1300	464	464	387	127	127
Mean	10.6 mIU/ml	26.8 mIU/ml	277.5 mIU/ml	12.7 mIU/ml	26.6 mIU/ml	280.7 mIU/ml
SD	1.41 mIU/ml	2.29 mIU/ml	17.59 mIU/ml	1.08 mIU/ml	1.69 mIU/ml	14.0 mIU/ml
CV	13.3%	8.6%	6.3%	8.5%	6.3%	5.0%

[a] Manual and Photon-ERA controls were different lot numbers with different expected values.

Table 3 Patient Correlation: Photon-ERA Compared to Manual Method

CK-MB (0–100 ng/ml)	
(Photon-ERA) = 0.98 (Manual) − 0.0 ng/ml	
$N = 63$	Mean (ERA) = 10.5 ng/ml
$r = 0.994$	Mean (manual) = 10.8 ng/ml
hCG (0–400 mIU/ml)	
(Photon-ERA) = 1.01 (Manual) − 0.5 mIU/ml	
$N = 30$	Mean (ERA) = 87.3 mIU/ml
$r = 0.989$	Mean (manual) = 86.7 mIU/ml

Table 4 Precision: CV of Duplicates, Photon-ERA and Manual

	Photon-ERA	Manual
Number with CV > 5%	10 (13.3% of total)	14 (18.7% of total)
Number with CV > 10%	1 (1.3% of total)	0 (0% of total)

summarizes a special study undertaken with the prolactin assay to compare the CV of duplicates for the Photon-ERA versus the equivalent manual method.

B. Operational

Hybritech recommends maintenance and performance verification procedures to be performed daily, weekly, and monthly. Daily maintenance consists of a warm boot of the computer, reagent refill, reagent priming and dispense volume check, and various housekeeping functions performed at startup at the beginning of the work day. Cleaning reagent and pipette lines, also part of daily maintenance, is performed at day's end. Total time for daily maintenance is approximately 20 min. Weekly maintenance consists primarily of changing peristaltic pump tubing and takes only 2–3 min. Monthly maintenance takes 30–45 min and consists of sample and reagent probe cleaning and an optical linearity check, along with additional housekeeping functions.

Since our laboratory had two Photon-ERAs used for higher-volume testing, analysis of the failure and frequency of repair record of the instruments should allow some insight into their ruggedness and reliability. The period covered by this analysis is from 2/89 to 2/90. During this time, there was a total of nine problems (six for one instrument, three for the other) serious enough to require a service call. Instrument problems may be indicated by error messages displayed on the computer screen. Even when no error message is displayed, the coefficient of variation of duplicates, using 10% as a general limit of acceptability, provides a sensitive indicator of a variety of instrument malfunctions. A breakdown of instrument malfunctions is given in Table 5. Malfunctions listed are those serious enough to result in instrument downtime or assay failure.

Analysis of instrument malfunctions indicates that the mechanism and sensors that control assay rack and probe alignment appear to be the weak link in the system. Specifically, the steps associated with bead washing seem to be most subject to error. Various minor problems, often

Table 5 Photon-ERA Service History

Malfunction	Frequency	
	Instrument 1	Instrument 2
Increased frequency of high CVs of duplicates	2	7
Bead wash errors	4	3
Instrument "not homed" (sensors indicate probes or racks not in initial "home" position at assay start)	3	1
Probe failure	1	5
Miscellaneous pipetting errors	0	3
Computer failures	1	0

associated with bead washing, result in approximately two runs per week being repeated per instrument.

It should be noted that not all instrument errors are of equal consequence, nor are all errors fatal to assay performance. Errors on the sample processing side, while relatively rare, are fatal in that the assay must be restarted and already pipetted assay tubes must be replaced with new tubes and antibody-coated beads. This is early in the assay processing sequence, however, and little time is lost. Errors occurring in the reaction processor side are more frequent and potentially more serious, since by this time several hours may already have been spent in performing the assay. If an error occurs either very early or late in the bead wash/read process, it is sometimes possible to continue the assay manually with final readings made on an automated spectrophotometer such as the Hybritech Photon. Failures in the middle of the wash/read generally require that the assay be repeated from the beginning. Run failures at this point tend to be stressful for the operator since by this time several hours have been invested in the assay. Result turn around time may also be affected.

Help in troubleshooting and correcting problems is available from several sources. We have found that rebooting the computer will often correct malfunctions by resetting the various mechanisms to their "home" or starting point. There are also several software routines that specifically reset error conditions or allow the various probe and rack movements to be exercised. Hybritech provides a 3-day operator training course, on-site repair by Hybritech service engineers, and a 24-h hotline for telephone consultation.

IV. CONCLUSION

A. Performance Compared to Evaluation Goals

We hoped to achieve several goals when the Photon-ERA was introduced into our laboratory:

1. Automation of an already familiar technology. The Tandem-E assays for CK-MB and hCG have been in use in our laboratory for several years. Both assay performance characteristics and clinical interpretation of results are well known.

2. Improvement in assay precision. Improvement in both overall assay precision and coefficient of variation (CV) of duplicates was observed, but the improvement was not as large as expected. This suggests that factors other than pipetting and timing limit overall precision. These factors may be reagent related, such as uniformity of antibody coating on the beads or antibody-conjugate stability. Since improvement in precision was not as great as expected, we were not able to accomplish another goal, that of reducing patient assay tube replicates. We felt that the change in precision did not warrant a change from current practice of duplicate analysis. Also, poor CV of duplicates is often the only indicator of declining instrument performance or malfunction.

3. Reduction of hands-on time for assay performance. Although the instrument does not achieve the ultimate goal of full walk-away operation, the automation of the pipetting and wash/read steps does provide significant saving of technologist time of up to 1 h per run. It should be noted, however, that automation of the Tandem-E immunoassays on the Photon-ERA does not significantly reduce the total time required to produce assay results. This is due to the fact that the greatest blocks of assay time, the incubation steps, are fixed by assay protocol and are the same for both automated and manual operation.

B. Summary

In summary, the strengths and weaknesses of the Photon-ERA in our laboratory were as follows:

1. Weaknesses

1. There appears to be an engineering weakness in the reaction processor, particularly the bead wash components, that results in a higher-than-expected malfunction rate.

2. There is essentially no reduction in total assay performance time.

3. The amount of reagent handling and preparation is greater than typical for an automated system.

4. Total walk-away operation is not possible. Pipetted assay racks must be moved on and off the instrument manually for the primary incubation.

5. Run size is limited to 60 assay tubes (including calibrators and controls).

2. Strengths

1. The Photon-ERA uses proven chemistries with a good record of performance.

2. The same assay may be run either automated or manually with complete equivalence of results.

3. Automation provides precise pipetting, accurate timing of assay events, and absolute standardization of assay protocol, regardless of operator.

4. Significant reduction in assay hands-on time.

5. Hybritech provides a good menu of tests for the ERA. Some like CEA, CK-MB, and prolactin are not commonly available on automated systems.

6. The system controller is a PC-compatible computer. When the Photon-ERA is not in use, this computer is available to the laboratory for other uses.

CHAPTER 21

SR1 Immunoassay System

Laurence M. Demers
Department of Pathology and Medicine,
The Milton S. Hershey Medical Center,
Pennsylvania State University, Hershey, Pennsylvania

I. INTRODUCTION

The Serono-Baker SR1 is a random-access, cartridge-based, bench-top, fully automated immunoassay system designed to provide technologists with walk-away immunoassay technology with minimal operator intervention. The basic reagent system utilizes a bar-coded, self-contained cartridge that includes all of the antibody reagents and calibrators necessary to carry out the assay following the addition of patient sample to the cartridge. The assays on the system include both "sandwich-based" immunoenzymetric assays (IEMA) for large protein molecules and "competitive" enzyme immunoassay (EIA) for small molecules like thyroid hormone and ovarian steroids. The system utilizes a magnetic, solid-phase separation technology and a common reaction signal for all assays based on the color development of phenolphthalein. The SR1 instrument itself is a dual-channel colorimeter that can accomodate up to 80 tests at a time on a continuous basis. The instrument generates a time to first result that ranges from 35 to 102 min, depending on the analyte to be measured. The stated throughput of the analyzer is 55 test results per hour and the on-board standard curve stability claimed by the manufacturer is a minimum of 30 days. The SR1 system has the flexible capability of performing in either a batch, profile, stat, or random access mode.

Immunoassay Automation: A Practical Guide

II. THE SR1 TOTAL SYSTEM

A. Instrumentation

The instrument associated with the SR1 system is basically a colorimeter with the capability of reading at several wavelengths including 490, 554, and 650 nm. The purpose of the multiple wavelengths is to first provide a reading of the primary phenolphthalein colorimetric signal at 554 nm with a secondary reading at 490 nm, which is 20% of the maximal absorbance reading for phenolphthalein. This secondary wavelength provides for an extension of linearity without sacrificing precision at the low end and is reflexed to automatically once a peak color development has been achieved at 554 nm. A specimen blank reading is also taken at 650 nm. This is essential in reducing background interference for each sample.

As indicated previously, the SR1 instrument is a self-contained unit (Fig. 1) capable of performing all the steps necessary to produce a dose measurement of a patient sample. All reactions take place in the self-contained cartridge. Each cartridge carries a bar-code label that contains a serial number, an identification number for the analyte, and specific calibrator information for each cartridge. The calibrator information allows for a specific reference for the data reduction of that particular analyte. Before the placement of each cartridge into the system, the opera-

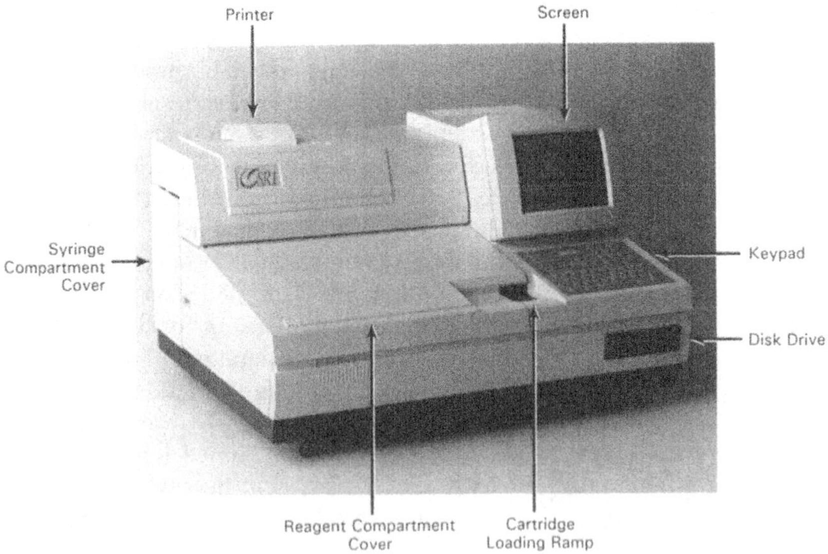

Figure 1 SR1 automated immunoassay instrument.

tor bar-code wands this information for each cartridge, which then registers that cartridge into the instrument.

The cartridges are loaded by the operator into the instrument by way of a small conveyer belt. Up to 11 cartridges will fit on the conveyer belt at one time. The conveyer belt automatically moves the cartridges into the center of the instrument where they are picked up by an extractor and transfered from the conveyer belt to a heated carousel where the pipetting, reagent transfers, and reaction incubation take place. The carousel will hold 30 cartridges at one time. At the completion of the assay process, the cartridges are transferred to a common wash station where magnetic pulldown and photometer readings take place. Once the final color has been read, all liquids are aspirated from the cartridges and the cartridges are then automatically disposed into a solid waste bin within the instrument. The solid waste container is emptied every 45 cartridges, liquid waste every 90 cartridges. Common reagents for the color development used by the system are located within the instrument itself and are replaced with every 90 cartridges processed.

B. Reagents

The SR1 utilizes specially designed cartridges as shown in Fig. 2. This figure depicts the component parts inherent to the cartridge for carrying out a unit dose assay. There is a space for two samples, two specific reagents, and a calibrator compartment, two reaction chambers, and two optical windows through which the photometer readings occur. Each cartridge contains a single-point calibrator and two antibody reagents. The single-point calibrator is referenced to a five-point standard curve, which is stored in memory within the computer system. A full five-point calibration is performed on a monthly basis. The standard curve interpolation utilizes a four-parameter fit routine for data reduction purposes. The calibrator located within the cartridge is utilized each time the operation of the system occurs in a random access mode but only in the first cartridge when the system operates in a batch mode.

For illustrative purposes, Fig. 3 depicts the processing of the cartridge system in either batch, profile, or random access mode.

The cartridge-based antibody reagents are different depending on the type of immunoassay method employed for a particular analyte, whether a "sandwich" or "competitive" format. The direct IEMA utilizes two monoclonal antibodies, one labeled with the enzyme alkaline phosphatase and the other labeled with fluorescein isothiocyanate (FITC). The competitive EIA, on the other hand, only utilizes one antibody, which is labeled with alkaline phosphatase. An FITC label form of the hormone to be

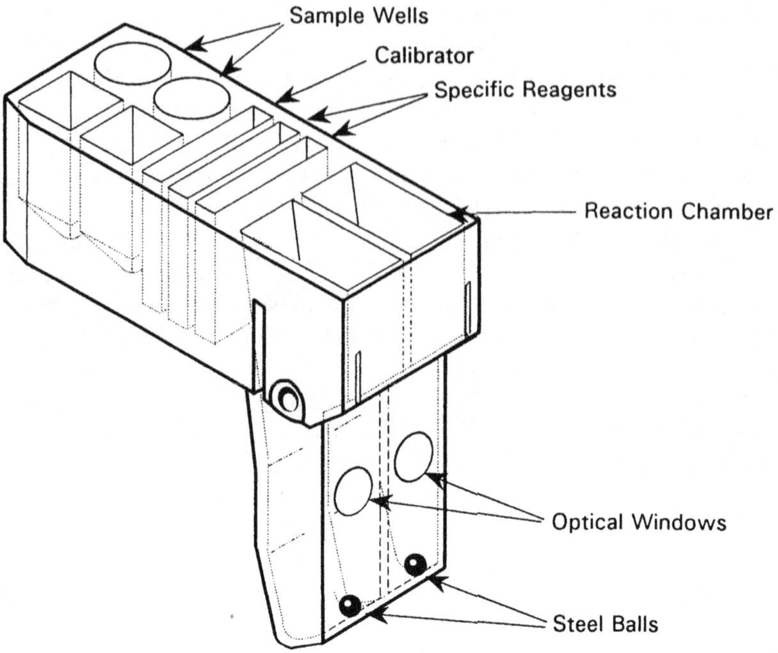

Figure 2 SR1 cartridge.

measured is then included in the other reagent well in the cartridge for the competitive EIA.

The bound-from-free separation process uses a paramagnetic microparticle separation reagent that consists of magnetic particles coated with anti-FITC antibody. The antibody is specific for FITC. In IEMA type assays (Fig. 4), the antigen–antibody complexes (containing equal amounts of hormone and enzyme) as well as unreacted excess FITC-labeled antibody combine with the magnetic separation reagent. In EIA type assays (Fig. 5) the magnetic particle separation reagent combines with all the FITC-labeled hormone, both free and combined with the enzyme-labeled antibody.

The substrate for the enzyme alkaline phosphatase used in these assays is phenolphthalein monophosphate. Free phenolphthalein is released in proportion to the amount of enzyme present and the intensity of the color development is then related to the concentration of the hormone present in the sample. In IEMA assays, the more color developed, the more hormone in the sample. In EIA assays, the more color developed, the lower the amount of hormone in the sample.

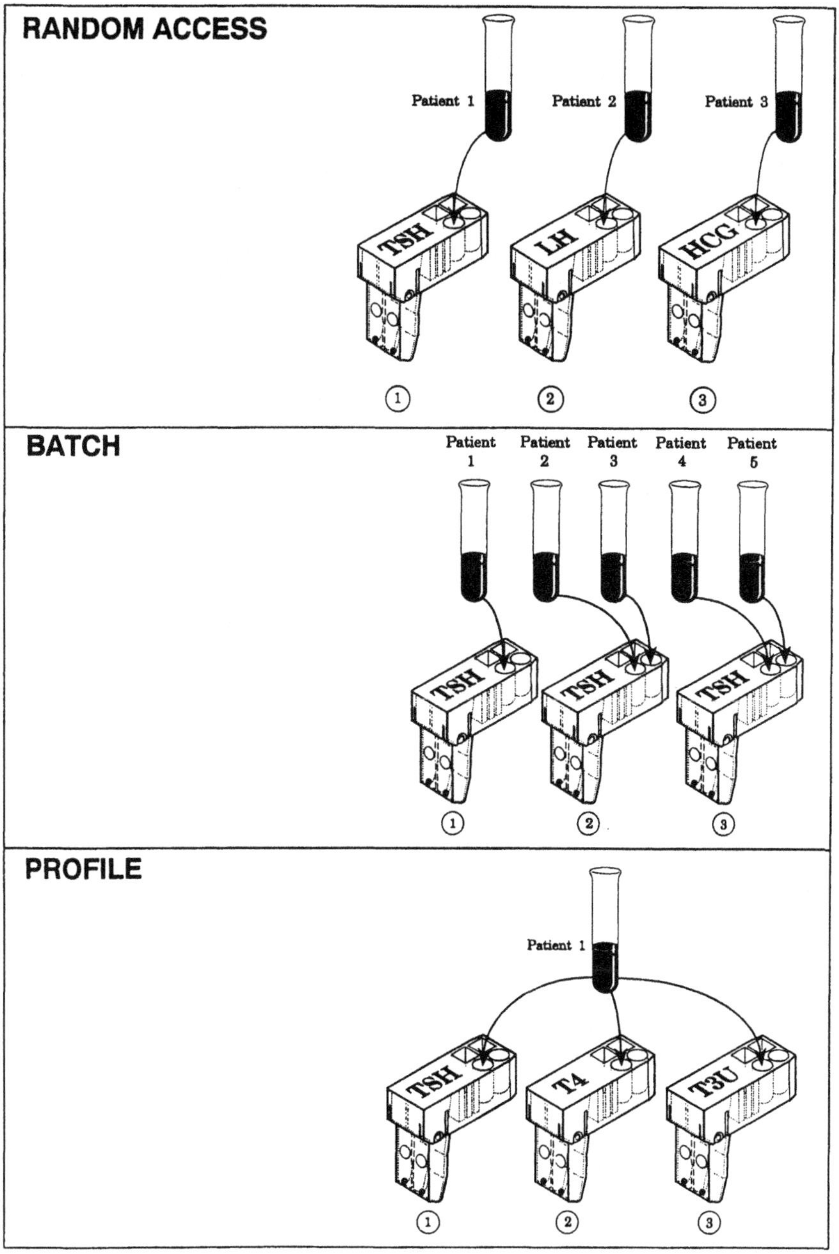

Figure 3 SR1 cartridge used in random access, batch, or profile modes.

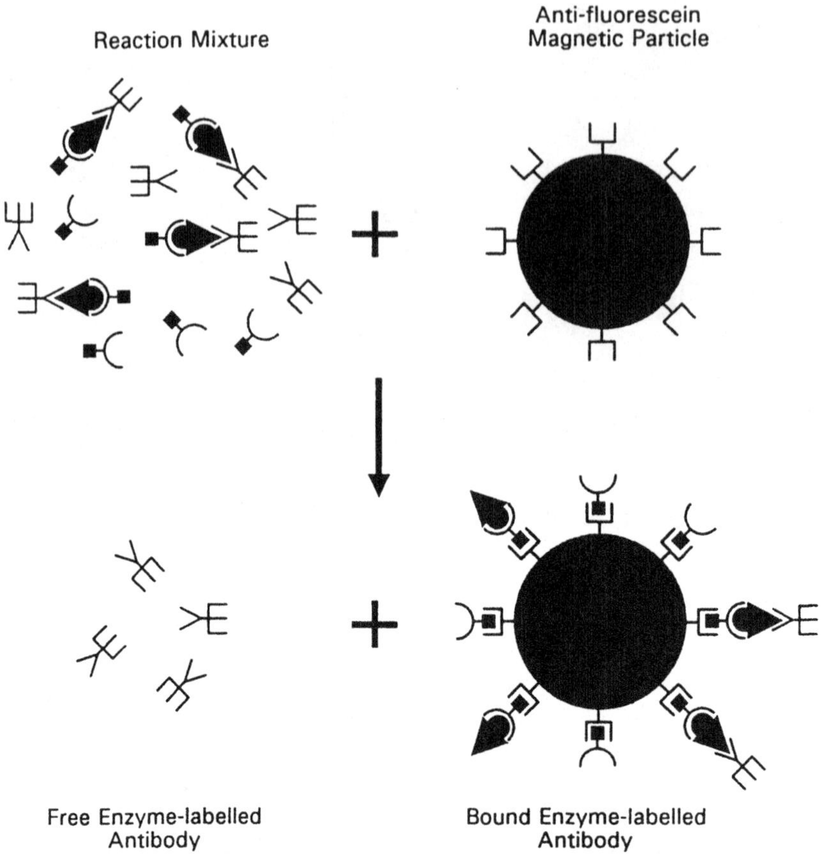

Figure 4 IEMA separation reaction.

The system operation is obviously influenced by whether the assays are to be performed as random access or batch or whether an IEMA or EIA method is desired. The following summarizes the operation in these various modes.

Random Access

1. Transfer patient sample into well A.
2. Read bar-code data by wand and enter patient ID (optional).
3. Place cartridge on conveyer.

Batch Mode

1. Transfer single patient sample into well A of first cartridge.
2. Transfer two patient samples into wells A and B for rest of batch.

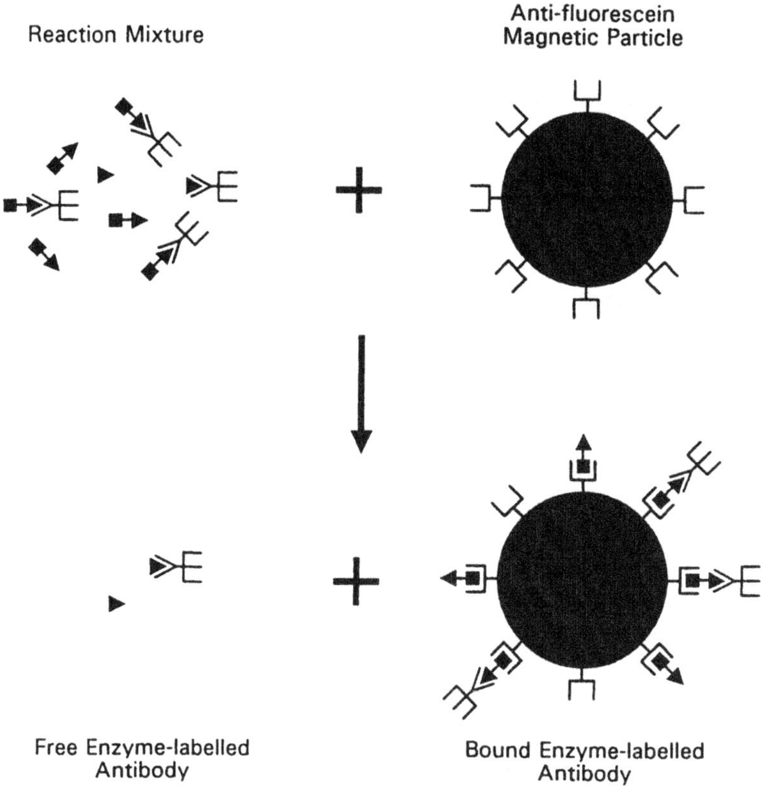

Figure 5 EIA separation reaction.

3. Read barcode data by wand into worklist and if desired enter patient ID, and/or dilution.

4. Place cartridges on conveyer, taking care to load calibrator cartridge first.

IEMA Operation

1. Cartridge transfered onto carousel from conveyer belt.
2. Sample, FITC-labeled antibody (Ab), and E-Ab transferred to reaction well A.
3. Calibrator (first cartridge only with batch mode) or sample, FITC-Ab,and E-Ab transferred to reaction well B.
4. Cartridge incubated at 37°C on the carousel.
5. Anti-FITC-labeled magnetic solid phase added to wells A and B.
6. After incubation, magnet applied to isolate FITC complex.

7. Wells washed and phenolphthalein monophosphate added.
8. Cartridge is then mixed to release FITC complex to incubate with substrate.
9. An alkaline stop solution is then added, causing pink phenolphthalein color.
10. Magnet is then applied to remove solid phase out of suspension.
11. Photometer reads at 650, 554, and 490 nm.

EIA Operation

1. Cartridge transfered onto carousel from conveyer belt.
2. Sample, E-Ab, and FITC-labeled hormone transferred to reaction well A.
3. Calibrator (first cartridge only with batch mode) or sample, E-Ab, and FITC-labeled hormone transferred to reaction well B.
4. Cartridge incubated at 37°C on the carousel.
5. Separation and substrate incubation proceed as per IEMA.

III. SR1 PERFORMANCE

A. Technical Performance

The SR1 currently has the capacity to perform 10 different immunoassays with another seven procedures close to release (Table 1). The manufacturer has chosen to approach a more highly specialized test menu at the initial offering to target specialty clinics for unit dose testing support. This is evident by the introductory test menu, which focuses on fertility testing in support of infertility and *in vitro* fertilization programs at reproductive

Table 1 SR1 Test Menu

Currently available	1991 introduction
LH	Free T_4
FSH	Progesterone
hCG	Cortisol
Prolactin	B-12
Estradiol	Folate
Ferritin[a]	Testosterone
TSH[a]	CK-MB
T_3[a]	
T_4[a]	
T_3U[a]	

[a] Pending FDA Approval.

centers across the United States and Europe. There have been numerous evaluation and clinical studies performed in Europe with this system; however, the information available in the United States is presently limited to either the Serono-Baker site in Allentown, Pennsylvania, or to a few clinical laboratories like our own that are currently performing an evaluation of the system. From the manufacturer's viewpoint, the precision, accuracy, and comparison studies have been encouraging. A select example of the performance studies generated with the SR 1 is shown in Figs. 6 and 7 and Tables 2–6.

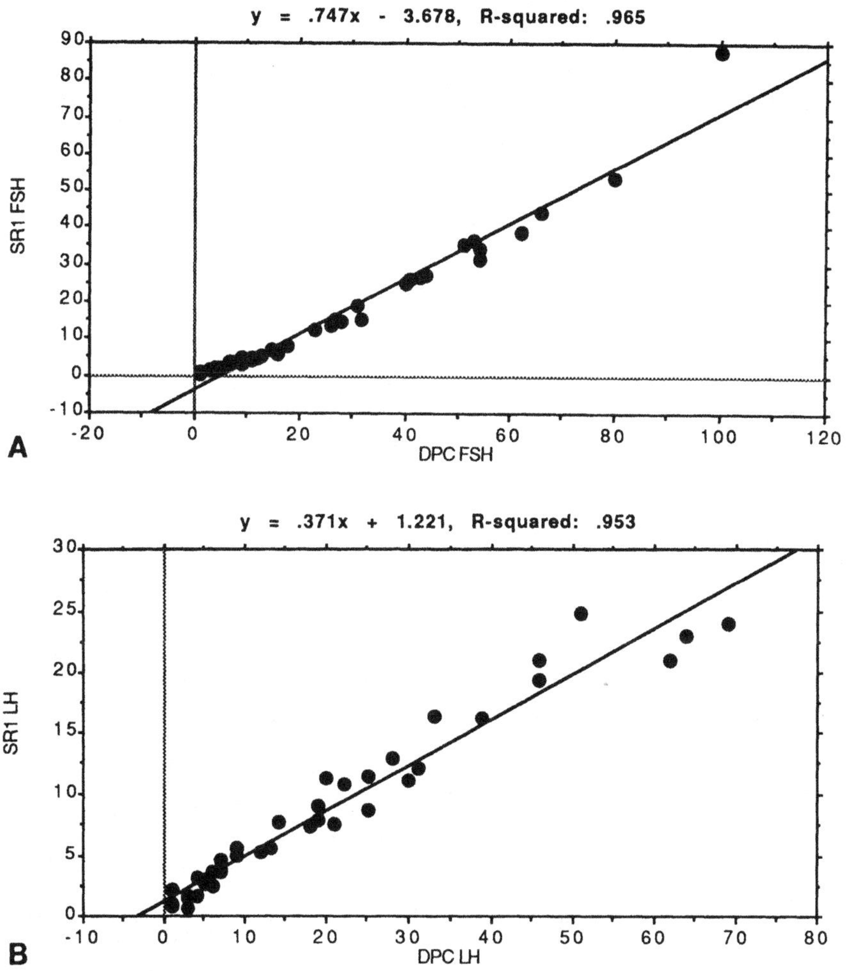

Figure 6 Comparison of (A) FSH and (B) LH results between the SR1 and Diagnostic Products Corporation (DPC) reagents.

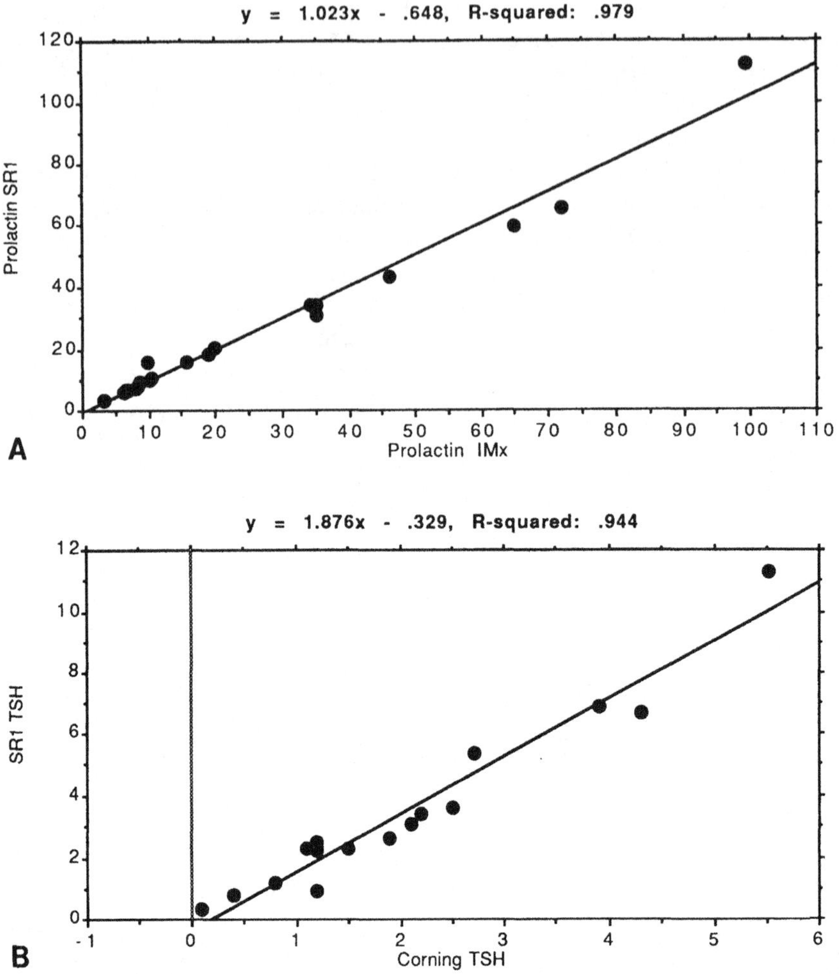

Figure 7 Comparison of (A) prolactin and (B) TSH results between the SR1 and DPC reagents.

To date the precision and accuracy results for the analytes tested have been impressive and suggest acceptable performance for the tests currently on the system. It should be noted, however, that most of the performance has been generated with the IEMA technology applied to large protein molecules like human chorionic gonadotropin (hCG) and thyroid-stimulating hormone (TSH). The proof of the pudding, so to speak, will come when the performances of the small-molecule assays like the steroids are evaluated.

Table 2 Assay Performance: Linearity on Dilution, hCG[a]

Dilution faction	*n*	Percent neat value	SD
1 in 2	12	101	5.1
1 in 4	12	102	7.2
1 in 8	12	98	7.0
1 in 16	12	93	12.0
Overall	**48**	**99**	**8.8**

[a] Twelve serum samples containing concentrations of hCG within the assay range (1–500 mIU/ml) were diluted 1 in 2, 1 in 4, 1 in 8, and 1 in 16 in zero standard matrix, then assayed to determine linearity on dilution. The study was performed on several instruments, and two batches of cartridges and common reagents, which were used in a crossover manner. The average percent neat value was 99%, which indicates a correct reagent matrix for the assay.

In our laboratory, we have now had the chance to evaluate and compare four protein hormone assays with the SR1. The comparison results, which are essentially summarized by the scattergrams noted in Figs. 6 and 7, appear to be quite acceptable for the four protein hormones

Table 3 Assay Performance: Linearity on Further Dilution, hCG[a]

Dilution factor	*n*	Percent neat value	SD
1 in 200	5	102	2.3
1 in 400	5	102	5.0
1 in 800	5	99	4.0
1 in 1000	4	100	2.6
1 in 1600	5	101	2.3
1 in 2000	4	99	3.3
1 in 4000	4	97	3.7
1 in 8000	4	104	8.0
Overall	**36**	**100**	**4.3**

[a] Serum samples containing concentrations of hCG above the assay range (>500 mIU/ml) were diluted 1 in 200, 1 in 400, 1 in 800, 1 in 1000, 1 in 1600, 1 in 2000, 1 in 4000, and 1 in 8000, in SR1 hCG diluent, then assayed on the SR1 system to determine linearity on dilution. The study was performed on several instruments, and two batches of cartridges and common reagents, which were used in a crossover manner. The average percent neat value was 100%.

Table 4 Assay Performance: Accuracy, hCG[a]

hCG added (mIU/ml)	*n*	Mean percent recovery	SD
20.2	5	104	14.1
41.7	5	99	5.5
81.7	5	98	9.6
162.1	5	92	8.4
260.5	5	94	1.1
Overall	**25**	**97**	**9.3**

[a] Accuracy is a measure of how close the SR1 measurement of hCG comes to the real level of hCG present in the serum sample. Accuracy is determined by adding known quantities of hCG to serum samples which have low levels of hCG, assaying the serum and determining the recovery of the amount added. Five patient samples were used to determine the accuracy of the assay. The amounts of hCG added were selected to cover the range of the assay. The study was performed on several instruments, and two batches of cartridges and common reagents, which were used in a crossover manner. Recovery of added hCG averaged 97%.

tested. The correlation statistics compare favorably well to established radioimmunoassay (RIA) and microparticle capture enzyme immunoassay (MEIA) methods in our laboratory. The results we generated are still rather limited but our overall impression is that the SR1 does produce accurate and reasonably precise results for the gonadotropins follicle-stimulating hormone (FSH) and luteinizing hormone (LH) and for pro-

Table 5 Assay Performance: Linearity on Dilution, TSH[a]

Dilution factor	*n*	Percent neat value	SD
1 in 2	16	99.7	3.3
1 in 4	16	97.7	4.8
1 in 8	16	96.9	3.8
1 in 16	16	97.8	7.5
1 in 32	16	99.4	9.3
Overall	**80**	**98.3**	**5.7**

[a] Sixteen serum samples containing concentrations of TSH within the assay range (0.05–50 μIU/ml) were diluted 1 in 2, 1 in 4, 1 in 8, 1 in 16, and 1 in 32 in zero standard matrix, then assayed to determine linearity on dilution. The study was performed on several instruments, using two batches of cartridges and common reagents. The average percent neat value was 98%, which indicates a correct reagent matrix for the assay.

Table 6 Assay Performance: Accuracy, TSH[a]

TSH added (μIU/ml)	*n*	Mean percent recovery	SD
1.94	4	100.9	9.3
4.75	4	117.6	11.1
15.47	4	97.8	14.8
26.42	4	108.2	6.1
37.68	4	103.6	5.8
Overall	**20**	**105.6**	**7.7**

[a] Accuracy is a measure of how close the SR1 measurement of TSH comes to the real level of TSH present in the serum sample. Accuracy is determined by adding known quantities of TSH to serum samples that have low levels of TSH, assaying the serum, and determining the recovery of the amount added. Four patient samples were used to determine the accuracy of the assay. The amounts of TSH added were selected to cover the range of the assay. The study was performed on several instruments, using two batches of cartridges and common reagents. Recovery of added TSH averaged 106%.

lactin. We did note a minor discrepancy with the absolute levels of the gonadotropins when compared to Diagnostic Products Corporation radioimmunoassay reagents. However, although the mean values were lower by the SR1 method, the SR1 gonadotropin reagents are referenced to the same international reference preparations as for the DPC reagents in a one-to-one relationship. DPC uses a factor that inflates the absolute numbers by about 40% for purposes of standard concentration assignment. Thus a systematic bias was observed, although a high degree of correlation was obtained for the gonadotropin assays.

B. Instrument and Reagent Performance

Overall, the technologists found the SR1 to be user friendly with a minimum of training required to competently operate the system. They likened its use to the Dupont ACA in that one simply has to place a patient sample into the sample well of the cartridge, place the cartridge into the system, activate the system via the computer terminal, and wait for the result. On-board calibration of the standard curve, calibration of each cartridge, and a lack of sample or reagent preparation time reduce the technologist effort in operating the system. The system operates quite well in a random access mode with a "one-test-at-a-time" output much along the lines of the ACA. The size of the instrument is also a favorable consideration in that it only occupies a small amount of bench-top space. There is no need for water or waste hookup, and the instrument can be placed into any small specialty clinic laboratory or physician's office laboratory without the need for extensive remodeling. The instrument does generate a continuous low-level sound, particularly during the magnetic particle mixing phase. The sound, however, does not appear to be that obstrusive to the technologists working in the area. The instrument itself has not experienced any significant down time in our hands, and the maintenance requirements are quite minimal to maintain the system.

The operator controls the instrument via an easy-to-use computer keyboard that is part of the unit. The display terminal is easy to read and alerts the operator at the start of a run about common reagent inventory, waste disposal needs, and instrument status before commencing a run. The computer has a few attractive, built-in features for quality assurance monitoring that could facilitate the workload and quality control paperwork for the small laboratory.

As for the reagent cartridge, everything is self-contained and the bar-code wand introduces the cartridge into the system in terms of analyte and calibrator information. The operator only has to enter the patient ID and provide dilution factors when applicable. Working with the cartridges could become an issue in some laboratories in that unlike tubes, they do not fit into a standard tube rack and cannot be simply lined up to add the patient sample. A special cartridge rack, however, is supplied by the manufacturer to hold the cartridges during specimen addition, which does provide some help. Another problem spot with the cartridge could be with the patient sample addition step. The well port where one places the patient sample is quite small and requires a concerted effort for proper sample placement, particularly when two different patients are sharing the same cartridge as with a batch assay. Sample entry into the system is also somewhat limited in the sense that individual sample pipetting to each cartridge is required. A built-in carousel entry for multiple samples would be more desirable for the higher-volume laboratory.

C. System Costs

Although the reagent costs are expected to be competitive with other competitive immunoassay reagents ($2–4/test), the reagent cost figures have not been finalized for this system in the United States. As expected of a system of this size and capability, the unit will most likely be sold along the lines of reagent rental rather than through outright purchase of the instrument. This is particularly important to parts of the intended audience for this system, that is, specialty clinics and physician offices where capital equipment outlay is difficult to obtain. The university hospital laboratory supporting an *in vitro* fertilization program and fertility clinic will also see an appeal from this type of system to individually support these programs at the practice site.

IV. CONCLUSIONS

The Serono-Baker SR1 is a bench-top immunoassay analyzer that should fit a niche in the small to medium clinical laboratory with demands of up to 200–300 tests/day for the test menu supported by this system. Advantages of the SR1 include its random access capability for the small-volume user who heretofore had to send out tests like LH, FSH, and prolactin because of a lack of commitment to RIA. The complete self-sufficiency of the system makes it an ideal walk-away unit (ACA-like) with minimal operator intervention once the cartridges have been placed on the system. The time to first result is another appealing advantage of this system that will attract the infertility specialists who require daily estradiol levels as part of infertility treatment and monitoring. The clinicians working in this area now must wait almost a full working day before an RIA-based estradiol result can be generated.

In terms of technologist acceptance and the user friendliness of the instrument, the SR1 has immediate appeal. Most technologists working with the system achieved competency in running the system within 1 day of operation. The low maintenance requirements of the system are an additional positive feature of the SR1 commented upon by the technologists.

From a technical perspective, the liquid-based technology employing a dual monoclonal antibody principle is very attractive and imparts the kind of specificity desired in immunoassay methodology. In addition, the extended linearity created by the innovative second wavelength reading could be a plus, although this principle has not been fully tested in the practicing, clinical immunoassay laboratory. The blanking of each sample to reduce matrix interference effects is also an obvious advantage of this system and imparts an important degree to the sensitivity of the methods on the unit.

Test menu is another consideration. It is clear that this instrument is initially targeted for specialized laboratory testing needs and for the small- to medium-volume clinical laboratory. Everyone likes to see thyroid hormones as part of an automated immunoasssay system; however, not too many analyzers also have a focus on fertility tests support such as the SR1 has.

From the disadvantages viewpoint, there are a few considerations that should be discussed. The sample entry mode as alluded to is not that convenient in the handling of cartridges, and the pipetting of sample into a small sample well is somewhat restrictive. For the small laboratory handling only a few samples at a time this could be just a minor problem. For the busy, high-volume clinical laboratory, this could be a nuisance and a source of technologist error.

Although the reagents have a positive ID capability, the sample ID must be entered into the system by the operator. Although not a major problem, this could lead to a potential source of error. The relatively large sample volume required for most of the assays is another potential problem area that could arise, particularly when supporting a pediatric unit. The average sample volume is 200 μl, which could be prohibitive with some of the pediatric thyroid test needs.

As far as sample throughput is concerned, the output per hour is relatively modest with the SR1; however, throughput is only important in the medium- to large-volume laboratory. Throughput is undoubtedly a nonissue in the small clinic laboratory environment or in the physician office setting, where samples appear one at a time.

The final disadvantage would be the question regarding the proven sensitivity of this colorimetric-based immunassay technology. Most immunoassayists would agree that the closest signal to isotopic decay in terms of sensitivity is either chemiluminescence or time-resolved fluorescence. When one dwells in the realm of nanogram to picogram per milliliter sensitivity, such as we require with estradiol and progesterone measurements, a big question mark arises as to whether the phenolphthalein-based colorimetric signal is sensitive and strong enough to reproduce consistently at the nanogram/picogram level. Clinical trials will certainly be forthcoming to validate and test the sensitivity question with the SR1 as it finds its way into more clinical laboratories. The manufacturer appears confident that the sensitivity issue will not be a problem and that by virtue of the blanking and two wavelength reading capability of the analyzer, the system should be able to operate effectively at the nanogram to picogram level of sensitivity.

CHAPTER 22

STRATUS II IMMUNOASSAY SYSTEM

Stephen E. Kahn and Edward W. Bermes, Jr.
Departments of Pathology and Biochemistry,
Loyola University Medical Center, Maywood, Illinois

I. INTRODUCTION

The Stratus II immunoassay system is an automated immunoassay analyzer manufactured by Baxter Diagnostics, Inc., or BDI (Miami, Florida). The unique analytical features of the original Stratus as well as those of the innovative technique employed, radial partition immunoassay, were first reported to clinical laboratorians in 1982 (Giegel *et al.,* 1982). In 1983, Stratus was released to the clinical laboratory market by American Dade, which was then a Division of American Hospital Supply (both companies being subsequently acquired by Baxter Healthcare Corporation, which was recently reorganized as BDI). The introductory test menu of the Stratus was not extensive, consisting of assays for eight therapeutic drugs and thyroxine. But the instrument utilized a solid-phase fluorescent enzyme-labeling methodology that provided an innovative alternative to radioimmunoassay and other nonisotopic immunoassay methods.

In 1989, BDI introduced the Stratus II immunoassay system. This was a fully automated batch immunoassay analyzer that, unlike the earlier Stratus model, had a dilutor module built into the main frame of the analyzer. A strong corporate commitment to research and development has been sustained throughout the life history of Stratus and Stratus II. In

Immunoassay Automation: A Practical Guide

the past 10 years, the menu has evolved to 27 tests for measurement of large and small molecules in the areas of therapeutic drug monitoring, reproductive endocrinology, thyroid function, general endocrinology, cardiac disease, anemia, and the allergic response.

Also in 1989, BDI announced a joint venture with Hybritech, Inc. (San Diego, California). A focus of this joint venture was to adapt several Hybritech assays, particularly tumor markers in the oncology area, to the Stratus II. Incorporation of these tests into an already broad test menu on Stratus II and future Stratus models should benefit both corporate partners in this joint venture. Most importantly, the expanded test menu resulting from this joint venture should provide present and future Stratus users with a substantial degree of flexibility in work-load organization and testing configuration for their laboratories.

II. SYSTEM DESCRIPTION

A. Instrumentation

1. System Overview

The Stratus II Immunoassay System is a batch/STAT processing bench-top instrument and is diagrammatically illustrated in Fig. 1. Stratus II performs fluorometric immunoassay tests on plastic disposable reagent/matrix filter paper slides or "tabs" for each patient specimen, calibrator, or control material. Stratus II contains a 30-position sample carousel, tab magazine and feed subsystem, transport mechanisms, three fluid transfer subsystems, a front-surface fluorometric optical system, tab disposal, data input keyboard, display, printer plus power supplies, dilutor module, computer, and an exterior housing for all of the components. The Stratus did not house an on-board dilutor module (Heller *et al.,* 1984).

Designed as a bench-top immunoassay analyzer, Stratus II has compact dimensions. The analyzer is approximately 46.4 cm high (with carousel cover), 48.3 cm deep, and 91.5 cm wide (Plaut and McLellan, 1991). Additionally, approximately 5 cm in depth is required for the rear fan housing while an additional 15 cm in width is required for distilled water and buffer bottles. Stratus II operates on 120 VAC or 220 VAC power, generates minimal heat, operates over an ambient temperature range from 22 to 32°C, and requires no special plumbing facilities.

General details of the Stratus II subsystems are described in the following section. Full details of system description and complete operational characteristics are located in the Operator's Manual for the Stratus II Fluorometric Analyzer (Baxter Healthcare Corporation, Miami, Florida, 1989).

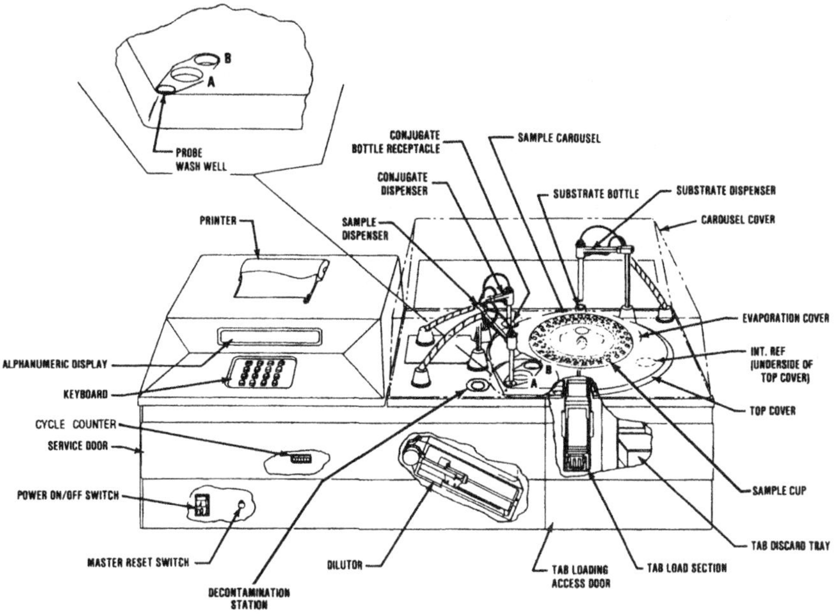

Figure 1 The Stratus II immunoassay system. From the Stratus II Immunoassay System Operator's Manual (1989, Figure 3-1, p. 3-4, Baxter Diagnostics, Inc., Miami, Florida).

2. Subsystem Description

a. Transport System, Sample Carousel, and Heating System Patient specimens are loaded in sample cups on the sample, or inner, carousel (Fig. 1). The minimum specimen volume is 0.2 ml. Reagent tabs are stored in the tab loading section and are discarded in the tab discard tray after use. Up to 30 tabs for a single assay can be loaded at one time for batch analyses. A stepper motor transport system moves the top tab around the outer carousel, indexing the tab to different stations in a clockwise motion. Tabs can be continuously loaded and discarded during a batch run. Unused tabs should not be stored on-board the analyzer and should be returned to the refrigerator after a batch run. In a synchronic motion, the transport system rotates the inner sample carousel with the outer tab carousel. This allows up to 30 patient samples to be loaded on the inner carousel, while 10 tabs are processed on the outer carousel.

In the tab transport system, a dual heating system is employed to maintain the tab at appropriate temperatures. The first heating system uses resistance heating elements to bring up the tab temperature (38 ± 0.5°C) to a level close to that required for reading of the reaction rate. The second heating system, located at the front-face fluorescent optical head, uses a thermoelectric solid-state device to maintain a constant temperature, 40 ± 0.5°C, during the reaction measurement period (Giegel *et al.*, 1982; Heller *et al.*, 1984; Plaut and McLellan, 1991).

b. Fluid Handling Systems The three dispensing stations utilized for fluid handling on the Stratus II are the sample dispenser, conjugate dispenser and substrate dispenser (Fig. 1). At the sample dispenser, a probe wash station (or well) allows the sample dispenser tip to be washed after each patient sample transfer to minimize carryover. A decontamination station is also included at this location for any assays that require additional cleaning of the sample probe. At the conjugate dispenser, enzyme-labeled conjugate can be added to the tab in sequential fashion after the patient sample. Enzyme-labeled conjugate can also be dispensed at the sample dispenser. A substrate dispenser is used for the substrate/wash reagent, which washes unbound antigen or antibody from the central matrix of the tab and also generates a reaction rate through the addition of substrate.

All of the Stratus II assays are either competitive, sequential saturation, or sandwich immunoassays. The enzyme-labeled conjugate is dispensed at the sample dispense station if the assay is a competitive immunoassay. If the assay is a sequential saturation or sandwich assay, the enzyme-labeled conjugate is dispensed at the conjugate dispenser. That is, sequential and sandwich assays add conjugate after the sample and use all three dispense stations. Competitive assays add conjugate with the sample (and do not use the conjugate dispense station). Since all assays require a substrate wash solution, this station is always used. Any requirements for placement of the various reagent bottles at specific dispense stations are clearly described in the protocols for each assay provided by the manufacturer. Liquid level sensors also verify proper placement of reagents for each test protocol.

With the Stratus, any assay steps to predilute the patient specimen had to be performed with a separate dilutor prior to placing the specimen on the analyzer. But Stratus II has an on-board, programmable dilutor module (Fig. 1). In addition to automatically diluting patient samples for some assays, the on-board dilutor in Stratus II provides a means for washing the sample probe in every assay. Customized wash protocols can be programmed for specific assays, which can be useful if the potential for carryover is high. The dilutor provides a mechanism for mixing sample, conjugate, and/or diluent as the specific test protocol requires. It can dispense enzyme-labeled conjugate and generally serves as the aspiration/discharge mechanism for the sample dispenser. The dilutor can perform serial dilutions. Nine different dilution protocols can be programmed and stored in the analyzer. For each serial dilution performed, an additional sample cup is used (for example, 10 specimens that require a second serial dilution would use 20 sample cup spaces on the 30 position carousel).

Liquid level sensors are used at all three dispense stations and are a permanent part of the aspiration probes. These sensors serve a twofold purpose. Use of level sensors minimizes the penetration of the probes into the reagents or sample. Additionally, the level sensors provide a mechanism to determine if sufficient reagents are available to perform a programmed batch run. Before initiating a batch run, these sensors perform an inventory check to verify that reagents are located in their proper positions. If the reagents are not detected in the appropriate location, a message is displayed on the alphanumeric display (as shown in Fig. 1) to alert the operator of the problem.

c. Fluorometric Optical System The Stratus II read station employs a front surface fluorometer to measure reaction rates (Giegel *et al.*, 1982; Heller *et al.*, 1984). To maintain a constant temperature and minimize reaction drift due to thermal effects, all fluorometer components are fitted within a temperature-controlled enclosure. These components include the low-pressure mercury lamp, excitation filter, emission filter, dichroic mirror, reference diode, and photomultiplier (PMT) detector. A Hoya U-360 ultraviolet transmitting filter is used at the excitation stage and a 450-nm filter is used for emission wavelength transmission to a conventional photomultiplier tube.

Excitation light strikes the underside of the tab and the emitted fluorescence is read. There are two zones of fluorescent reactivity on the tab—a central circle and a peripheral ring. Antibody-bound conjugate due to the presence of the antigen of interest is localized in the center of the filter tab. Unbound conjugate is eluted, or radially partitioned, to the outside of the measurement zone. Emitted light from the central tab reaction site is converted to electrical signals by the PMT and processed through an electronic analog-to-digital conversion network. The microprocessor stores 100 kinetic fluorescent readings at 0.2-s intervals (Heller *et al.*, 1984). Since a kinetic measurement is employed rather than an end-point measurement, background fluorescence does not result in significant interference.

Reaction rate emission signals are compared to those of stored standard curves. These previously stored rates will have been obtained from appropriate blank samples and multiple levels of calibrators. Stratus II also houses an internal reference, which is activated at the beginning of each measurement cycle to adjust system gain. This internal reference is used as a diagnostic component to verify optical/electronics system operation. Digitized signals are shown on the visual display and printed on paper tape, but an RS-232 output permits transmission of measured data to an off-line computer system at the end of each batch run.

d. Microprocessor, Key Pad, and Printer The operator interacts with the Stratus II through the 16-character key pad and the 20-character alphanumeric display (Fig. 1). The Stratus II is operated by an Intel 8088

16-bit microprocessor (De Cresce and Lifshitz, 1990). There is 512 kB of random access memory (RAM), 512 kB of read only memory (ROM), and a battery backed-up RAM to maintain calibration data and control lot data. Battery backed-up microchips store keyboard assay parameters, sample profile steps, and other user-defined information. Relevant parameters on available assays are programmed into the Stratus II prior to shipment. But the user can exercise the option of keying in additional assays because Stratus II can store as many as 100 separate test protocols.

Use of the microprocessor provides the capability to monitor important operational parameters such as reference voltages and temperatures (Giegel *et al.*, 1982). If any of these parameters drift outside of acceptable limits, a flagged message is displayed to the operator. The operator views a series of prompts in the alphanumeric display at the beginning of each test run to ensure proper analyzer setup. Interactive routines are also utilized for stepping through each phase of instrument calibration with the operator until the calibration is complete.

There is storage of patient results for one test run, which can be retrieved by sequence number if the printer fails. With each new test run, patient results from the previous run are automatically purged. Hard-copy results of assay data, diagnostic readings, and calibration curves are printed on a 10-cm-wide, 40-character alphanumeric thermal printer. Due to the presence of an RS-232 serial port, there is also the capability to transfer data from the Stratus II to a host computer for permanent data storage.

B. Principles of Analysis and Measurement

1. Immunoassay and Separation Methodology

Available methods on the Stratus II are either competitive, sequential saturation, or sandwich immunoassays. As of June 1991, there were 27 assays available on Stratus II. These assays, the general assay classes, and the corresponding immunoassay methodology employed are listed in Table 1. Competitive or sequential saturation immunoassays are employed for measurement of low-molecular-weight molecules such as therapeutic drugs, thyroid hormones, and cortisol. The sandwich immunoassay method is employed for measurement of high-molecular-weight molecules such as polypeptide hormones, creatine kinase MB (CK-MB), immunoglobulin E (IgE), and ferritin.

The separation methodology is radial partition immunoassay (Giegel *et al.*, 1982). This method is a hybrid of chromatographic and solid-phase enzyme immunoassay techniques. The reaction tabs contain a preimmobilized antibody raised against the antigen of interest. When the sample

Table 1 Stratus II Immunoassay System Test Menu[a,b]

Assay category	Analyte	Type of immunoassay utilized
Therapeutic drugs	Amikacin	Competitive
	Carbamazepine	Competitive
	Digitoxin	Sequential saturation
	Digoxin	Sequential saturation
	Gentamicin	Competitive
	Lidocaine	Competitive
	Phenobarbital	Competitive
	Phenytoin	Competitive
	Primidone	Competitive
	Procainamide	Competitive
	N-Acetyl procainamide	Competitive
	Quinidine	Competitive
	Theophylline	Competitive
	Tobramycin	Competitive
Reproductive endocrinology	Human chorionic Gonadotropin (hCG)	Sandwich
	Human follicle-stimulating hormone (hFSH)	Sandwich
	Human luteinizing hormone (hLH)	Sandwich
	Prolactin (PRL)	Sandwich
Thyroid function assays	Total T_3	Sequential saturation
	Total T_4	Sequential saturation
	Free T_4	Sequential saturation
	Human thyroid-stimulating hormone (hTSH)	Sandwich
	Thyroid uptake (TU)	Sequential saturation
Other assays	CK-MB	Sandwich
	Cortisol	Competitive
	Ferritin	Sandwich
	IgE	Sandwich

[a] Available test menu as of June 1991.
[b] Assays under development that are due to be released in mid 1991 are listed at the end of this chapter.

antigen is added, the antigen binds to the immobilized antibody. Once other steps in the reaction sequence have occurred (which vary depending on the immunoassay methodology employed), unbound enzyme-labeled antigen is radially eluted (or partitioned) to the periphery of the reaction tab, forming a second "ring" of reactivity around the reaction zone in the center of the tab.

For competitive immunoassays, the sample antigen of interest is premixed with the enzyme-labeled antigen conjugate and is spotted on the center portion of the reaction tab, which contains preimmobilized antibody. Sample antigen and enzyme-labeled antigen compete for binding sites on the antibody molecule. When substrate/wash solution is applied, unbound conjugate is washed from the central reaction zone through radial partition elution. Since substrate is included with the wash solution, the enzymatic reaction occurs simultaneously with the wash.

For sequential saturation immunoassays, the sample antigen of interest is prediluted and is spotted on the center portion of the reaction tab, which contains preimmobilized antibody. After sample antigen binds to the immobilized antibody, the enzyme-labeled antigen conjugate is added and binds to unoccupied antibody binding sites. Substrate/wash solution is applied, unbound conjugate is radially washed from the central reaction zone, and the enzymatic reaction is initiated.

For sandwich immunoassays, the undiluted sample antigen of interest is spotted onto the center portion of the reaction tab, which contains preimmobilized antibody. Generally, antibodies employed for the various sandwich assays are monoclonal. After a short incubation period, a conjugate consisting of an enzyme-labeled second monoclonal antibody is added. This forms an antibody/antigen/labeled antibody sandwich. The second antibody is directed against a different epitope, that is, different antigenic sites, than the first antibody. Substrate/wash solution is applied, unbound labeled antibody is radially washed from the central reaction zone, and the enzymatic reaction is initiated.

2. Enzymatic/Fluorescence Detection Methodology

As an example of the enzymatic/fluorescence detection methodology employed, the analytical basis of the detection for the Stratus II CK-MB assay is diagrammatically illustrated in Fig. 2. The first antibody is a murine monoclonal anti-CKMB IgG preimmobilized onto the surface of the reaction tab by Fc fragment-specific goat antisera to murine IgG. After patient sample is added and CK-MB is bound to the immobilized antibody, enzyme-labeled anti-CK-B conjugate is added to form a sandwich around the CK-MB antigen. This second antibody/enzyme-labeled conjugate is calf intestinal alkaline phosphatase covalently linked to murine monoclonal anti-CK-BB Fab′. The substrate/wash solution contains 4-methylumbelliferyl phosphate, which serves as the alkaline phosphatase substrate. After the enzymatic reaction has occurred, the rate of chromagen formation is measured. As illustrated in Fig. 2, 4-methylumbelliferone can be detected by front-face fluorometry in the center of the reaction tab (antibody-bound antigen or CK-MB). A second ring of reac-

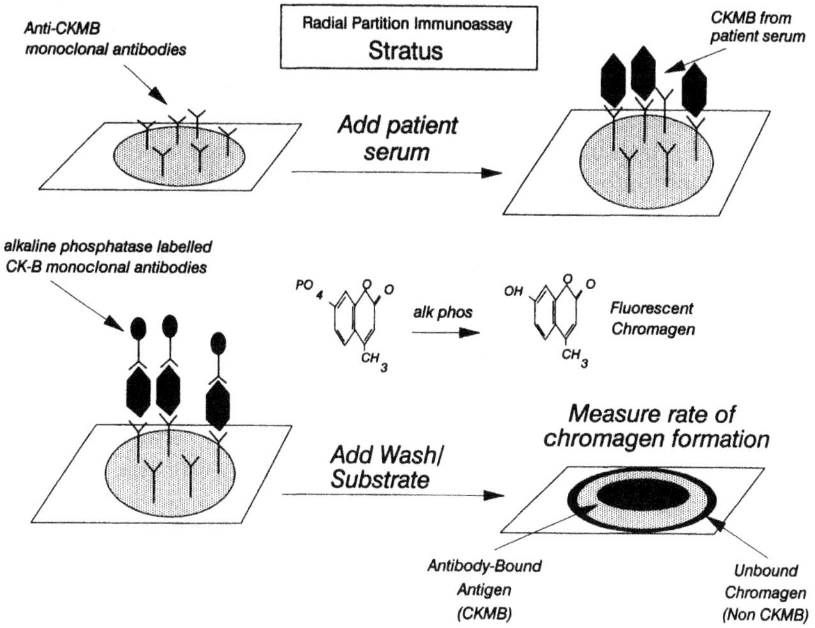

Figure 2 Radial partition immunoassay of CK-MB. CK-MB is measured by a sandwich immunoassay in which the antigen is bound by a preimmobilized anti-CKMB monoclonal antibody and an alkaline phosphatase–labeled anti-CKB monoclonal antibody. Addition of substrate/wash solution results in the formation of the fluorescent chromagen, 4-methylumbelliferone. Antibody-bound antigen is separated from unbound chromagen by radial partition elution.

tivity, due to unbound 4-methylumbelliferone (non-CK-MB), is also present, but is excluded from the reaction measurement.

3. Calibration and Data Reduction Methodology

On Stratus II, calibration materials are supplied at six different levels for each assay. The calibration points utilized are a zero-level calibrator and five levels of analyte spanning the technical range of the particular assay. Depending on the specific assay, calibration materials are typically stable, once opened, for 90 or 120 days at 2–8°C. While customers may achieve longer calibration curve stability, the manufacturer guarantees a 14-day interval for all assays.

During calibration, measured calibrator rates are coarse-screened, according to internal criteria, to eliminate unacceptable combinations and outliers (Heller *et al.*, 1984). The data for assays are fitted to the functional relationship illustrated in Eq. (1) (Giegel *et al.*, 1982):

$$R = \frac{(\mathrm{A} - \mathrm{D})}{1 + (X/C)^{B}} + D \quad (1)$$

where R is the rate of change or relative fluorescence and X is the analyte concentration, and A, B, C, and D are parameters determined during the calibration. During calibration routines, a log-logit transformation is applied to linearize Eq. (1) (Giegel *et al.*, 1982). The best-fitting values of A, B, C, and D are determined by linear regression, and an iterative procedure to converge on the best value of D is employed. CAL parameters are stored in memory until recalibration is required (Heller *et al.*, 1984).

III. PERFORMANCE

A. Technical Performance of Stratus II Assays

1. Summary

A summary of analytical parameters relevant to Stratus II assay performance is provided in Table 2. All of the information in this table has been compiled from the technical protocols accompanying each assay kit. Numerous reports have been published on the technical performance of the majority of Stratus and Stratus II assays listed in Table 2. In several instances, reports in the literature are method performance characteristics published by the scientific R & D staff of BDI. The information summarized in the subsequent technical sections is provided to give an overview of the expected technical performance reported for Stratus II assays.

For the majority of assays, mildly hemolyzed or lipemic samples are acceptable. Whenever possible, severely hemolyzed samples should not be used for Stratus II assays. If the manufacturer notes more specific information for a particular assay, this information is summarized in the "Special comments" column in Table 2. In the majority of assay protocols, the manufacturer notes that the presence of patient antibodies to *Escherichia coli* alkaline phosphatase may result in unexpected patient values. The expected incidence of this antibody in patient specimens is extremely low.

2. Therapeutic Drug Assays

Providing the assay capabilities to monitor levels of therapeutic drugs was one original design goal of the Stratus. Indeed, eight of nine initial assays released when the instrument was introduced in 1983 were therapeutic drugs. Since that time, Stratus and Stratus II have been proven to be reliable analyzers for measurement of the majority of commonly monitored therapeutic drugs.

Radial partition immunoassay has been reported to be a viable approach for measurement of certain aminoglycoside antibiotics. The gentamicin and amikacin assays have been demonstrated to correlate well with both radioimmunoassay (RIA) and other enzyme immunoassay (EIA)

Table 2 Technical Parameters of Stratus II Immunoassays[a]

Assay	Technical range	Sensitivity[b]	Special comments
Amikacin	0–64 μg/ml	<1 μg/ml	None[c]
Carbamazepine	0–20 μg/ml	0.1 μg/ml	None
Digitoxin	0–60 ng/ml	1.0 ng/ml	<10% Cross-reactivity list[d]
Digoxin	0–4 ng/ml	0.3 ng/ml	<0.1% Cross-reactivity list[d]
Gentamicin	0–16 μg/ml	0.1 μg/ml	<0.1% Cross-reactivity list[d]
Lidocaine	0–12 μg/ml	0.1 μg/ml	None
Phenobarbital	0–60 μg/ml	0.3 μg/ml	<3.0% Cross-reactivity list[d] Mephobarbital interferes
Phenytoin	0–40 μg/ml	0.5 μg/ml	<1.0% Cross-reactivity list[d]
Primidone	0–20 μg/ml	0.2 μg/ml	25% Cross-reactivity list[d]
Procainamide	0–16 μg/ml	0.1 μg/ml	10% Cross-reactivity list[d]
N-Acetyl procainamide	0–32 μg/ml	0.2 μg/ml	20% Cross-reactivity list[d]
Quinidine	0–8 μg/ml	0.1 μg/ml	<30% Cross-reactivity list[d]
Theophylline	0–40 μg/ml	0.1 μg/ml	<2% Cross-reactivity list[d] Uremia may cause high results
Tobramycin	0–16 μg/ml	0.2 μg/ml	<15% Cross-reactivity list[d]
hCG	0–500 mIU/ml	1.9 mIU/ml	None
hFSH	0–150 mIU/ml	0.3 mIU/ml	<0.5% for hLH <0.01% for hTSH <0.001% for hCG[e]
hLH	0–200 mIU/ml	0.3 mIU/ml	<0.0003% for hCG <0.001% for hFSH <0.02% for hTSH[e]
Prolactin	0–350 ng/ml	0.4 ng/ml	<0.01% Cross-reactivity list[d]
Total T_3	0–8 ng/ml	0.16 ng/ml	Triiodothyroacetic acid interferes; <0.4% cross-reactivity list[d]
Total T_4	0–25 μg/dl	0.5 μg/dl	D-Thyroxine interferes; <0.1% cross-reactivity list[d]
Free T_4	Varies with lot	0.1 ng/dl	D-Thyroxine interferes; <0.1% cross-reactivity list[d]
hTSH	0–50 μIU/ml	0.1 μIU/ml	<0.03% hFSH <0.01% hLH
T Uptake	1–100%	1%	None
CK-MB	0–125 ng/ml	0.4 ng/ml	None
Cortisol	0–50 μg/dl	0.1 μg/dl	Prednisolone, prednisone, and 6-alpha-methylprednisolone interfere; refer to <1.0% cross-reactivity list[d]
Ferritin	0–800 ng/ml	0.7 ng/ml	None
IgE	0–1000 IU/ml	2 IU/ml	None

[a] Information compiled from Stratus II Immunoassay protocols provided by manufacturer.
[b] Minimum detectable limit of analyte (95% confidence interval) according to manufacturer.
[c] The assay listed is highly specific for the analyte listed unless described otherwise in this column.
[d] Refer to individual test protocol for a list of compounds that have been tested by the manufacturer and shown to be cross-reactive at less than the percentage listed in this column.
[e] Percentages expressed as the average picomoles per liter analyte to produce a given response divided by the picomoles per liter of cross-reactant required to give the same response.

methods (Evans *et al.*, 1984; Sheiman *et al.*, 1985). Performance of a proposed plasma vancomycin assay also demonstrated acceptable agreement to a commercial assay (Monticello *et al.*, 1988), while reported interrun imprecision of the vancomycin assay was in the range of 5–9%. However, this assay was not commercially available at the time of publication of this chapter.

Several abstracts have been published briefly describing the performance of the Stratus and Stratus II for antiepileptic drugs. Generally, there is good agreement between Stratus II assays and homogenous EIA or high-performance liquid chromatography (HPLC) for carbamazepine, phenobarbital, phenytoin, and primidone (Sheiman *et al.*, 1983, 1984; Rugg *et al.*, 1984). Stratus II has been reported to be a precise, accurate, and rapid method for the determination of carbamazepine, phenobarbital, phenytoin, and primidone (Nadkarni *et al.*, 1990). Depending on the analyte level tested, interrun imprecision has been demonstrated to be in the range of 4–8%.

Numerous reports of the performance of Stratus and Stratus II in the quantitation of cardioactive drugs have also appeared. The quinidine assay demonstrated good agreement with EIA or fluorescence polarization immunoassay (FPIA) (Leung *et al.*, 1985). Interrun imprecision of the lidocaine assay was reported to be less than 10% at three levels spanning the technical range of the assay (Rugg *et al.*, 1983). The Stratus digoxin assay demonstrated acceptable agreement with an RIA method (Cilessen *et al.*, 1986). Interrun imprecision of the digoxin and digitoxin assays has been reported to range from 3 to 7% (Cilissen *et al.*, 1986; Phillips *et al.*, 1990a). Compared to RIA or FPIA, the Stratus digoxin method was shown to have only minimal interference from endogenous digoxinlike substances in a study of specimens from low-birthweight infants (Ng *et al.*, 1985). One report cited good precision and throughput for three automated digoxin methods including the Stratus (Clark *et al.*, 1986). However, all three automated methods demonstrated problems of standardization and lot-to-lot reagent variation (Clark *et al.*, 1986).

A recent report cites excellent correlation and agreement of the Stratus theophylline method with HPLC, EMIT, or FPIA (Welch *et al.*, 1990). Recoveries of theophylline spiked into serum were acceptable and the method did not demonstrate significant interference from icterus, hemolysis, lipemia, or uremia. However, the level of interfering substances, which is of particular interest for the uremic specimens, was not reported in this abstract. Interrun imprecision was less than 5% at all levels of theophylline tested (Welch *et al.*, 1990).

3. Reproductive Endocrinology Assays

The principal Stratus II reproductive endocrine assay is probably human choriogonadotropin (hCG), but basic performance characteristics of three other reproductive endocrine tests available have also been reported. For hLH, hFSH, and prolactin, interrun imprecision is less than 10% (Flaa *et al.*, 1988; Leung *et al.*, 1988; Mahmood *et al.*, 1989). Each of these assays demonstrated acceptable agreement to RIA and, most importantly, did not demonstrate any appreciable cross-reactivity with other pituitary polypeptide hormones with similar structural features.

Performance characteristics of the Stratus hCG method were first reported in 1986 (Rogers *et al.*, 1986a; Rugg *et al.*, 1986a; Beinlich and Carpenter, 1987). The hCG method is a dual-monoclonal antibody sandwich assay that detects the intact, native hCG polypeptide. The assay was shown to detect both highly purified and crude preparations of hCG while retaining a high degree of specificity (Rugg *et al.*, 1986a). Excellent correlation of results was demonstrated between the Stratus hCG method and RIA or EIA methods. Interrun imprecision of this automated hCG method was typically less than 5%. Of note was the absence of a high-dose "hook effect" with the hCG assay, since radial elution washes unbound sample components to the periphery of the tab, allowing sandwich formation to proceed without inhibition at high antigen concentrations (Rugg *et al.*, 1986a).

Rogers *et al.* reported rare spuriously elevated values of hCG on Stratus (Rogers *et al.*, 1986a). In response to this evidence, the manufacturer made modifications to the enzyme reagent. This was prompted by a study suggesting that a factor in discordant patient samples, likely an immunoglobulin, could form a sandwich in the absence of hCG (Rugg *et al.*, 1986b).

It has also been shown that spurious high hCG results can occur from carryover after a high level specimen. This carryover may be in the range of 0.03% (Ryan and McKenzie, 1986; Peltyszyn *et al.*, 1989). While this could result in a false positive pregnancy specimen when a negative sample follows a very high sample, this can be easily assessed by the operator when performing an hCG either in the batch mode or run as a stat. If necessary, the potentially positive specimen can be reassayed for verification. The Stratus hCG method has been used on urine specimens by one group after pretreatment of the tab with Stratus serum sample diluent (van den Berg *et al.*, 1990). Additional studies are required to validate the use of the Stratus for urinary hCG measurements.

4. Thyroid Function Assays

Automation of thyroid function assays is particularly useful due to the typically high numbers of tests laboratories are required to perform. Several reports have been published evaluating the total thyroxine assay on the Stratus (Mc Carthy *et al.*, 1984; Soto *et al.*, 1986; Stahlschmidt *et al.*, 1988). Good correlations have been demonstrated to RIA and interrun imprecision is typically in the range of 4–7%. One report cited increased imprecision of 12% at low T_4 values (4.2 μg/dl) and loss of linearity beyond a T_4 level of 20 μg/dl (Stahlschmidt *et al.*, 1988).

Reports have also indicated acceptable performance of the Stratus T_3 assay with respect to correlation to RIA and imprecision (Morejon *et al.*, 1988; Elin *et al.*, 1990). Results from RIA comparisons for both the T_4 and T_3 assays demonstrate somewhat different linear regression parameters. Through a two-way analysis of variance, it has been reported that proportional and systematic biases clearly exist between four common T_3 methods including Stratus (Elin *et al.*, 1990). This suggests that careful validation of the T_3 reference range is essential when switching from one T_3 method to another. Acceptable performance of the thyroxine binding capacity method has also been reported (Morejon and Soto, 1984).

A free thyroxine assay has also been described which appears to be a viable alternative to classical RIA methods (Smith *et al.*, 1987; Sapin *et al.*, 1988; Perdrisot *et al.*, 1989). This assay required manual predilution with the Stratus, but this step is now part of the Stratus II automated protocol. The Stratus free thyroxine assay demonstrated excellent agreement when compared to RIA and a low-end sensitivity of 0.1 ng/dl. Interrun imprecision was reported to be high, 28%, at the low end of the free thyroxine range (Sapin *et al.*, 1988). This is likely not clinically significant and imprecision at all other levels of free thyroxine was generally less than 10%.

Several studies have been reported on the performance of the Stratus thyrotropin (hTSH) assay (Rugg *et al.*, 1988; Sacks *et al.*, 1988; Wong and Hutchins, 1988; Sgoutas *et al.*, 1989). The hTSH assay is a sandwich assay employing two monoclonal antibodies specific for the intact hTSH molecule. This assay is not an ultrasensitive TSH assay, but compares favorably with other sensitive TSH methods. The lower limit of detection for this assay is 0.1 μIU/ml. Comparison of Stratus hTSH results to results from various RIA methods demonstrated good correlation and agreement. One report suggested "matrix effects" as a reason for observed differences in a subset of hospitalized patient results between the Stratus hTSH method and other methods (Sgoutas *et al.*, 1989). Interrun imprecision of the hTSH assay was 4% at 0.5 μIU/ml and 12% at 0.3 μIU/ml (Rugg *et al.*, 1988).

5. CK-MB Assay

The Stratus CK-MB mass-based method was first described in 1987 (Goodnow *et al.*, 1987). This two-site monoclonal antibody sandwich method has become a widely used technique for automated measurement of CK-MB. Numerous reports have been published on performance of the Stratus CK-MB method. In 1990 alone, more than a dozen posters reporting, in part, on performance characteristics of the Stratus CKMB method were presented at the XIV International Congress of Clinical Chemistry in San Francisco, California. The following technical information summarizes the findings from these and several other reports.

The Stratus CK-MB assay is linear from approximately 2 to 125 ng/ml (Butch *et al.*, 1989a,b). Minimum sensitivity of the assay is 0.4 ng/ml (Wu *et al.*, 1989). Generally, interrun imprecision ranged from 7 to 13% at normal CKMB levels and 4 to 8% at elevated CK-MB levels (Butch *et al.*, 1989b; Wu *et al.*, 1989; Bermes *et al.*, 1990; Heenie *et al.*, 1990). Elevated levels of bilirubin, triglycerides, and creatinine do not result in interference (Butch *et al.*, 1989a). The method is specific for CK-MB being free from interference due to CK-BB or macro CK (Bermes *et al.*, 1990; Sachs *et al.*, 1990).

The method compared favorably with other mass-based CK-MB immunoassays (Goodnow *et al.*, 1987; Christenson *et al.*, 1989; Wu *et al.*, 1989; Bermes *et al.*, 1990; Chapelle and Allaf, 1990). Stratus CK-MB correlated well with electrophoresis and other activity-based methods, but clearly requires a normal range appropriate to mass-based CK-MB assays (Christenson *et al.*, 1989; Bermes *et al.*, 1990). This point will be discussed further in the section on clinical performance.

6. Ferritin, Cortisol, and IgE Assays

Radial partition immunoassay has demonstrated analytical acceptability for measurement of serum ferritin levels (Goodnow *et al.*, 1986; Singh *et al.*, 1988; Vernet *et al.*, 1989; Mee *et al.*, 1990). The assay demonstrated excellent correlation and good agreement with other EIA and RIA methods. Interrun imprecision was typically less than 5%.

Stratus immunoassay methods for serum cortisol and IgE have also demonstrated acceptable parameters for analytical performance (Castillo *et al.*, 1984; Rogers *et al.*, 1986b; Phillips *et al.*, 1990b). The cortisol assay demonstrated good agreement to RIA, and interrun imprecision of this assay was 5–10%. Interrun imprecision for the IgE method was less than 4% at all levels tested.

B. Clinical Performance Aspects of Selected Stratus II Assays

Providing the necessary service capabilities to meet clinical demands of every laboratory operation continues to be a primary challenge for health care professionals. The automation of a broad menu of analytically reliable immunoassays on the Stratus II offers a number of advantages in providing laboratory services. Some of these capabilities are due to the innovative radial partition immunoassay method. A major advantage is the minimal amount of time from placement of a specimen on the analyzer until the first result is generated. This interval is 8 min. Due to radial partitioning, separation of bound from unbound ligand requires much less time in comparison to other heterogeneous immunoassays and most other immunoassay instruments.

The ability of Stratus II to actually provide a "stat" test result is of a particular clinical relevance. This feature can be highly effective in improving stat turnaround times (Peltyszyn *et al.*, 1989). This feature is important for assays of therapeutic drugs or intact hCG. Stat CK-MB analyses are not generally advisable because clinical judgement should not be based on a single CK-MB result. Still, many laboratorians may have to provide a stat CK-MB assay to meet the clinical demands unique to their own institutions. The Stratus II CK-MB assay is well suited to meet this need or to provide, in a timely manner, sequential CK-MB results during a 2–6 h period. Stat thyroid function tests are rarely appropriate, if ever. But in some institutions, rare requests may occur on the second or third shift when a patient is suspected to be in "thyroid storm."

Digoxin was one of the first assays offered on the Stratus. The Stratus II continues to offer a stat digoxin capability, which can, at times, be clinically necessary. Even though the initial Stratus digoxin protocol required a manual predilution, the automation of this test was a distinct improvement over many costly and time-consuming RIA digoxin procedures. Additionally, endogenous digoxinlike substances (EDLS) will cross-react in many digoxin procedures to give incorrect results for digoxin levels. In a study of the effects of EDLS interference on digoxin levels of low-birthweight infants, the Stratus assay demonstrated superior specificity compared to RIA and FPIA methods (Ng *et al.*, 1985).

Requirements for stat hCG levels continue to be significant in the emergency patient population. Verification of pregnancy may be necessary if the clinical history suggests this possibility, if an ectopic pregnancy is suspected, or if additional diagnostic procedures need to be performed that may cause harm to the unborn child (Rogers *et al.*, 1986a). The provision of a stat quantitative serum hCG assay on Stratus II meets these needs. Furthermore, the ability to quantitate serial serum hCG levels, stat, may be required to identify an ectopic pregnancy by assessment of the "doubling time" for serum hCG levels.

According to the manufacturer, the hCG assay can exhibit 0.02–0.08% carryover. While very small, this level can cause a false positive result in an otherwise negative specimen if the preceding elevated specimen is greater than 5000 mIU/ml. A built-in diagnostic flag on the analyzer alerts the operator if a second specimen has followed a first specimen with a very high hCG level. The manufacturer recommends repeating analysis on the second specimen to verify the correct hCG level.

Serum hCG levels can be elevated in a variety of conditions. The Stratus II hCG method detects the intact molecule, but may not consistently detect hCG fragments such as the beta subunit. Therefore, comparison of hCG levels in patients with trophoblastic tumors may demonstrate confusing results between the Stratus II and other methods such as RIA. Another use of hCG measurements has been suggested by a study of samples from 12 females in the second trimester of pregnancy (Spiekerman, 1990). These patients ultimately gave birth to babies suffering from Down's syndrome, and seven of 12 patients demonstrated increased hCG levels over two times the median value cutoff (2 MOM). Further studies are required to elucidate the role of hCG measurements in this clinical situation.

The initial Stratus TSH assay was only a "sensitive" method, but an "ultrasensitive" TSH assay will be released in mid 1991. There has been disagreement as to whether the older TSH assay met proposed criteria for analytic performance and clinical utility (Rugg *et al.*, 1988; Sgoutas *et al.*, 1989). One study suggested that while the Stratus TSH assay generally correlated well with an RIA procedure, some discrepancies were apparent in results from hospitalized patients who were clinically euthyroid (Sacks *et al.*, 1988). An additional study by this group reported increased TSH values in patients with liver-function abnormalities (Sacks *et al.*, 1990). Only a portion of these patients had elevated alkaline phosphatase levels, so the probability that this could be due to interference by a high-molecular-weight alkaline phosphatase isoenzyme was considered to be low (Butch *et al.*, 1989b).

The first TSH assay has been reported to be reliable for TRH stimulation procedures, but the investigators emphasized the importance of each laboratory determining their own reference intervals (Marcial *et al.*, 1988). Another study reported the results of using the sensitive TSH assay for monitoring treatment with levothyroxine (Watts, 1989). The TSH assay on the Stratus was sufficiently sensitive to discriminate truly low TSH levels from the lower range of normal without the need for further stimulation testing (Watts, 1989).

The manufacturer plans to release a second generation Stratus TSH assay in mid 1991. This test is an ultrasensitive TSH assay and will probably replace the current TSH method at some future time. Assuming that the new assay meets the analytical and clinical requirements for an ultrasensitive TSH method, this test should be the required complement to Stratus II assays for the assessment of thyroid function. The offering of a full menu of thyroid function tests makes the Stratus II a strong candidate for automation of these typically high-volume procedures.

The CK-MB assay is a critical procedure in the evaluation of many patients, especially those who may have had an acute myocardial infarction (AMI). Any CK-MB method must meet stringent criteria for clinical utility. In addition to reliable results, there must be a mechanism for correctly assessing an elevated CK-MB to achieve optimum diagnostic sensitivity and diagnostic specificity. Due to the high volume of CKMB tests ordered in our institution, this assay is probably one of the most important tests provided by the laboratory. Our laboratory performs approximately 25,000 tests per year using the Stratus II for CK-MB measurement. This assay was chosen because it meets our stringent requirements for analytical, clinical, and operational performance.

While all mass-based CK-MB assays have the same difficulties, a recent study cited the elevated false positive rate in Stratus CK-MB levels by using the CK-MB value alone as a diagnostic parameter (Rosecrans *et al.*, 1989). Mass-based CK-MB assays are more sensitive than activity-based measurements. Since CK-MB is located in tissues other than heart, additional measures may be required to provide diagnostically useful results. Optimal diagnostic specificity can be achieved by calculation of a relative index value or RIV (Wu *et al.*, 1989; Apple *et al.*, 1990; Bermes *et al.*, 1990). This calculation is performed by dividing the CK-MB value (in ng/ml) by the total CK value (in IU/l) and multiplying by 100. Because the units of the two results are different, we prefer to refer to this index as a relative index value rather than a percentage of total CK activity.

Our CKMB patient population predominantly consists of patients with various cardiac disorders, AMI, trauma, or those individuals who are pre- or postoperative coronary bypass patients. In this patient population, we have found that roughly 95% of the AMI patients will have RIV greater than 3.0 during the first 36 h after onset of chest pain (Bermes *et al.*, 1990). Roughly 95% of the remaining patients will not have RIV greater than 3.0. Although this does not represent a community hospital patient population, these percentages would approach 100% in this type of institution with appropriate use of the RIV. A threshold RIV of 3.0 should not be generalized to every clinical setting. Depending on the patient population and the method for total CK analysis, RIV values from 2.0 to 5.0 may be appropriate.

The reference range for the Stratus CK-MB method should also be determined in each laboratory's patient population. In a population of patients with a high incidence of cardiac disease, the upper reference interval has been reported to be in the range of 5–7 ng/ml (Wu *et al.*, 1989; Apple *et al.*, 1990; Bermes *et al.*, 1990). However, in a general patient population, without noncardiac disease, this upper reference interval may fall within the range of 2–4 ng/ml (Sachs *et al.*, 1990).

There were initial reports of rare spuriously high CK-MB values, which were attributed to the presence of high-molecular-weight alkaline phosphatase in the serum of certain patients with obstructive liver disease (Butch *et al.*, 1989b). However, this problem has been eliminated by the manufacturer with a reformulation of the CK-MB substrate/wash solution (Butch *et al.*, 1989b).

C. Operational Performance of the Stratus II

The use of the Stratus and now Stratus II has grown throughout recent years, suggesting that many customers have been satisfied with the operational advantages this immunoassay analyzer offers to the user. Stratus and Stratus II have been used in our laboratory for several years. The use of the Stratus II for CK-MB testing has proved invaluable in our laboratory setting. Technical staff members have found these instruments to be relatively easy to operate and reliable. Initially, our laboratory conducted clinical trials on several of the assays previously discussed. The hCG and IgE methods were also put into routine use for 3 years. Our current use of the Stratus and Stratus II has focused on these assays because we have been satisfied with methods previously used in our laboratory for therapeutic drugs and thyroid testing.

Our laboratory is fortunate to have no demands for stat CK-MB testing. Both our clinical and laboratory staff have been satisfied with the CK-MB service provided. The laboratory performs four batch runs per day at roughly 10 a.m., 3 p.m., 9 p.m., and 2 a.m. In our experience with CK-MB, calibration curve stability of 14 days has also been a reliable feature. Stability of substrate wash, sample diluent, and calibrators is generally guaranteed for 4–6 months by the manufacturer. The stability of the conjugate reagent and the assay tabs is shorter, 1–2 months. Assay kits are designed to perform 120 tests. In rare instances, a low-volume user may have to consider this fact in conjunction with the frequency of quality control and calibration analyses to assess if there is any likelihood of reagent wastage.

In addition to the stat capability and short time to first result, maximum instrument throughput is approximately 60 tests/h. The preventative maintenance procedures on the Stratus II require minimal amounts of time. These routines focus on analyzer hygiene as well as mechanical alignment and serve to minimize analytical system imprecision (Plaut and McLellan, 1991). Daily maintenance procedures require 15 min of system operation, but not operator, time. Weekly maintenance procedures require 20 min of operator time while monthly maintenance procedures require only 5 min of operator time (Plaut and McLellan, 1991). An attractive feature is that any positional realignment of the probes can be directed by the operator, using the keypad.

D. Economic Aspects of Stratus II

As of mid 1991, the list price of Stratus II was $58,500. This is a competitive price compared to other similar automated immunoassay analyzers. In certain instances, BDI may discount this price depending on various issues unique to each prospective customer institution. Lease or reagent rental agreements may also be negotiated. While the original Stratus lists for $42,500, prospective customers would be wise to choose a Stratus II acquisition, given the improvements in sample handling and interactive routines on the newer model.

The following list prices for reagent kits are cost per test values based on dividing the total list price, as of mid 1991, by 120 tests per kit. Each of the following costs are list prices for direct reagent costs only. Assays in the therapeutic drug category are $3.36 per test. Digitoxin costs are $4.23 per test. The T_4 and TU costs are $3.18 per test. TSH, T_3 , and free T_4 costs range from $4.58 to $5.00 per test. Reproductive endocrine assay costs are $5.08 per test. Cortisol costs are $4.32 per test. IgE costs are $4.09 per test. Ferritin costs are $4.49 per test. CK-MB costs are $6.32 per test. As with the instrument costs, discounts on these prices may be available from the manufacturer, depending on the total work-load volume and general scope of BDI products used by a particular customer.

There are two additional cost features worth mentioning. The Stratus II is a "walk-away" instrument. It requires reduced amount of labor time compared to other more conventional immunoassay technologies and even other automated immunoassay analyzers. Utilization of the Stratus II should free up additional technologist time, which can be used for staff to perform other work in the laboratory. The degree of impact that this feature has would depend on the particular institutional setting and the type of methodology Stratus II might replace.

The stat capability of the Stratus II can provide additional cost savings to the institution. The best example of this impact is in the reduction of time patients may spend in a coronary care unit due to the increased availability of a rapid CK-MB test. It is worth repeating that a single negative CK-MB test should not be used to rule out sending a patient to the coronary care unit. However, increased frequency of CK-MB testing should help reduce the amount of time that patients may spend in the unit unnecessarily. A recent report has estimated that in a community hospital, the increased availability of CK-MB results provided by the Stratus

CKMB test, compared to electrophoresis, may save the institution as much as $96,000 per year (Apple *et al.*, 1990).

IV. CONCLUSIONS

As a result of the joint venture between BDI and Hybritech, it is anticipated that the Stratus II test menu will include prostate-specific antigen (PSA), carcinoembryonic antigen (CEA), and alpha-fetoprotein (AFP) by mid 1991. Other assays planned for release in mid 1991 are the ultrasensitive TSH assay, estradiol, and B12/folate. Later in 1991, prospective Stratus II customers will have the option of acquiring the Stratus Intellect. This model will house an on-board microcomputer broadening the software capabilities of the Stratus II, particularly in the areas of data reduction and user-defined modifications. The option to purchase an upgrade to the Stratus Intellect will also be available to present Stratus II customers.

It appears reasonable to expect that the Stratus II will continue to be one of the most widely used automated immunoassay analyzers. Stratus II offers the clinical laboratory a unique combination of broad test menu and numerous operational advantages that are difficult to obtain with other types of immunoassay equipment.

REFERENCES

Apple, F. S., Preese, L. M., Riley, L., Gerken, K. L., and Van Lente, F. (1990). Financial impact of a rapid CK-MB-specific immunoassay on the diagnosis of myocardial infarction. *Arch. Pathol. Lab. Med.* **114,** 1017–1020.

Beinlich, C. J., and Carpenter, R. H. (1987). Automated and manual quantitative assays of choriogonadotropin in serum compared. *Clin. Chem.* **33**(1), 167–169.

Bermes, E. W., Kahn, S. E., Jandreski, M. A., Augustine, G., and Khan, I. (1990). Analytical and clinical comparison of four methods for determination of the MB isoenzyme of creatine kinase. *Clin. Chem.* **36**(6), 1130.

Butch, A., Brown, W., Koenig, J., Hinds, B., Kessler, G., and Scott, M. (1989a). Evaluation of an automated CK-MB mass assay. *Clin. Chem.* **35**(6), 1107.

Butch, A. W., Goodnow, T. T., Brown, W. S., McClellan, A., Kessler, G., and Scott, M. G. (1989b). Stratus automated creatine kinase-MB assay evaluated: Identification and elimination of falsely increased results with a high-molecular-mass form of alkaline phosphatase. *Clin. Chem.* **35**(10), 2048–2053.

Castillo, M., Linne, A., and Soto, A. (1984). A radial partition immunoassay for cortisol. *Clin. Chem.* **30**(6), 1042.

Chapelle, J-P., and Allaf, M. E. (1990). Automated quantification of creatine kinase MB isoenzyme in serum by radial partition immunoassay with use of the Stratus analyzer. *Clin. Chem.* **36**(1), 99–101.

Christenson, R. H., Toffaletti, J., Ohman, M., Clemmensen, P. M., and Wagner, G. S. (1989). Four assays for creatine kinase MB compared. *Clin. Chem.* **35**(6), 1124.

Cilissen, J., Hooymans, P. M., and Merkus, F. W. H. M. (1986). Modified fluorescence polarization immunoassay compared with radial partition immunoassay and a radioimmunoassay for digoxin. *Clin. Chem.* **32**(11), 2100.

Clark, D. R., Inloes, R. L., Kalman, S. M., and Sussman, H. H. (1986). Abbott TDx, Dade Stratus, and Du Pont aca automated digoxin immunoassays compared with a reference radioimmunoassay method. *Clin. Chem.* **32**(2), 381–385.

De Cresce, R., and Lifshitz, M. S. (1990). Profile of the Stratus II. *The Instrument Report* **2**(8), 1–8.

Elin, R. J., Glickman, J., Ruddel, M., and Zweig, M. (1990). Comparison of four methods for the determination of triiodothyronine (T_3). *Clin. Chem.* **36**(6), 1147.

Evans, S., Leung, K., Tokarski, R., Knight, W., and Giegel, J. (1984). Radial partition immunoassay: Monitoring gentamicin levels in serum and plasma. *Clin. Chem.* **30**(6), 1025.

Flaa, C., Rodriguez, L., Leung, K., Dawson, S., and Rugg, J. (1988). Radial partition immunoassay: Quantifying hFSH levels in human serum or plasma. *Clin. Chem.* **34**(6), 1221.

Giegel, J. L., Brotherton, M. M., Cronin, P., D'Aquino, M., Evans, S., Heller, Z. H., Knight, W. S., Krishnan, K., and Sheiman, M. (1982). Radial partition immunoassay. *Clin. Chem.* **28**(9), 1894–1898.

Goodnow, T., LeBlanc, M., Koski, K., Welsh, M., Leung, K., Charie, L., and Evans, S. (1987). Radial partition immunoassay: Quantitating CKMB levels in human serum. *Clin. Chem.* **33**(6), 988.

Goodnow, T., Timmons, R., Koski, K., Soto, A., Kennedy, S., and Evans, S. (1986). Radial partition immunoassay: Monitoring ferritin levels in serum and plasma. *Clin. Chem.* **32**(6), 1143.

Heenie, L., Sims, J., Cummings, C., Plaut, D., and McLellan, W. (1990). Comparison of Stratus and Embria methods for serum CKMB. *Clin. Chem.* **36**(6), 1133.

Heller, Z. H., D'Aquino, M., Alvite, A., Becker, J., Cronin, P., Giegel, J., Hatch, W. P., and Intengan, F. S. (1984). Design principles of the Stratus fluorometric immunoassay instrument. *Biomed. Sci. Instrum.* **20,** 63–72.

Leung, K., Dawson, S. R., and Rugg, J. A. (1988). A rapid automated radial partition immunoassay for the measurement of human lutropin. *Clin. Chem.* **34**(6), 1221.

Leung, K., Evans, S., Fabian, B., Knight, W., and Giegel, J. (1985). Radial partition immunoassay: monitoring quinidine levels in serum and plasma. *Clin. Chem.* **31**(6), 927.

Mahmood, N., Srebro, S., Mc Carthy, M., Brotherton, M., Hunter, T., and DeMarco, C. (1989). Rapid automated determination of total prolactin on the Stratus analyzer. *Clin. Chem.* **35**(6), 1095.

Marcial, G., Carlson, J., Mitchell, G., Raymond, A., Herrero, L., and Trundle, D. (1988). Comparison of TSH response to TRH stimulation using ultrasensitive and routine TSH assays. *Clin. Chem.* **34**(6), 1210.

McCarthy, M., Oeser, T. H., Collins, S., Kahn, S. E., and Bermes, E. W. (1984). Evaluation of the Stratus immunoassay system in the determination of serum T_4 levels. *Clin. Chem.* **30**(6), 1039.

Mee, A. V., Tandory, J., Uchimaru, D., Garces, B., and Wong, P. Y. (1990). Comparison of Baxter's Stratus II system and Abbott's IMx system for the determination of serum ferritin. *Clin. Chem.* **36**(6), 1102.

Monticello, J. E., Smith, D., Hunter, T., Singh, P., Manes, M., and Soto, A. (1988). Radial partition immunoassay: A rapid, automated determination of serum or plasma vancomycin. *Clin. Chem.* **34**(6), 1257.

Morejon, C. B., Soto, A., Timmons, R., Delgado, J., Singh, P., Ni, W. C., and Hunter, T. (1988). Radial partition immunoassay for triiodothyronine. *Clin. Chem.* **34**(6), 1213.

Morejon, C. B., and Soto, A. R. (1984). Enzyme radial partition immunoassay for thyroxine binding capacity. *Clin. Chem.* **30**(6), 1037–1038.

Nadkarni, S. R., Tymeson, C., Howell, R., and Rey, A. (1990). Clinical evaluation of the Stratus II immunoassay system for quantitative determination of antiepileptic drug levels. *Clin. Chem.* **36**(6), 1037.

Ng, P. K., LeGatt, D., Coates, J., and Collins-Nakai, R. L. (1985). Measuring endogenous digoxin-like substance and exogenous digoxin in the serum of low-birth-weight infants. *Am. J. Hosp. Pharm.* **42,** 1977–1979.

Peltyszyn, S., Alexander, L., Mercer, W., Nouri, N., and Wimmer, C. (1989). Evaluation of the Baxter Dade Stratus as a stat methodology for human chorionic gonadotropin (hCG), digoxin and digitoxin. *Clin. Chem.* **35**(6), 1111.

Perdrisot, R., Bounaud, M-P., Bounaud, J.-Y., and Jallet, P. (1989). Four nonisotopic immunoassays for free thyroxin evaluated. *Clin. Chem.* **35**(1), 115–120.

Phillips, R. N., Nadkarni, S., Howell, R., and Rey, A. (1990a). Hospital laboratory evaluation of the Stratus II immunoassay system for digoxin and digitoxin in human serum. *Clin. Chem.* **36**(6), 1028–1029.

Phillips, R. N., Nadkarni, S., Howell, R., and Rey, A. (1990b). Clinical evaluation of the Stratus II immunoassay system for IgE, ferritin and theophylline. *Clin. Chem.* **36**(6), 1187.

Plaut, D. S., and McLellan, W. N. (1991). The Baxter Diagnostics Inc., Dade Stratus II automated fluorometric immunoassay system. *J. Clin. Immunoas.* **14**(2), 120–125.

Rogers, L. C., Kahn, S. E., Oeser, T. H., and Bermes, E. W. (1986a). The Stratus immunofluorometric assay system evaluated for quantifying human choriogonadotropin in serum. *Clin. Chem.* **32**(7), 1402–1404.

Rogers, L. C., Kahn, S. E., Oeser, T. H., and Bermes, E. W. (1986b). The Stratus immunofluorometric assay system evaluated for measuring serum cortisol. *Clin. Chem.* **32**(8), 1588.

Rosecrans, R., Buttita, D., Oiley, A., and Serna, F. (1989). Evaluation of the Dade Stratus for the determination of CKMB. *Clin. Chem.* **35**(6), 1090.

Rugg, J. A., Rigl, C. T., Leung, K., Lamar, S. L., Welsh, M., LeBlanc, M., and Evans, S. A. (1986a). Radial partition immunoassay applied to automated quantitation of human choriogonadotropin with use of two monoclonal antibodies. *Clin. Chem.* **32**(10), 1844–1848.

Rugg, J. A., Soto, A. R., and Castillo, M. J. (1983). A radial partition immunoassay for lidocaine. *Clin. Chem.* **29**(6), 1273.

Rugg, J. A., Flaa, C. W., Dawson, S. R., Rigl, C. T., Leung, K. S., and Evans, S. A. (1988). Automated quantification of thyrotropin by radial partition immunoassay. *Clin. Chem.* **34**(1), 118–122.

Rugg, J. A., Leung, K., Singh, P., Lamar, S. L., Tokarski, R., Flaa, C. W., Brotherton, M., and Evans, S. A. (1986b). Radial partition immunoassay for hCG: Resolution of one source of discordant patient values. *Clin. Chem.* **32**(6), 1167–1168.

Rugg, J., Rigl, T., Soto, A., and Castillo, M. (1984). A radial partition immunoassay for monitoring serum or plasma carbamazepine. *Clin. Chem.* **30**(6), 1023–1024.

Ryan, F. J., and McKenzie, C. (1986). Dade Stratus hCG method evaluated. *Clin. Chem.* **32**(6), 1168.

Sachs, E., Sachs, B., and Bernstein, L. H. (1990). Evaluation of CK-MB with the Dade Stratus analyzer. *Clin Chem.* **36**(6), 1187.

Sacks, D. B., Lim, M. M., Parvin, C. A., and Kessler, G. (1990). Interference in an automated radial partition fluorescent immunoassay of thyrotropin associated with liver-function abnormalities. *Clin. Chem.* **36**(7), 1343–1345.

Sacks, D., Lim, R., Valdes, R., and Kessler, G. (1988). Efficacy of sensitive thyrotropin (TSH) measurements in the assessment of thyroid dysfunction in a hospitalized population. *Clin. Chem.* **34**(6), 1211.

Sapin, R., Gasser, F., and Schlienger, J. L. (1988). "Stratus" fluorometric enzyme immunoassay system evaluated for determination of free thyroxin. *Clin. Chem.* **34**(10), 2159–2160.

Sgoutas, D. S., Barton, E. G., Hammarstrom, M., Pete, P. M., and Sgoutas, S. A. (1989). Four sensitive thyrotropin assays critically evaluated and compared. *Clin. Chem.* **35**(8), 1785–1789.

Sheiman, M., Srebro, S., Tokarski, R., Knight, W., and Giegel, J. (1985). Radial partition immunoassay: Monitoring amikacin levels in serum and plasma. *Clin. Chem.* **31**(6), 933.

Sheiman, M., Mahmood, N., Fabian, B., Knight, W., and Giegel, J. (1984). Radial partition immunoassay: Monitoring phenytoin levels in serum and plasma. *Clin. Chem.* **30**(6), 1021.

Sheiman, M., Srebro, S., Knight, W., and Giegel, J. (1983). Radial partition immunoassay: Monitoring phenobarbital levels in serum and plasma. *Clin. Chem.* **29**(6), 1239.

Singh, J., Pang, E., Lucco, L., Dudley, A. W., Diaz, S. R., Mayfield, C., Dimanina, L., Kulig, K., and Carreras, L. I. (1988). Evaluation of Dade Stratus for measurement of serum ferritin. *Clin. Chem.* **34**(6), 1276.

Smith, D., Soto, A., Chivite, J., Gil, P., Singh, P., and Ni., W. C. (1987). Radial partition immunoassay for free thyroxine. *Clin. Chem.* **33**(6), 885.

Soto, A., Morejon, C., Delgado, J., Chivite, J., Gil, P., Singh, P., and Ni, W. C. (1986). Radial partition immunoassay for thyroxine. *Clin. Chem.* **32**(6), 1165.

Spiekerman, M. (1990). Comparison of hCG median values on second trimester pregnancy samples using Hybritech Tandem-E EIA and Baxter Dade Stratus fluorometric EIA methodology. *Clin. Chem.* **36**(6), 1084.

Stahlschmidt, G. E., Smith, C. H., Miller, R. E., and Landt, M. (1988). Stratus fluorometric enzyme immunoassay system evaluated for determination of total thyroxin. *Clin. Chem.* **34**(2), 433–434.

Van den Berg, R. J., Segers, M. F. G., and Thomas, C. M. G. (1990). The Stratus automated immunofluorometric assay system: A modification for measuring urinary human choriogonadotropin. *Clin. Chem.* **36**(4), 697.

Vernet, M., Revenant, M-C., Bied, A., Naudin, C., Jauneau, M., Olivier, F., and Ruiz, J-C. (1989). Rapid determination of ferritin in serum by the "Stratus" fluoroenzymoimmunometric assay. *Clin. Chem.* **35**(4), 672–673.

Watts, N. B. (1989). Use of a sensitive thyrotropin assay for monitoring treatment with levothyroxine. *Arch. Intern. Med.* **149,** 309–312.

Welch, C., Dunham, S., Labruzzo, C., Burford, D., and Nadkarni, S. (1990). Theophylline analysis utilizing the Stratus immunoassay system. *Clin. Chem.* **36**(6), 1039–1040.

Wong, H. T., and Hutchins, S. (1988). Comparison of the hTSH using Stratus immunoassay system and Corning Immunophase RIA method. *Clin. Chem.* **34**(6), 1178.

Wu, A. H. B., Gornet, T. G., Harker, C. C., and Chen, H-L. (1989). Role of rapid immunoassays for urgent ("stat") determinations of creatine kinase isoenzyme MB. *Clin. Chem.* **35**(8), 1752–1756.

CHAPTER 23

TDx Systems

Steven H. Y. Wong
Department of Pathology (Laboratory Medicine),
Clinical Chemistry Division,
The Johns Hopkins University School of Medicine,
Baltimore, Maryland

I. INTRODUCTION

TDx systems have enhanced and redefined clinical laboratory drug measurements, and are now regarded as the "benchmark" methodology in the specialty of therapeutic drug monitoring (TDM) and toxicology. Such recognition by laboratory scientists is attributable to the sound scientific principles, instrumentational design, and outstanding level of support by the manufacturer. As with any clinical instrumentation, its advantages would also be accompanied by disadvantages, which are, according to this author's judgment, relatively minor. In parallel with the theme of this book, this chapter focuses on the practical aspects of TDx systems. The following is a brief summary of the evolution of TDx systems. Readers are encouraged to turn to original references for detailed discussions (Jolley, 1981; Jolley *et al.*, 1981).

The original TDx systems were designed primarily for TDM. The principle was based on fluorescence polarization immunoassay (FPIA), described in more detail in the section on system description. Using this principle, scientists (Jolley *et al.*, 1981) at the Abbott Laboratory introduced the immunoanalyzer at the 1981 annual meeting of the American Association for Clinical Chemistry (AACC) at Kansas City, Missouri. The name TDx was to signify the application of the immunoanalyzer for TDM as denoted by TD, while x would imply therapeutic drugs as part of the logo of Rx from the field of pharmacy. The key features included reagents

Immunoassay Automation: A Practical Guide

manufactured by Abbott Laboratory, the immunoanalyzer manufactured and serviced by the company, and educational support in the maintenance. After its initial introduction, the users' experiences were reviewed in publications as well as in the meeting abstracts since the 1983 AACC annual meeting. The list of drugs steadily expanded from theophylline, antiepileptics, antiarrhythmics, antimicrobials, and others. The emphasis up to the mid 1980s was centered around TDM. With the emerging substance abuse testing, TDx systems were developed to also incorporate the analysis of illicit drugs such as cocaine metabolite, cannabinoids, opiates, amphetamines, phencyclidine, and others. In completing the capability of total drug measurement, another methodology, radiative energy attenuation (REA), was also incorporated for the measurement of ethanol and other low-molecular-weight analytes, as shown by Table 1. From these systems, two other analyzers were engendered, ADx and IMx. Since its introduction in the early 1980s, TDx systems have become, as shown by the survey results of the College of American Pathologists and the American Association for Clinical Chemistry, the most utilized drug analyzers in the American clinical laboratory.

Thus, the current status of TDx systems, after over 8 years of widespread clinical laboratory experience, may be characterized as mature—reliable, efficient for low to moderate test volume, and flexible with the application of unit dose and the latest addition of TDxFLx. With the updating easily performed by switching "Rev." (revision) provided by Abbott, the users have been satisfied with the addition of tests and/or revision of data manipulation, and various instrumentation adjustment. The more detailed technical description of some of the adjustments will be given in the later section under Technical Performance. As a result of the desire to have flexibility, the latest update centers around performing multiple assays in a single run. With the TDx systems characterized as mature, the focus of this chapter in presenting practical aspects will be:

1. To describe (a) the instrumentational configurations of various TDx systems and (b) the methodologies and principles of FPIA and REA, with focus on the reagents utilized.

2. To assess the performances of the systems from the technical, clinical, operational, and economical points of views, with particular references to selected analytes from published literature from 1985 to 1990. Earlier developments may be referred to previous reviews (Blecka, 1983; Wong, 1984).

3. To draw conclusions on the current status and possible future needs and developments.

Table 1 TDx Drug and Chemistry Assays

Therapeutic drugs	Abused drugs (urine)	Specific proteins
Antiarrhythmics	Amphetamine/methamphetamine II	C-Reactive protein
Disopyramide	Amphetamine class (urine)	IgA, IgG, IgM
Flecainide	Barbiturates (urine)	Transferrin
Lidocaine	Barbiturates (serum)	**Pregnancy detection/management**
N-Acetylprocainamide (NAPA)	Benzodiazepines (urine)	Fetal lung maturity (FLM)
Procainamide	Benzodiazepines (serum)	Free estriol
Quinidine	Cocaine metabolite	Total estriol
Antiasthmatics	Cannabinoids	**New assays**
Theophylline II	Methadone	LITES Lithium
Antibiotics	Opiates	MEGX
Amikacin	Phencyclidine II (PCP)	MHPG
Gentamicin	**Toxicology**	
Kanamycin	Acetaminophen	
Netilmicin	Ethanol (serum, urine, whole blood)	
Streptomycin	Salicylate	
Tobramycin	Tricyclic antidepressants	
Vancomycin	**Chemistries**	
Anticonvulsants	Amylase II	
Carbamazepine	REA BUN	
Free carbamazepine	REA cholesterol	
Ethosuximide	HDL cholesterol	
Phenobarbital II	Creatinine	
Phenytoin	REA glucose	
Free phenytoin	REA iron/TIBC	
Primidone	REA lactic acid	
Valproic acid	REA LDH	
Free valproic acid	Triglycerides	
Antineoplastics	REA uric acid	
Methotrexate	**Biogenic amines**	
Cardiac Glycosides	5-HIAA (urine)	
Digitoxin	**Transplant diagnostics**	
Digoxin II	Cyclosporine and metabolites (serum plasma, whole blood)	
Digoxin NXT	Cyclosporine trending software	
Hormones		
Cortisol (serum, urine)		
T_4 Plus		
T-Uptake		
Total T_3 plus		

II. SYSTEM DESCRIPTION

A. Instrumentation

TDx systems are based on two different principles—fluorescence polarization immunoassay (FPIA) for therapeutic and illicit drugs and metabolites (Blecka, 1983; Jolley *et al.*, 1981; Wong, 1984), and radiative energy attentuation for ethanol (Cary *et al.*, 1984). The instrumentation is the same, as shown by Fig. 1, the major components of the analyzer. In changing the "Rev board" for updating purposes, the back of the analyzer can be easily opened for that, and other adjustment purposes. Of most interest to the analyst, the major components shown on Fig. 1 should function correctly as indicated by the specific recommendations by Abbott Laboratories. In case of malfunctioning, the self-diagnostic and, if needed, the available service phone usually allow timely identification and correction of the problems. In describing the instrumentation, it is helpful to go from the left side of Figure 1 to the right side in following the operational sequence.

Starting on the left, the first component is the buffer reservoir, supplied by the company in a disposable bottle. The inlet to the buffer is easily inserted so as to almost reach the bottom. When starting a new bottle, prime the pump tubing and syringe to avoid trapping air bubbles, since these affect the accuracy of the assay. These air bubbles are visible in the pumping lines and the glass syringes. For the actual assay, the buffer is

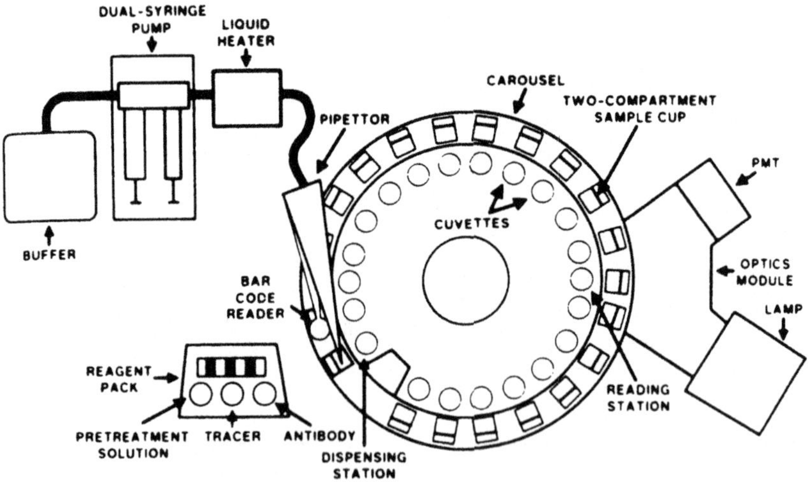

Figure 1 Major components of the totally automated benchtop TDx.

drawn by the dual syringe pump for sample dilution and transfer purposes. Thus, the correct function of the dual syringe also affects the accuracy and precision of the assay. Since there is multiple movement associated with each assay, the moving parts and syringes are subjected to normal "wear and tear," requiring periodic replacement. Buffer temperature is maintained at 30°C by the liquid heater and is delivered to the robotic arm with a bar-code reader. Typically, the bar-coded reagent pack would contain three to four vials, with antibody, tracer, and pretreatment solution. The robotic arm, equipped with two level sensors, sequentially pipettes pretreatment solution, tracer, and antibody into the reaction wells of the sample cups loaded inside the carousel.

Prior to loading the carousel into the TDx, 50-μl aliquots of calibrators, quality controls, and patient samples are pipetted into the sample wells of the sample cartridges, without any air bubbles as they affect pipetting accuracy. The first sample cartridges are placed sequentially with the matching number of cuvettes. Care is taken to ensure that the cuvettes are placed with opening upward, by either visual inspection or by rubbing a finger over the openings. Finally, the liquid levels of the samples are visually checked against the side marker. Then the carousel is placed inside the instrument compartment, as shown by Fig. 2. The caps of the appropriate reagent pack are opened, and the films, if present, are then quickly punctured so that the level sensors of the robotic arm are not "misled" into an incorrect position for pipetting. The pack is then placed

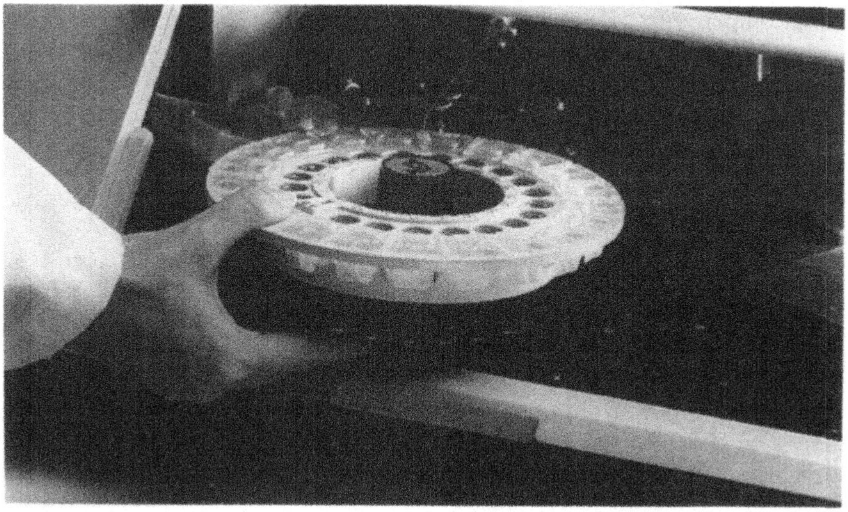

Figure 2 TDx carousel.

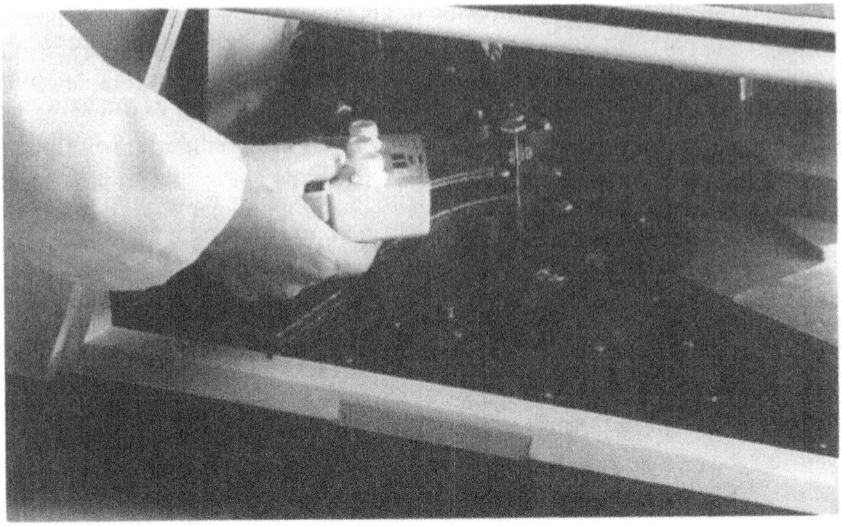

Figure 3 TDx reagent pack with bar coding.

inside the compartment, as shown by Fig. 3. The assay is initiated by pushing the "Run" button, as shown by Fig. 4.

The scanner of the robotic arm then reads the bar code, signaling the instrument to perform the necessary self-diagnostics: reading sample level, reagent quantity, the appropriate number of cuvettes, and the cuvette temperature by the infrared source placed on the optics module on the right side of the compartment as shown in Fig. 1. After passing these tests, the name of the reagent, such as theophylline, is displayed. TDx then

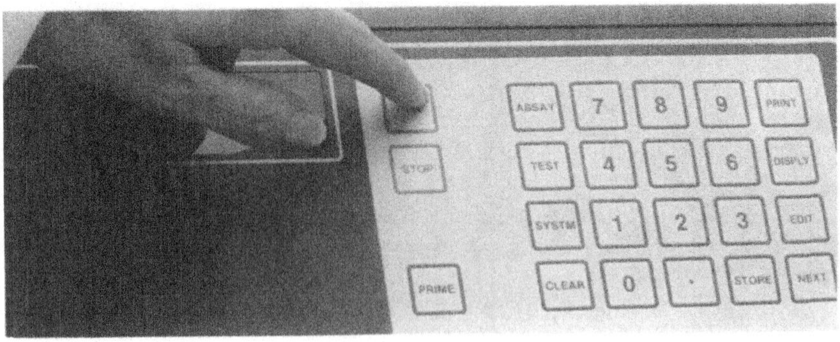

Figure 4 TDx run panel.

performs either the fluorescence polarization immunoassay or the radiative attenuation assay by dispensing the appropriate reagents from the pack, performing the photometric measurements, and the necessary computations as described in the following section on principles and methods.

B. Principles and Methods

1. Fluorescence Polarization Immunoassay

a. Principle Perrin (1926) described fluorescence polarization, followed by the Weber (1953) and Dandliker *et al.* (1973) applications in biologic and immunoassays systems. Jolley (1981) demonstrated the theoretical and operational details of the commercially available TDx systems using FPIA for drug monitoring. The two major factors are the competitive binding, and the dipolarity and fluorescent capacity of the drug analytes.

As with other competitive binding immunoassays, the drug molecules from a patient serum and drug molecules (tracers) labeled with fluorescein compete for the limited binding sites of the antibody (i.e., immunoglobulin) molecules. With low patient drug concentration, the greater number of binding sites is occupied by the tracer molecules. The reverse situation applies for high patient drug concentration. The extent of this binding is measured by the fluorescence polarization, governed by the dipolarity and fluorescent capacity.

For the molecules within the path of a beam of polarized incident light, their dipoles being parallel to the light, absorption will occur, followed by emission of a beam of polarized light. The polarity of the emitted light is parallel to the light-emitting molecular dipoles. In quantifying the degree of polarization, P, the following equation may be used:

$$P = (I_{vv} - I_{hv})/(I_{vv} + I_{hv}) \tag{1}$$

where I_{vv} is the intensity of the vertical component of the emitted light (525–550 nm), followed by sample excitation by a vertically 485 nm polarized light, and I_{hv} is the intensity of the vertical component of the emitted light, followed by sample excitation by a horizontally polarized light.

Polarization depends on the fluorescence lifetime and rotational relaxation time of the fluorescent molecules. For small molecules such as fluorescein, the rotational relaxation time is short, about 1 ns, and for large molecules such as immunoglobulins, about 100 ns. For patient serum with low drug concentration with resultant low free tracer concentrations, most of the tracer would be bound to the large antibodies. This decreases the rate of rotation of the fluorescein-labeled antibody, resulting in increased rotational relaxation time and a high degree of fluorescence polarization.

For serum with high drug concentrations, most of the tracer would be unbound, resulting in "normal" rotational relaxation time and a low degree of fluorescence polarization.

b. Competitive Binding The instrument may begin the assay by using the "equilibrium mode," that is, allowing the reaction equilibrium to occur for the antibody-bound and free drug molecules in the assay solution. At first, the robotic arm transfers 20 μl from each of the sample wells into the dilution well, followed by adding about 700 μl of buffer. After completing all the samples, 10–25 μl of these sample–buffer mixtures, 25 μl of the pretreatment solution, and an additional volume of buffer are transferred into the corresponding sample curvettes. The sample pretreatment solution ensures complete drug dissociation from protein. "Blank" measurements are performed by the optics module and stored in the instrument's memory. Then, 25 μl of the antibody reagent and tracer is transferred from the reagent pack, followed by buffer into the cuvette. These mixtures are incubated at 35°C for 3 min, followed by photometric measurements.

c. Fluorescence Polarization Excitation of the samples is actuated by vertically and horizontally polarized light beams of 485 nm. The intensity of the emitted vertical component is measured between 525 and 550 nm. The principle of these measurements will be explained later on in the following section. Together these three measurements and the blank readings are used for automatic computation of specimen concentration.

d. Equilibrium versus Nonequilibrium Modes For most of the TDx therapeutic and illicit drug measurement, the assays are performed in equilibrium mode as described above. The tracer molecules have low binding affinities for serum proteins, minimizing nonspecific binding. With the application of high-affinity antibodies, small sample volumes of 1–2 μl are used for competitive binding. Nonequilibrium mode is used for low-concentration drugs such as digoxin.

e. Unit Dose To allow multiple assays in a single run, unit dose reagent packs are placed in a unit dose "UD" carousel as shown in Fig. 5. The reagents are similar to those in the regular TDx reagent packs. Each of the unit dose reagents may be accompanied by the quality control and patient samples. The bar code of the reagent packs instructs TDx as to what assay(s) are needed. Depending on the configurations, a maximum of 6–10 assays may be performed on a single patient sample.

f. Random Access To offer further flexibility, TDx has been recently modified, as TDxFLx, to hold up to eight reagent kits as shown in Fig. 6. The bar-coded reagents wedges would be placed in the left side of the compartment, where a single reagent pack is usually placed for the regular TDx. The system is then programmed for a customized run for enhanced flexibility. Automated data input is provided through a bar-code wand or "gun." According to Abbott Laboratories, this new analyzer may

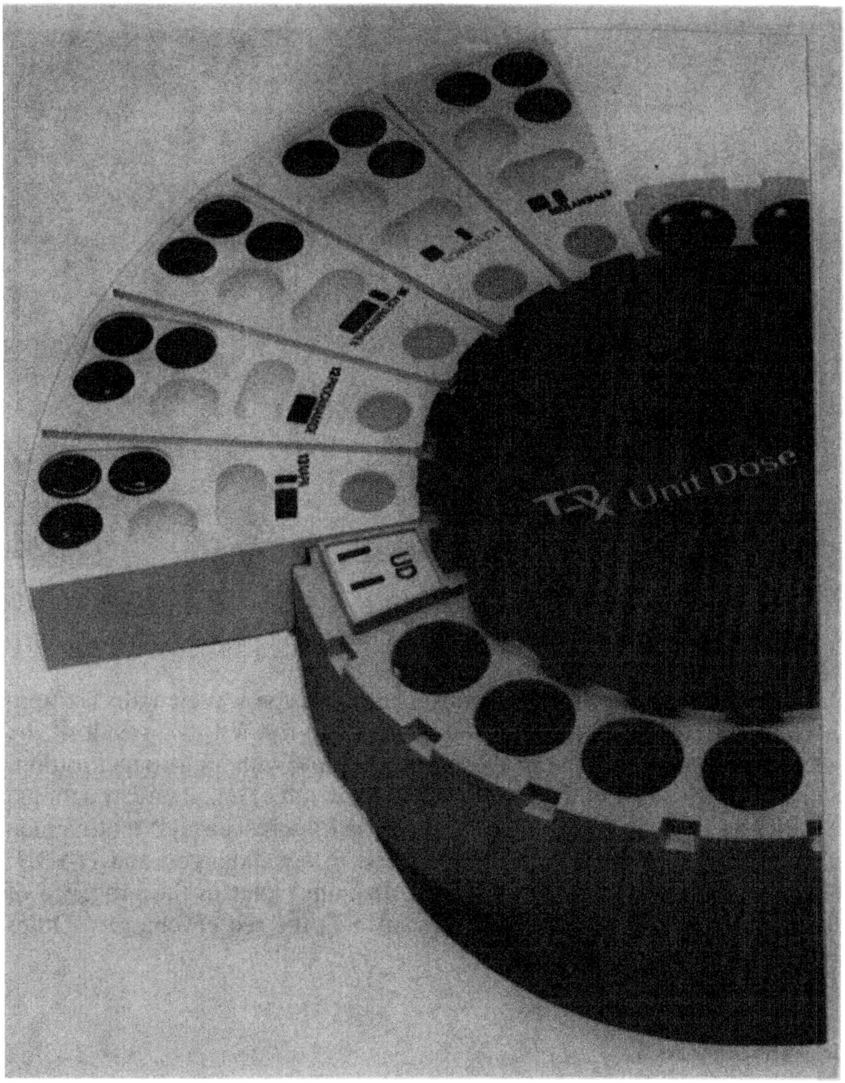

Figure 5 TDx unit close reagent packs and carousel.

be used for FPIA, REA, and other modes of immunodiagnostic technologies in the future.

2. Radiative Energy Attentuation

The principle is based on the measured fluorescence intensity of the fluorophore in solution, proportional to the absorbance of the solution.

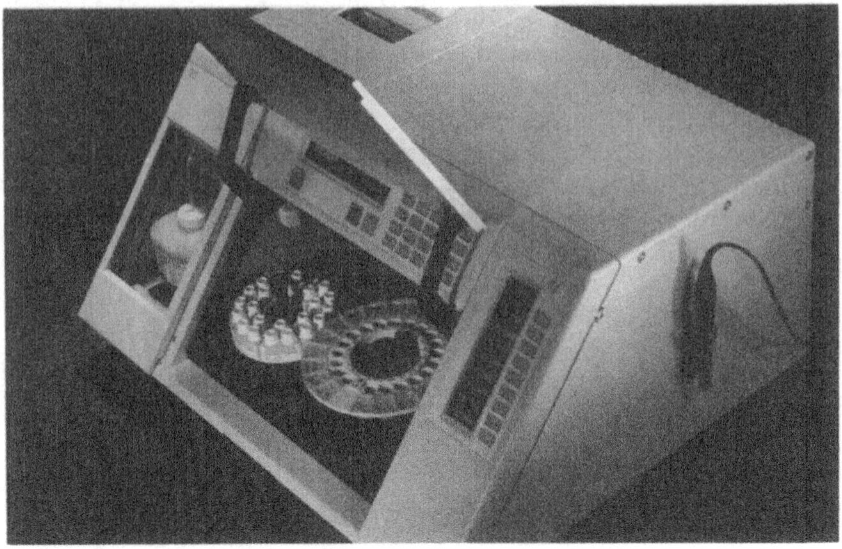

Figure 6 TDxFLx.

The absorbance of both the excitation and emission wavelengths is attentuated by the concentration of red chromogen formed as a result of the enzymatic reactions of the analyte. For a sample with high concentration, a large amount of chromogen is formed as a result of enzymatic reactions, resulting in large attentuation and decreased fluorescense. Nicotinamide adenine dinucleotide (NAD) is converted to acetaldehyde and NADH. Then NADH reacts with iodonitrotetrazolium violet in the presence of diaphorase to form NAD and formazan-INT, the red chromogen. Other REA assays are listed in Table 1.

III. PERFORMANCE

The performance of TDx systems for TDM and Clinical Toxicology is discussed in two main parts: (a) the College of American Pathologists Surveys (1989 and 1990), and (b) the individual/drug group testing. This latter section will address the technical and clinical performance. Further, because the majority of the TDx tests have been introduced for some time, the emphasis of this section will focus on recent developments, novel technical information, and interesting findings including cross-reactivity. With this arbitrary approach, the readers are thus encouraged to refer to the instrument manuals, and past literature such as the informative *Clini-*

cal Chemistry and *Journal of Analytical Toxicology* on the general performance characteristics as the tests were introduced in the earlier 1980s.

Performance characteristics according to the surveys of the College of American Pathologists are outlined in Tables 2 and 3.

A. Performance of Selected Analytes/Drugs/Drug Groups

In this section, the discussion will be arranged according to Tables 2 and 3, starting with antiarrhythmics. As proposed at the beginning of this section, it is not meant to encompass all the analytes.

1. Therapeutic Drug Monitoring

a. Antiarrhythmics Flecainide FPIA measurements were compared with HPLC assay using 400 μl of serum for a solid-phase extraction protocol (Webb *et al.*, 1989). To increase cost-effectiveness, these extraction columns were used up to 40 times. For 25 patient samples, the linear regression analysis showed that FPIA = 1.01 HPLC + 0.058 with r = 0.9856. The means for three controls by HPLC were 0.21, 0.74, and 1.29, respectively, as compared to the corresponding FPIA measurements: 0.15, 0.65, and 1.14.

Total and free quinidine were assayed by both HPLC and FPIA, showing that for total quinidine, FPIA = 0.956 HPLC + 0.234, r = 0.993, and for free qunidine, FPIA = 1.126 HPLC + 0.064, r = 0.917 (Chen *et al.*, 1988). Further, free quinidine was not affected by 3-hydroxyquinidine. FPIA was shown to offer rapid assays of both total and free quinidine.

b. Antiepileptics By mixing serum containing both phenobarbital and pentobarbital with NaOH and heating at 90°C, phenobarbital was "destroyed" (Sobeski *et al.*, 1990). After neutralizing the mixture with HCl, pentobarbital may be measured by using the TDx barbiturate assay. Both precision and recovery were comparable to other TDx drug assays. The following barbiturates showed none or minimal interference: allobarbital, barbital, barbituric acid, hexobartial, mephobarbital, amobarbital, aprobarbital, butabital, and secobarbital. The authors concluded this to be a fast and convenient way to measure pentobarbital on a 24-h basis. By making use of the immuno-crossreactivity of FPIA drugs of abuse assay for barbiturates, rapid assay of pentobarbital was possible in the range of 0.5–3.0 mg/l, with dilution of about 20-fold for measurement of concentrations up to 20 mg/l (Wells and Napper, 1988). Interassay coefficient of variation ranged from 2.5 to 3.9%. This modified assay was suggested for pentobarbital measurement if that is the only drug present.

Table 2 Performance of TDx Systems by FPIA for TDM[a]

Drugs and metabolites	Linear range (mg/l)	Sensitivity (mg/l)	Calibration stability (weeks)	CAP		FPIA		
				Target	*n*	Mean	*n*	SD
Antiarrhythmics								
Disopyramide	0.0–20.0	0.1	4	4.0	230	4.07	175	0.20
Flecainide	0.0–1.50	0.1	—	0.52	69	0.59	62	0.03
Lidocaine	0.0–10.0	0.1	4	4.0	630	4.18	441	0.19
Procainamide	0.0–20.0	0.2	4	8.0	966	7.07	655	0.34
N-Acetyl procainamide	0.0–30.0	0.2	4	16.0	946	13.53	638	0.58
Quinidine	0.0–8.0	0.1	4	3.0	2544	3.09	1600	0.18
Antiasthmatics								
Theophylline	0.0–40.0	0.4	4	5.0	4330	4.75	2182	0.29
Caffeine (?)								
Antiepileptics								
Carbamazepine	0.0–20.0	0.5	4	5.0	2909	5.02	1796	0.29
Ethosuximide	0.0–150.0	0.6	4	60.0	245	59.23	166	3.83
Free carbamazepine	0.0–6.0	0.1	—	1.30	37	1.30	30	0.10
Phenobarbital	0.0–80.0	0.8	4	9.5	3741	9.35	2175	0.41

Phenytoin	0.0–40.0	0.8	3	8.3	4171	9.07	2336	0.39
Free phenytoin	0.0–4.0	0.02	4	0.99	86	1.00	70	0.10
Primidone	0.0–24.0	0.2	4	9.0	1185	8.79	713	0.45
Valproic acid	0.0–150.0	0.7	4	60.0	869	49.30	598	2.37
Free valproic acid	0.0–25.0	0.1	—	4.88	31	4.92	26	0.47
Antimicrobials								
Amikacin	0.0–50.0	0.6		18.3	577	17.58	464	0.71
Gentamicin	0.0–10.0	0.3		5.4	3277	5.11	2042	0.28
Kanamycin	0.0–50.0	0.4						
Nitilmicin	0.0–10.0	0.1						
Tobramycin	0.0–10.0	0.2		3.8	2162	3.80	1421	0.18
Vancomycin	0.0–100.0	0.6		9.8	774	9.88	712	0.67
Cardiac glyosides								
Digoxin	0.0–5.0 ng/ml	0.2 ng/ml	4	0.34	3519	0.40	2005	0.09
Others								
Acetaminophen	0.0–2000	0.8	4	120.9	2626	111.4	1475	5.60
Methotrexate	0.0–1.0	0.01 uM/L	4	2.50	242	2.361	213	0.180
Salicylate (mg/dl)	0.0–800	5.0	4	6.5	2624	7.30	905	0.50

[a] Survey data are based on the Set ZT-C 1990 of the College of American Pathologists (CAP).

Table 3 Performance of TDx Systems by FPIA and REA for Toxicology[a]

Drugs and metabolite	Set	Range (μg/ml)	Sensitivity (μg/ml)	Analyzed concentration (μg/ml)	CAP all methods %	CAP all methods *n*	FPIA %	FPIA *n*
Amphetamine group	UTB-04(90)	0–6	0.1	—	99.3	947	99.6	273
		(Amph. class assay as *d,l*-amph.)						
Amphetamine		0–8	0.1	1	89.5	409	83.9	31
		(Amph. II assay as *d*-amph.)						
Methamphetamine		—	—	3	97.2	390	96.4	28
Amphetamine group	UTB-05(90)	(Same as above)		1	41.8	885	5.9	221
Antidepressants	UTB-05(90)	0–1	0.02	—	97.4	303	97.6	41
		(Antidep. class assay as imipramine)						
Amitriptyline		0–1	0.02	2	97.8	369	100	5
Nortriptyline		0–1	0.02	2	97.3	367	100	5
Antidepressants	UTC-08(90)	0–1	0.02	—	90.2	287	97.7	44
Desipramine		0–1	0.02	3	91.3	345	80	5
Barbiturate group	UTB-05(90)	0–2	0.06	—	96.0	988	97.5	284
		(Barbiturates as secobarbital)						
Barbiturate (butalbital)		(Same as above)		2	76.9	13	71.0	214

Benzodiazepine group	UTA-03(89)	0–2.4 (Benzodiazepines as nordiazepam)	0.04	3(0.3)[b]	26.8	832	52.3	266
Cannabinoids	UTA-03(90)	0–150 ng/ml (As 11-*nor*-delta-8-THC-9-carboxylic acid)	10	120	94.9	1015	97.2	360
Cocaine and/or metabolites	UTA-01(89)	0–5	0.03	—	97.0	896	96.4	280
Benzoylecgonine				2	—	—	—	—
Ecgonine methyl ester				1	—	—	—	—
Ethanol	UTA-01(90)	0–300 mg/dl	10	20	36.9	575	38.1	147
Methadone	UTA-01(89)	0–4 (As methadone)	0.1	1	99.3	549	83.3	6
Methadone metabolite				2	—	—	—	—
Opiate group	UTA-92(90)	0–0.1000 (Opiate as morphine)	0.025	—	99.2	1048	99.7	334
Codeine				5	97.3	414	100	41
Morphine and metabolite				2	22.3	377	25.0	36
Phencyclidine	UTA-03(90)	0–0.500	0.005	0.7	97.4	89.4	98.2	273
Phenylpropanolamine	UTB-06(90)	(Same as amph. group)		6	87.7	349	88.9	9

[a] Survey data based on sets of UTA-1989, and UTA and UTB-1990 of the College of American Pathologists (CAP).

[b] Supposedly prepared at 3, but confirmed by reference lab to be 0.3.

For the estimation of total and free phenytoin and carbamazepine, comparison of HPLC and FPIA yielded similar results (Maas *et al.*, 1988). Further, carbamazepine epoxide did not interfere with FPIA of carbamazepine. Due to the possible spurious effect of the blood collection device of some tube, the effect of postcollection storage time inside the gel tube was evaluated for four antiepileptics—carbamazepine, phenobarbital, phenytoin, and valproic acid (Wong *et al.*, 1983). By comparison to a reference tube, the concentrations up to 24 h were similar, as determined by FPIA.

c. Antimicrobials To enhance the monitoring of genamicin or netilmicin in serum of neonatal and pediatric patients, blood was initially collected onto filter paper and subsequently extracted by phosphate buffer (Fujimoto *et al.*, 1989). This extract, with recovery up to 90%, was then assayed by FPIA. The dried sample in filter paper was stable at ambient temperature for up to eight days. This technique would be valuable for pharmacokinetic study of the above patient groups. Astromicin is an aminoglycoside antibiotic for treating infections due to gram-negative bacteria (Uematsu, 1988). FPIA was linear from 0.31 to 25 mg/l, with between-run coefficients of variations up to 2.74%. No cross-reactivity was observed with other aminoglycosides. Comparison with HPLC showed that FPIA = 0.96HPLC + 0.48, $R = 0.966$. The assay was not affected by hemolysis and hyperbilirubinemia.

d. Digoxin Cross-reactivity was observed in digoxin II assay of samples from patients on high-dose canrenoate, while high-dose spironolactone may also show similar interference (Stone *et al.*, 1988). Digoxin-like immunoreactive factors (DLIF) have been shown to be detected by FPIA and other immunoassays in some patients, including pediatrics, neonates, pregnant women, and patients with liver and kidney dysfunctions (Christenson *et al.*, 1987). Using the manufacturer's method of protein precipitation with 5-sulfosalicyclic acid (SSA), 91% of clinically defined patients not receiving digoxin showed cross-reactivity in FPIA. These included pregnant women, renal-dialysis patients, and noenates. However, after ultrafiltration, no cross-reactivity was observed. Contrary to this earlier study, by using centrifugal ultrafiltration of the serum, a reduction, but not elimination, of DLIF interference was shown in the monitoring of both infant and neonates samples (Crisan *et al.*, 1989). A bias of 0.35 ng/ml was demonstrated. For another patient group—volume expanded and/or hypertensive—ultrafiltration was helpful to differentiate the discrepancy caused by DLIS, since this step would separate DLIS bound to protein, allowing the measurement of free digoxin without much interference (Dasgupta *et al.*, 1989). Thus, the measurement of both total and free digoxin by FPIA may be useful for the above patient groups. Interference from DLIF and canrenoate may be lowered by using TCA precipitation after methylene chloride extraction, while solid-phase extraction using C-18 cartidges would be useful to remove digoxin metabolites (Giesbrecht and Verjee, 1990). Thus, for renal patients, the above techniques would enhance specificity of digoxin monitoring for either TDx and EMIT digoxin assay. Decreasing digoxin QC values were attributed to degradation of reagent, speculated to be caused by evaporation from an open kit at 37°C (Bacaj *et al.*, 1990). The rates of decay for two kits were estimated to be −0.05 and −0.02 μg/l per day. The decay may be minimized by recapping the kit as soon as possible.

Digibind (Burroughs Wellcome) has been used for treatment of digoxin toxicity. Since the binding is similar to immunoassay antibodies, it may interfere with FPIA of digoxin. Rainey (1989) demonstrated the variable results of digoxin monitoring in the presence of a clinically relevant concentration of Digibind by various immunoanalyzers. For FPIA using digoxin II using dilution protocol, total digoxin levels were comparable to traditional methods. For this patient group, clinical evaluation would be the rational approach for patient treatment.

e. Cyclosporine FPIA for cyclosporine and metabolites was shown to be a reliable, simpler, and less hazardous assay (Sanghvi *et al.*, 1988). After collecting patient blood using ethylenediamine tetraacetic acid (EDTA) as anticoagulant and allowing equilibration at room temperature for 2 h, plasma was separated and transferred at room temperature. Then, cyclosporine assay was performed in a similar manner as the other FPIA drug assays, with calibration range up to 1000 μg/l. When compared to RIA, precision studies showed improved between-run CVs ranged from 4.4 to 9.5%. When compared to RIA by Sandoz, the linear regression showed FPIA = 1.72RIA + 61.8, r = 0.884 for n = 408. Metabolites M17 and M1, which exhibit immunosuppressive activity, may account for the greater scatter of observed high values as a result of potential cross-reactivity. This was demonstrated to be in the following descending order (Lensmeyer *et al.*, 1988): M17>18>21>25>302-218>MUNDF1>8>26>, ranging from 75 to 0.6%. The upper calibration of 1000 μg/l and possible reagent evaporation were noted as concerns. In another study comparing with HPLC for 131 samples from heart and kidney transplant patients, regression analysis showed FPIA = 3.92HPLC+ 93.37, r = 0.756. Using the new monoclonal antibodies RIA methods, linear regression showed FPIA = 0.77RIA (monoclonal) + 125, r = 0.95. This was confirmed by another study (Schroeder *et al.*, 1988a, 1988b). Similar observations were made for cyclosporine whole blood assay by FPIA versus RIA and HPLC. The procedure involved mixing 25 μl of whole blood with pretreatment agent, followed by centrifugation and transferring the supernatant. Using the FPIA assay for serum cyclosporine, the cyclosporine/metabolites concentrations of patients with normal BUN and creatinine values ranged from 97 to 550 μg/l, while those of patient showing nephrotoxicity ranged from 150 to 379 μg/l (Alexander, 1988). In comparing three polyclonal antibodies immunoassays of serum cyclosporine (Abbott, Inc., Star, and Sandoz), acceptable correlations were observed, with improved precision and labor effectiveness for the first two assays (Vogt and Welsch, 1988). Whole-blood cyclosporine samples were measured by either preparing a hemolysate or by dilution with TDx buffer. Both were mixed with ammonium acetate for protein precipitation and their supernatants were then assayed by FPIA. By comparison of 70 patient samples, FPIA overestimated by about 10%, while the ease of measurement was a major advantage: 50 min for FPIA, versus 5–6 h for RIAs.

f. Others For rapid and accurate liver function test, the FPIA of a lidocaine metabolite, MEGX, was measured for patients (pretransplant donors and posttransplant recipients) (Littlefield *et al.*, 1988). After administering the test dose of 1 mg/kg, blood was drawn at 15 min and serum was assayed for MEGX. Calibration range was from 0 to 250 μg/l, with a sensitivity of 15 μg/l, and acceptable between-run coefficient of variation (CV) of 3.44% (Oellerich *et al.*, 1987, 1989). By measuring the MEGX, prognostic information about patient selection may be based on the concentrations. In comparison to a normal subject with a median concentration of 73 μg/l, the transplant patients' concentrations of MEGX were significantly lower. Further, in transplant patients surviving more than 120 days, the median MEGX concentrations were higher: 19 versus <3 for adults, and 37 versus <3 for children.

We next consider salicylate (Sarma *et al.*, 1985). Due to the structural similarity of diflunisal with salicylate, significant cross-reactivity was observed for both the enzymatic assay and FPIA, estimated to be 59–63% and 230%, respectively. Thus, it would be important to note that in case of monitoring an arthritic patient medicated with diflunisal, an alternative method, such as HPLC, may be needed.

In monitoring patients on high-dose methotrexate, serial dilution is performed as 1 : 1, 1 : 10, 1 : 100, and 1 : 1000. Recently, the latter two protocols yielded quality control values persistently higher than acceptable limits (Weigand and Wong, 1990). This problem is being solved by manual dilution, and is being investigated by the manufacturer.

g. Pediatric Protocol In reducing the sample size requirement for monitoring of pediatric and neonatal patients, FPIA was modified to utilize as little as 20 μl of serum for the monitoring of phenobarbital, theophylline, carbamazepine, gentamicin, and tobramycin (Wong *et al.*, 1986). This was easily achieved by modifying the pipetting sequence as follows: pipette 20-μl aliquot of patients' sera directly into the dilution wells of the cartridge, while 70-μl aliquots of TDx buffer were pipetted into sample wells.

Between-run precision ranged up to 7%. For the above five drugs, the concentrations were well correlated to those by the normal protocol. Linear regression studies showed slopes ranged from 0.910 to 1.0116, and $r = 0.988\text{–}0.999$.

h. Alternative Reagents Three alternative reagent suppliers included Innotron, Canam, and Colony (Harsha *et al.*, 1988; Kampa and Jarzabek, 1986; Kapke and Bustamante, 1986). These reagents were tested for phenobarbital, phenytoin, gentamicin, tobramycin, and theophylline, showing satisfactory performance. In a latter evaluation of gentamicin reagent by Colony for 39 patients, the regression analysis showed that Colony = 0.961(Abbott) + 0.107. The authors concluded that the alternative reagent is suitable for clinical monitoring (Jones and Lehn, 1987).

2. Testing for Drugs of Abuse

a. Cocaine Metabolite Since meconium has been suggested to be more sensitive for detecting fetal exposure to maternal drug abuse, FPIA of illicit drugs/metabolites in meconium may serve as an useful adjunct in patient management (Boctor *et al.*, 1990). Prior to the assay, meconium was extracted with methanol. Aliquots were then mixed with TDx buffers and assayed for cocaine metabolite. Another study demonstrated the detection of cocaine and benzoylecgonine in meconium by using solid-phase extraction and gas chromatography/mass spectroscopy (GC/MS) analysis (Clark *et al.*, 1990). After methanolic extraction, the transferred supernatant was evaporated, and reconstituted in methylene chloride/isopropanol for solid-phase extraction for subsequent GC/MS analysis. Using the above procedure, cocaine was identified in one baby's meconium, negative by both TDx and EMIT. The positive meconium sample for cocaine and benzoylecgonine by TDx was confirmed by GC/MS (Ostrea *et al.*, 1989). After the above methanolic extraction, meconium spiked with amphetamine, benzoylecgonine, morphine glucronide, and 11-*nor*-COOH-9 THC, was analyzed by both TDx and EMIT (Rosenzweig, 1990). Results from nine specimens from cocaine babies showed that TDx was a more sensitive screening technique.

b. Tetrahydrocannabinoids By comparing 1500 urine samples positive for cannabinoids by an enzyme method, FPIA for Delta-8 and Delta-9 and GC/MS showed that the two FPIA methods were similar (Peat *et al.*, 1989). For samples with a concentration of 15 μg/l by GC/MS, Delta-8 and Delta-9 FPIA showed 59 and 51 μg/l, respectively.

c. Amphetamines The original FPIA amphetamines would detect amphetamines, methamphetamines, and other amines such as phenylpropanolamine, methylenedioxymethamphetamine (MDMA), and methylenedioxyamphetamine (MDA). More recently, a more specific amphetamine II FPIA assay is able to differentiate amphetamine and methamphetamine from the amphetaminelike compounds.

d. Benzodiazepines Acceptable comparison was shown by FPIA, EMIT, and GC of about 415 samples (Kiang and Backes, 1987). The dynamic range was 40–2400 μg/l, showing between-run CV of 4.1% at 200 μg/l. (Kapp *et al.*, 1988). TLC was compared to FPIA for the monitoring of drug-free urine with added bromazepam (BA) and oxazepam (OX). The practical sensitivity by TLC for BA and OX were 0.2 and 0.06 mg/l, respectively, and for FPIA, 0.07 and 0.02 mg/l. TLC was proposed to be able to distinguish these from other benzodiazepines.

e. Methadone The FPIA is semiquantitative, with a dynamic range from 0.15–4.0 mg/l and sensitivity of 0.10 mg/l (Thacker *et al.*, 1989). Comparison studies with GC/MS and EMIT showed similar results.

f. Phencyclidine Thimerosal, a stabilizer, and unidentified metabolites of dextromethorphan interfered with this assay.

g. Opiates Since poppy seeds have been shown to contain morphine, urine from a consumer of poppy seed food preparations would show a positive urine screening by FPIA. In order to differentiate this group from heroin users, the presence of the heroin metabolite, 6-monoacetyl morphine would be a useful indicator. This may be quantified by using gas chromatography/mass spectrometry.

h. Barbiturates A newly developed TDx assay for detection of toxic concentrations of barbiturates in serum or plasma was described, with detection range of 0 to 40 mg/l and sensitivity of 0.7 mg/l (Hu *et al.*, 1990). Calibration stability, precision, and recovery were comparable to other TDx drug assays. From 115 samples shown to be positive by GC/MS for barbiturates, nine negatives were shown by TDx, and these were therapeutic or subtherapeutic. The authors confirmed its efficacy for toxic concentrations.

i. Combined Cocaine Metabolite/Opiate Screening Equal amount of antisera and derivatives were added for the combined assay (Kampa, 1989). Other modifications included mixed calibrators, changing parameters on the opiate channel, and threshold set at 100 μg/l. For a total of 117 samples, 35 were positive for the combined drugs and 82 were negative. Precision shown by between-run studies ranged from 8.39 to 14.94%. This approach may shorten technologist time and reagent cost, but confirmation of each drug should follow.

j. MTDx In enhancing throughput, four TDx's were integrated and controlled by an IBM PS/2 with the appropriate software (Black and Cook, 1989). By using a unitized sample ring and sequentially moving the ring to each analyzer, 338 urine samples were assayed for amphetamines, barbiturates, benzodiazepines, cannabinoids, cocaine metabolite, opiates, and phencyclidine. For 68 samples per day, setup and operating time was lowered from 140 to 40 min, with similar reduction in data collection from 60 to 15 min. The software eliminated 120 min of labor per day. This system was precise and efficient.

3. Routine and Special Chemistry Analytes

a. Thyroxin (T_4) Spuriously high T_4 results were observed for 14 samples of some patients (Law *et al.*, 1988). In comparison, the EMIT and RIA yielded comparable results for these samples. The spuriously high results may be due to high serum background fluorescence such as from endogenous fluorescent substances, which may be present in uremic and normal plasma and also in some elderly patient >60 years of age.

b. Fetal Lung Maturity The relative concentrations of surfactant and albumin in amniotic fluid was measured by FPIA and compared to lecithin/sphingomyelin (L/S) ratios and phosphatidylglycerol (Russell *el al.*, 1989). For selected samples, 312 out of a total of 695 chosen within 3 days of delivery, 24 developed respiratory distress syndrome and seven developed transient tachypnea. In setting a surfactant/albumin level of 50 mg/g, the sensitivity was 0.96 and the specificity was 0.88 for all samples, while the L/S ratios showed a sensitivity of 0.96 and a specificity of 0.83. Due to the significant disagreement with predicted L/S ratios, a combination of the two tests might improve sensitivity and specificity.

c. Urinary MHPG This principle metabolite of norepinephrine in the central nervous system (CNS) may provide information for classification of depression and in predicting response to tricyclic antidepressant therapy (Chou *et al.*, 1988). Prior to FPIA, hydrolysis of urine was performed by using glusulase at 56°C for 3 h, followed by addition of HC1, NaC1, and Florisil. The mixture was centrifuged and the supernatant was assayed by FPIA. When compared to an HPLC assay for 90 samples, the linear regression showed FPIA = 1.4415HPLC + 0.0049, r = 0.9172. Between-run CV was 8.6% for 0.50-mg/l concentrations.

d. Urinary VMA Neural crest tumors such as pheochromocytomas and neuroblastomas would result in elevated urinary concentrations of vanillylmandelic acid (VMA), a metabolite of both epinephrine and norepinephrine (Mellor *et al.*, 1989; Mellor and Gallacher, 1990). Based on the authors' previous publication for the production and characterization of high-titer specific antibodies to VMA and label, a program was developed for using TDx for determination of VMA. FPIA by TDx was demonstrated for a concentration scope of 0.3–200 mg/l with a sensitivity of 0.3 mg/l. Between-run CV was 7.8%, and recoveries were 96–100%. Correlation with the Pisano *et al.* (1962) method showed a slope of 1.08, intercept of 0.49 mg/l, and r = 0.998.

e. Urinary Free Cortisol After extraction of 60 urine samples with methylene chloride, the samples were analyzed by FPIA, RIA, and HPLC

(Gupta *et al.*, 1988). Between-run CV ranged up to 9% for FPIA. Linear regression showed FPIA is comparable with HPLC (slope = 0.91), while RIA overestimated, possibly due to cross-reactivity.

f. Urinary Phenylacetylglutamine Urinary phenylacetic acid may be useful in the treatment of depressive disorders, since depressed patients' urinary concentrations are lower (70 mg/24 h versus normal of 140 mg/24 h) (Ghanbari *et al.*, 1988). Aliquots of urine, containing mainly phenylaceylglutamine, may be assayed by FPIA. When compared to GC/MS, correlation coefficient was 0.95. No known interference had been observed.

g. Paraquat A bipyridinium herbicide, if ingested, would result in fatalities. The FPIA digoxin II was modified, supplemented by prepared antiserum and fluorescent label (Colbert and Coxon, 1988). The calibration range was from 25 to 1800 μg/l, with a sensitivity of 3 μg/l. Comparison with another method for 19 samples showed an acceptable correlation coefficient of 0.96.

C. Economics

Since its introduction, FPIA and REA by using TDx systems have been shown to be reliable with a typical turnaround time of about 10–20 min. The performance of the assays by technologists requires careful pipetting, without much effort in parameter setting and other details. In short, it is a truly automated immunoanalyzer. Thus, the cost associated with personnel is relatively low. Typically, a technologist would be able to utilize multiple TDx systems at the same time. The actual cost of the reagent varies according to the test and hospital setting, ranging from several dollars per test to the more expensive, such as the Unit Dose reagent and the recently introduced monoclonal cyclosporine, of more than $10.00 per test. Further, with the introduction of TDxFLx, allowing multiple assays at the same time, and MTDx, for multiple illicit drug screening as described in the previous sections, the efficiency is further enhanced. The exact role of TDx systems thus depends on the need of the particular hospital, such as TAT requirements and staffing level.

IV. THE FUTURE

The TDx systems have greatly enhanced the specialty of therapeutic drug monitoring and toxicology. The instrument has been shown to be reliable. The TDx reagents for both therapeutic and illicit drugs/metabolites have satisfied the criteria set by laboratorians. Interference problems of several assays have been duly recognized, possibly addressed by using alternative methodologies. With the advent of TDxFLx, flexibility in the form of limited random assay is now possible. With MTDx, throughput is increased with patient data processing using PC.

REFERENCES

Alexander, R. L. (1988). Evaluation of a fluorescence polarization method for cyclosporine and its application in monitoring renal transplant recipients for nephrotoxicity. *Clin. Chem.* **34,** 1180.

Bacaj, P. J., Boyd, J. C., and Herold, D. A. (1990). Premature degradation of Abbott TDx reagents. *Clin. Chem.* **36,** 818.

Black, D., and Cook, L. (1898). Evaluation of the Abbott Laboratories MTDx™ drug analysis system. *Clin. Chem.* **35,** 1185.

Blecka, L. J. (1983). Fluorescence Polarization Immunoassay: A review of methodology and application in TDM. Continuing education and quality control programs, pp. 1–6. Washington, D.C.: American Association for Clinical Chemistry.

Boctor, F., Salfia, C., Horak, E., and Wong, S. H. Y. (1990). Measurement of a cocaine metabolite benzoylecogonine in meconium. *Ann. Clin. Lab. Sci.* **20,** 287–8.

Cary, P. L., Whitter, P. D., and Johnson, C. A. (1984). Abbott Radiation Energy Attenuation method for quantifying ethanol evaluated and compared with as liquid chromatography. *Clin. Chem.* **31,** 1867–1870.

Chen, B. H., Taylor, E. H., and Pappas, A. A. (1988). Determination of free quinidine by fluorescence polarization immunoassay. *Clin. Chem.* **34,** 1251.

Chou, P. P., King, B., Seemiller, B., Holmes, C., and Bailey, J. L. (1988). Evaluation of a fluorescent polarization immunoassay for the determination of urinary MHPG. *Clin. Chem.* **34,** 1218.

Christenson, R. H., Studenberg, S. D., Beck-Davis, S., and Sedor, F. A. (1987). Digoxin-like immunoreactivity eliminated from serum by centrifugal ultrafiltration before fluorescence polarization immunoassay of digoxin. *Clin. Chem.* **34,** 606–608.

Clark, G. D., Rosenzweig, I. B., and Raisys, V. A. (1990). Analysis of cocaine and benzoylecgonine in meconium of infants cocaine to cocaine dependent mothers. *Clin Chem.* **36,** 1022.

Colbert, D. L., and Coxon, R. E., (1988). Paraquat measured in serum with the Abbott TDx. *Clin. Chem.* **88,** 1948.

Crisan, D., Howrie, D. L., Fricker, F. J., and Lower, D. (1989). Digoxin-like immunoreactivity in neonates and infants minimized by centrifugal ultrafiltration and fluorescence polarization immunoassay. *Clin. Chem.* **35,** 1163–1164.

Dandliker, W. B., Kelly, R. J., Dandliker, J., Farquhar, J., and Levin, J. (1973). Fluorescence polarization immunoassay. Theory and experimental method. *Immunochemistry*. **10,** 219–227.

Dasgupta, A., Nakamura, A., Doria, L., and Dennen, D. (1989). Comparison of Free Digoxin and total digoxin: Extent of interference from digoxin-like immunoreactive substances (DLIS) in a fluorescence polarization assay. *Clin. Chem.* **35,** 323–324.

Fujimoto, T., Tsuda, Y., Tawa, R., and Hirose, S. (1989). Fluorescence polarization immunoassay of gentamicin or netilmicin in blood spotted on filter paper. *Clin. Chem.* **35,** 867–869.

Ghanbari, H., Roberts, B., Johnson, D., and Adamcyzk, M. (1988). Quantification of urinary phenylacetylglutamine (PAG) by FPIA using TDx. *Clin. Chem.* **34,** 1161.

Giesbrecht, E., and Verjee, Z. (1990). Improved measurement of serum digoxin. *Clin. Chem.* **36,** 1028.

Gupta, M. K., Pippenger, C. E., Seifarth, K., and Hahn, S. (1988). Measurement of urinary free cortisol by fluorescence polarization immunoassay (Abbott TDx): Comparison with RIA and HPLC. *Clin. Chem.* **34,** 1216.

Harsha, J., Munendra, S., Ramos, Y., and Dinovo, E. (1988). Evaluation of Colony reagents for theophylline and phenytoin using the Abbott TDx analyzer. *Clin. Chem.* **34,** 1261.

Hu, H-Y.Y., Wali, F., Grote, J., Backes, D., and Simpson, J. (1990). Fluorescence polarization immunoassay for detection of serum barbiturates. *Clin. Chem.* **36,** 1038.

Jolley, M. E. (1981). Fluorescence polarization immunoassay for the determination of therapeutic drug levels in human plasma. *J. Anal. Toxicol.* **5,** 236–240.

Jolley, M. E., Stroupe, S. D., Schwenzer, K. S., *et al.* (1981). Fluorescence polarization immunoassay. III. An automated system for therapeutic drug determination. *Clin. Chem.* **27,** 1575–1579.

Jones, J. E., and Lehn, R. (1987). Evaluation of Colony Gentamicin fluorescence polarization immunoassay. *Clin. Chem.* **33,** 955.

Kampa, I. S. (1989). Evaluation of a combined cocaine/opiate screening procedure on the Abbott Laboratories' TDx. *Clin. Chem.* **35,** 1115–6.

Kampa, I. S., and Jarzabek, J. I. (1986). A comprehensive evaluation of alternative fluorescent polarization reagents for use on the Abbott Laboratories TDx analyzer. *Clin. Chem.* **32,** 1054.

Kapke, G. F., and Bustamante, B. B. (1986). Comparison of Colony and Abbott theophylline fluorescence polarization immunoassays. *Clin. Chem.* **32,** 1054.

Kapp, S., Muller Th., and Sandow, U. (1988). Detection of 1,4-benzodiazepines with thin-layer chromatography (TLC) and fluorescence polarization (TDx). *Clin. Chem.* **34,** 1264.

Kiang, W., and Backes, D. (1987). Clinical evaluation of a TDx^R fluorescence polarization immunoassay (FPIA) for the detection of benzodiazepines in urine. *Clin. Chem.* **33,** 973.

Law, L. K., Cheung, C. K., and Swaminathan, R. (1988). Falsely high thyroxin results by fluorescence polarization in sera with high background fluorescence. *Clin. Chem.* **34,** 1918.

Lensmeyer, G. L., de Vos, D. J., Horswill, J. E., Rohde, D. A., Carlson, I. H., and Wiebe, D. A. (1988). Cross-reactivity study of cyclosporine metabolites with three commercial whole blood immunoassays. *Clin. Chem.* **34,** 1269.

Littlefield, M., Kolaczkowski, L., and Wang, P. (1988). Monoethylglycinexylidide (MEGX) determined by fluorescence polarization immunoassay (FPIA) as a liver function test. *Clin. Chem.* **34,** 1159.

Maas, M. C., Karcher, R. E., Epstein, E., and Kiechle, F. L. (1988). Comparison of fluorescence polarization immunoassay (Abbott-TDx) and high performance liquid chromatography (HPLC) for the quantitative determination of total and free phenytoin. *Clin. Chem.* **34,** 1253.

Mellor, G. W., and Gallacher, G. (1990). Fluorescence polarization immunoassay of urinary vanillylmendelic acid. *Clin. Chem.* **36,** 110–2.

Mellor, G. W., Gallacher, G., and Landon, J. (1989). Production and characterization of antibodies to vanillylmendelic acid *J. Immunol. Methods.* **118,** 101–7.

Oellerich, M., Raude, E., Burdelski, M., Schulz, M., Schmidt, F. W., Ring, B., and Lamesch, P. (1987). Monoethylglycinexylidide formation kinetics: a novel approach to assessment of liver function. *J. Clin. Chem. Clin. Biochem.* **25,** 845–853.

Oellerich, M., Burdelski, M., Lantz, H., Rodeck, B., and Duvell, J. (1989). Prognostic value of the MEAX liver function test in transplant candidates. *Clin. Chem.* **35,** 1135.

Peat, M. A., Pino, J. A., Caughlin, L., Noedel, M., and Peat, J. J. (1989). A comparison of Abbott TDx fluorescence polarization immunoassays for cannabinoids with gas chromatography-mass spectrometry. *Clin. Chem.* **34,** 1185.

Perrin, F. (1926). Polarization de la lumiere de fluorescence. Vie Moyenne de molecules dans l'etat excite. *J. Phys. Radium.* **7,** 390–401.

Pisano, J. J., Crout, J. R., Abraham, D. (1962). Determination of 3-methoxy-4-hydroxymandelic acid in urine. *Clin. Chem. Acta.* **7,** 285–91.
Rainey, P. M. (1989). Effects of digoxin immune Fab (ovine) on digoxin immunoassays. *Am. J. Clin. Pathol.* **92,** 779–786.
Rosenzweig, I. B., Clark, G. D., Thiersch, N. J., and Raiaya, V. A. (1990). Neonatal drugs of abuse screening in meconium. *Clin. Chem.* **36,** 1023.
Russell, J. C., Cooper, C. M., Ketchum, C. H., Torday, J. S., Richardson, D. K., Holt, J. A., Kaplan, L. S., Swanson, J. R., and Vie, W. M. (1989). Multicenter evaluation of TDx test for assessing fetal lung maturity. *Clin. Chem.* **35,** 1005–1010.
Sanghvi, A., Diven, W., Seltman, H., and Starzl, T. (1988). Abbott's fluorescence polarization immunoassay for cyclosporine and metabolites compared with the Sandoz "Sandimmune" RIA. *Clin. Chem.* **34,** 1904–1906.
Sarma, L., Wong, S. H. Y., and DellaFera, S. S. (1985). Diflunsal significantly interferes with salicylate measurements by FPIA and TDx and ACA methods. *Clin. Chem.* **31,** 1922–3.
Schroeder, T. J., Pesce, A. J., Hindenlang, L., Ruckrigl, D., Mauser, P., and Wadih, G. (1988a). Evaluation of TDx^R fluorescence polarization immunoassay (FPIA) for the monitoring of cyclosporine in whole blood. *Clin. Chem.* **34,** 1205.
Schroeder, T. J., Pesce, A., Mauser, P., Weibel, M., Hindenlang, L., and First, M. R. (1988b). Evaluation of the TDx^R fluorescent polarization immunoassay (FPIA) for the monitoring of cyclosporine in serum. *Clin. Chem.* **34,** 1261.
Sobeski, L. M., Earl, R. A., Timko, D. M., and Markin, R. S. (1990). Immunoassay of Pentobarbital in the presence of phenobarbital using the Abbott TDx^{TM}. *Clin. Chem.* **36,** 1037.
Stone, J., Bunting, P., and Soldin, S. J. (1988). Canrenoate interference with Abbott TDx digoxin II FPIA. *Clin. Chem.* **34,** 1252.
Thacker, S., Dubler, R., Wang, N., Walling, J., and Chiappeta, E. (1989). Development of a TDx/ADx fluorescence polarization immunoassay for the detection of methadone in human urine. *Clin. Chem.* **35,** 1176.
Uematsu, T., Ryuichi, S., Mizuno, A., Nishimoto, M., Nagashima, S., and Nakashima, M. (1988). A fluorescence polarization immunoassay evaluated for quantifying astromicin, a new aminoglycoside antibiotic. *Clin. Chem.* **34,** 1880–1882.
Vogt, W., and Welsch, I. (1988). Modified TDx^R assay for cyclosporine and metabolites, for use with whole-blood samples. *Clin. Chem.* **34,** 1459–1461.
Webb, G., Beierle, F., Berk, L., Hillock, R., and Eby, W. (1989). Flecainide: Comparison of fluorescence polarization technique with high performance liquid chromatography (HPLC). *Clin. Chem.* **35,** 1097.
Weber, G. (1953). Rotational brownian motion and polarization of the fluorescence of solution. *Adv. Protein Chem.* **8,** 415–459.
Wells, D. J., and Napper, J. C. (1988). Rapid quantitation of serum pentobarbital using the Abbott TDx^R abused drug assay for barbiturates. *Clin. Chem.* **34,** 1260.
Wiegand, T., and Wong, S. H. Y. (1990). Unpublished data. Drug Assay Laboratory Clinical Chemistry Division, Laboratory Medicine Dept., The Johns Hopkins Hospital.
Wong, S. H. Y., Pena, Y., Lin, F. C., and Narayanan, S. (1983). Assessment of evacuated serum separator gel blood collection tubes for antiepileptic monitoring by FPIA. *Clin. Chem.* **33,** 1017.
Wong, S. H. Y. (1984). The fluorescence polarization assay in TDM: Recent developments. *Lab. Manage.* **22,** 36–42.
Wong, S. H. Y., Donskoy, E., and Marzouk, N. (1986). A modified protocol of fluorescence polarization immunoassay (FPIA) for phenobarbital, theophylline, carbamazepine, gentamicin, and tobramycin. *Clin. Chem.* **32,** 1062.

CHAPTER 24

The Vista Immunoassay System

Thomas M. Li
Syva Company, San Jose, California

I. INTRODUCTION

The Vista Immunoassay System is a bench-top, fully automated multitest analyzer that offers random test selection. This system is designed for processing a broad immunodiagnostics work load in medium to large hospitals and laboratories. The instrument is manufactured by Hitachi and reagents are manufactured by Syva. The Vista system is a heterogeneous enzyme fluorescent immunoassay system utilizing chromium dioxide magnetic particles as solid phase and alkaline phosphatase as the enzyme label.

II. SYSTEM DESCRIPTION

A. Instrumentation

The instrument and layout are shown in Figs. 1 and 2. For simplicity and reliability, the Vista Immunoassay System features a single pipetting arm for dispensing samples and reagents with level-sensing capability. Sample addition, reagent addition, mixing, incubation, washing, and fluorescence measurements are totally automated. Multitest assay-specific reagent cartridges are stored on-board in a refrigerated carousel and are bar coded for automated testing and inventory management. These reagent cartridges are specially designed to assure precise dispensing of chromium dioxide particles. The instrument includes a sample wheel-reagent cartridge carousel, a particle mixer for consistent dispensing of magnetic particles, a

Immunoassay Automation: A Practical Guide

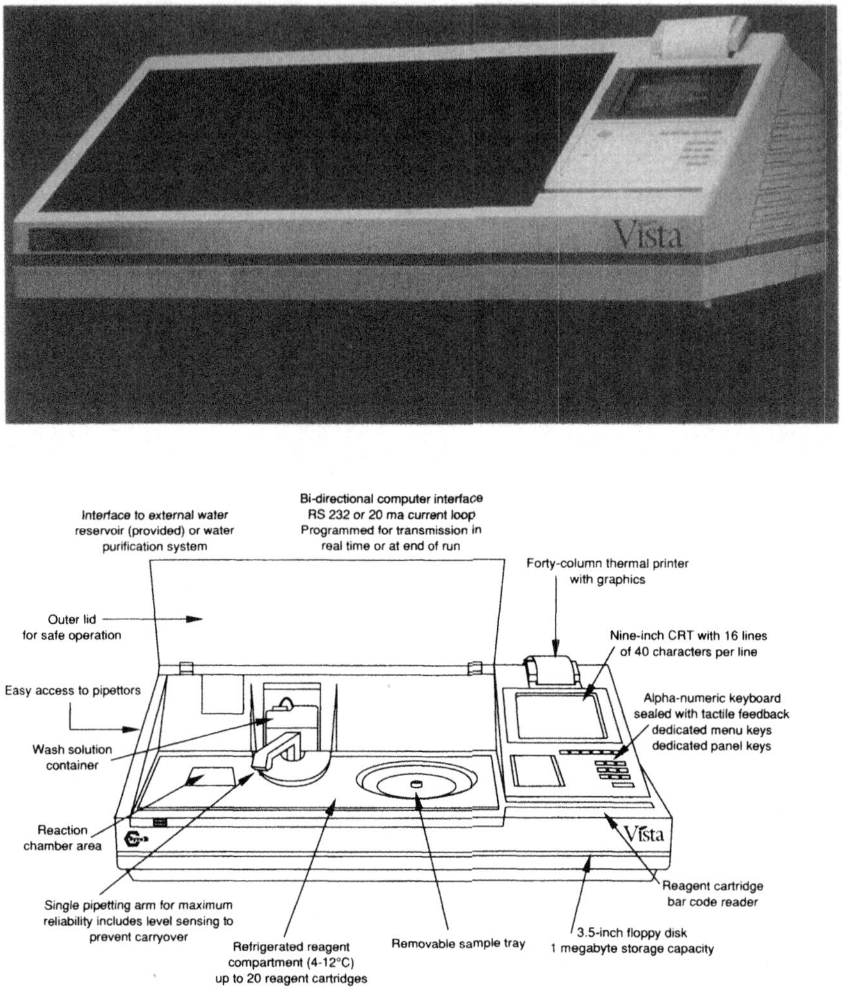

Figure 1 Major components of the Vista Immunoassay System.

pipetter/diluter, a fluorometer, a cuvette carousel, and a wash/separation station. Mixing, incubation, separation/wash, and fluorescence measurement steps are all automated in a single run through interleaving of the various method protocols. Up to a total of eight method protocols are allowed, thus providing great flexibility in assay design. Assay selection, parameter settings, or other communications are controlled through an alphanumeric keyboard and interactive cathode ray tube (CRT) display. Hard-copy results are reported by an on-board thermal printer. Assay

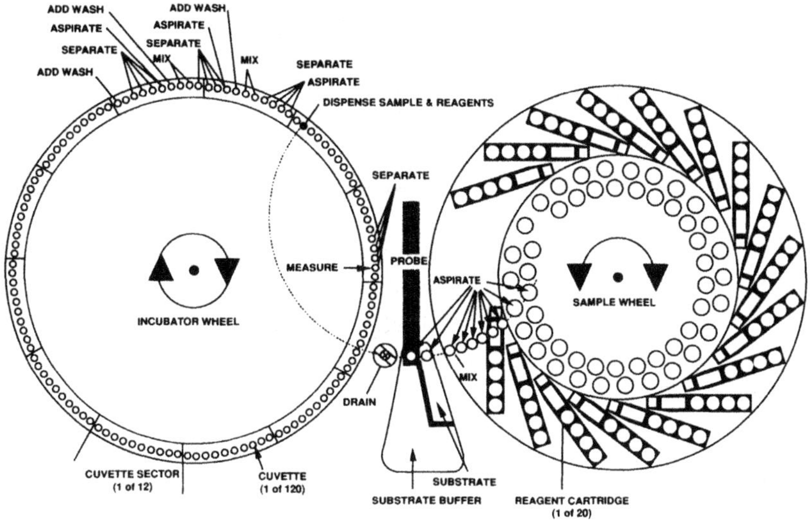

Figure 2 Top layout of the Vista Immunoassay System.

requests and results can also be transmitted via a bidirectional computer interface.

B. Reagents

The Vista Immunoassay System uses chromium dioxide magnetic particles as the solid support and alkaline phosphatase as the enzyme label. The advantages of chromium dioxide magnetic particles, including high surface area, easy dispersion, rapid analyte capture, and low nonspecific binding, have been described elsewhere (Birkmeyer *et al.,* 1987). For small-molecule assays, a heterogeneous competitive antibody-binding assay format is utilized in which the magnetic particles are coated with streptavidin and specific antibodies are biotinylated. For large-molecule assays, a heterogeneous antibody sandwich assay format is used. After the sample, reagent incubation, and washing steps, fluorescence is generated via the hydrolysis of 4-methylumbelliferone phosphate in diethanolamine buffer. In addition to the common substrate and diethanolamine buffer, the system also utilizes a common wash solution. The Vista Immunoassay System is designed to measure a wide variety of special chemistry analytes including thyroid, fertility, anemia, cancer markers, hepatitis, and antibody to human immunodeficiency virus tests.

III. SYSTEM AND ASSAY PERFORMANCE

We investigated the system pipetting and fluorescence measurement repeatability and found the total CV for the 4-methylumbelliferone pipetting and fluorescence measurement to be <1%. The fluorometer linear range was determined to be from 1 n*M* to 20 μ*M* 3-methylumbelliferone. Sample carryover was assessed using a human chorionic gonadotropin sample at 1×10^6 IU/l, and a 1–2 ppm sample carryover was obtained.

Typical within- and between-run precision for thyroxine, thyroxine-uptake, human chorionic gonadotropin, and thyroid stimulating hormone assays are shown in Table 1. Clinical sample correlation studies comparing the performance of the Vista carcinoembryonic antigen with Hybritech Tandem-EIA assay is shown in Fig. 3. The TSH assay sensitivity, defined by the amount of thyroid-stimulating hormone that is reliably distinguishable from the zero calibrator (2SD above the zero calibrator) was calculated for two different master lots to be 0.03 and 0.02 mIU/l. An example of calibration curve stability for the thyroxine assays and thyroid-stimulating hormone is shown in Figs. 4 and 5.

IV. DISCUSSION

The Vista Immunoassay System is designed to eliminate the need for multiple batch operation by offering random access for up to 19 different

Table 1 Typical Assay Precision for Thyroxine, Thyroxine Uptake, Human Chorionic Gonadotropin, and Thyroid-Stimulating Hormone Assay

Assay	Concentration	Within-run % CV	Between-run % CV
Thyroxine	4.7 μg/dl	1.6	3.6
	8.4 μg/dl	2.2	2.9
	14.2 μg/dl	3.0	3.0
	20.2 μg/dl	4.1	4.7
Thyroxine uptake	28.4%	3.3	4.1
	35.3%	1.9	2.1
	44.1%	0.5	1.3
	60.1%	1.2	1.8
hCG	5.1 mIU/ml	4.5	5.9
	26.0 mIU/ml	2.6	4.9
	199.3 mIU/ml	2.0	2.3
	436.5 mIU/ml	2.4	2.6
TSH	0.5 μIU/ml	2.8	3.7
	5.2 μIU/ml	0.7	1.6
	25.9 μIU/ml	0.8	2.5
	57.4 μIU/ml	2.2	2.5

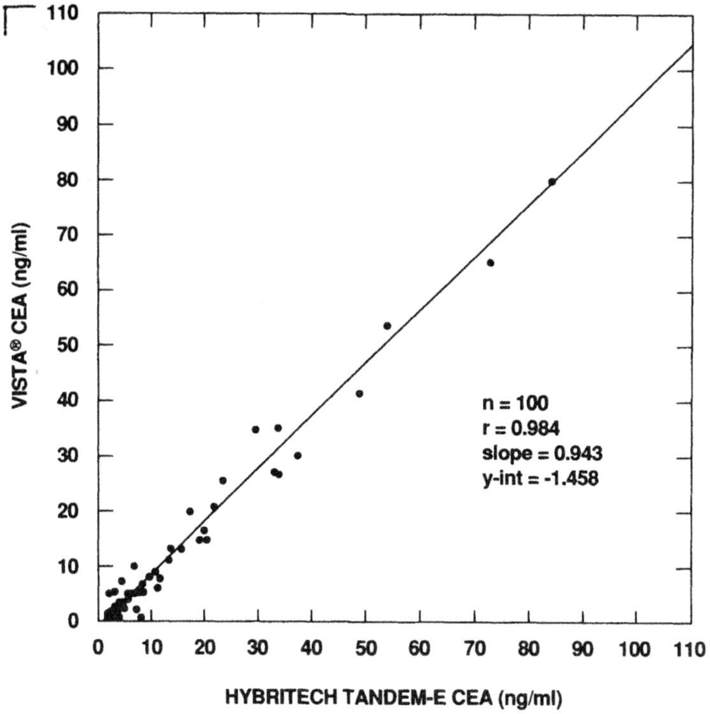

Figure 3 Clinical sample correlation: Vista carcinoembryonic antigen assay versus Hybritech Tandem-E.

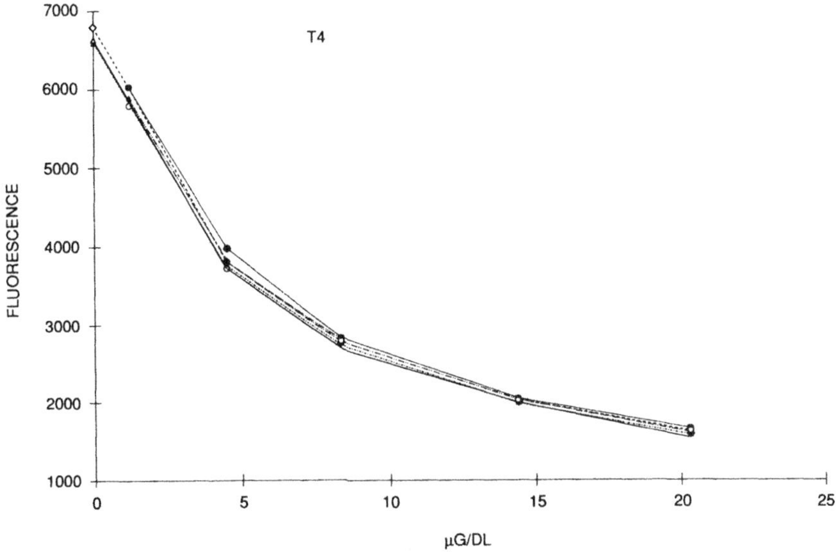

Figure 4 Thyroxine calibration curve stability. Calibration curves with five replicates at each concentration level were collected over 30 days.

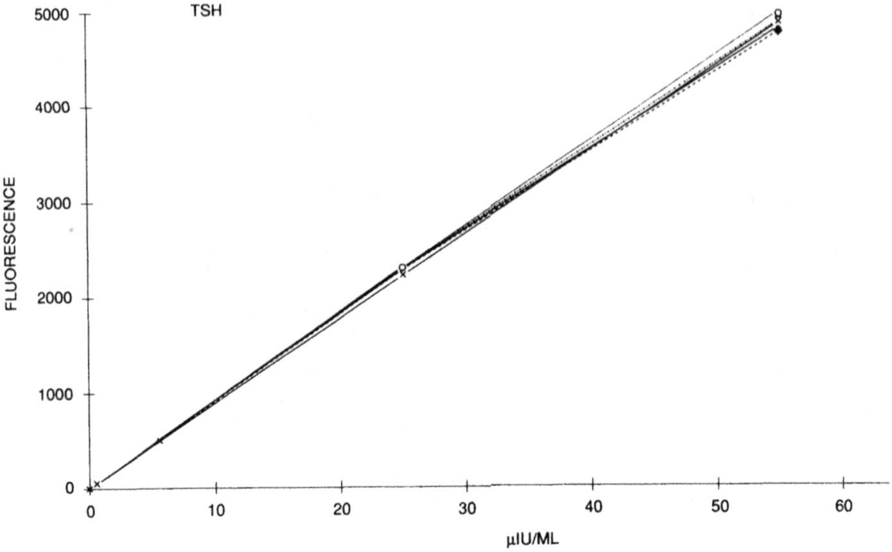

Figure 5 Thyroid-stimulating hormone calibration curve stability. Calibration curves with five replicates at each concentration level were collected over 30 days.

on-board assays. The user enters a sample number and can order single tests, panels, or profiles for each patient sample. Up to 50 samples at one time can be loaded onto the sample carousel and up to 19 different reagents can be on-board the instrument for any one run. Cartridges can be removed and replaced without affecting reagent inventory management. Thus any of up to 15 different methods can be selected on any sample without sample splitting.

The system is designed to be compatible with laboratory workflow. While the instrument is operating, the next run can be programmed. With automatic QC trend analysis and a bidirectional computer interface, record keeping is streamlined. A major economic advantage of the Vista system is total cost reduction. Total automation and nonisotopic assays replace time-consuming, labor-intensive manual methods and isotope handling. Consolidated testing reduces the technologist's time and the cost of operating multiple instruments or several runs. The broad test menu and multiple protocol capability reduce the turnaround time by eliminating the need to batch small volume tests or to send tests to a reference laboratory. The Vista reagent format is designed to be cost-effective and to increase laboratory productivity. The assay-specific cartridge holds sufficient reagents for 32 tests. With 100 tests per run, the Vista instrument is capable of processing in excess of 200 special chemistry tests per shift while providing extended walk-away time to the technologist. The Vista system also features extended curve storage capability to ensure accurate results without frequent and costly calibration.

REFERENCES

Richard C. Birkmeyer *et al.* (1987). Application of Novel Chromium Dioxide Magnetic Particles to Immunoassay Development. *Clin. Chem.* **33:** 1543–1547.

CHAPTER 25

Immunoassay Systems for the Physician's Office

Ronald H. Ng
Department of Pathology and Laboratory Medicine, Methodist Hospital of Indiana, Indianapolis, Indiana

I. INTRODUCTION

Traditional immunoassays are not suitable for use in the physician's office since they entail complicated manual procedures. Radioimmunoassays, for example, are incompatible with the physician office setting because of the radioactivity involved, whereas nonisotopic immunoassays still require adequate physical facility and a trained technologist to perform. Technique-dependent processes in immunoassays usually include numerous pipetting steps, timing and temperature control during incubation, separation of bound from free ligands, and detection of the bound fraction. However, recent advances in technology have made it simple and cost-effective for some immunoassays to be performed in the physician's office using small instruments. Completely automated or semiautomated procedures are performed with these systems.

In this chapter, I describe the operational features and analytical performance of various immunoassay systems available today for the physician's office.

II. ABBOTT VISION

A. Instrument Description

The Vision (Abbott Laboratories, Abbott Park, Illinois) is a "walk-away" or completely automated analyzer (52 cm wide, 44 cm high, 52 cm deep; approximately 32 kg) (Schultz *et al.*, 1985; Ng, 1986). The instrument consists of a built-in centrifuge, photometer, and microprocessor with keyboard and liquid crystal display panel. The system is based on two-dimensional centrifugation of plastic test packs, one for each test result. Each test pack contains prepackaged reagents and a separation device for use with the analyzer's centrifuge to separate plasma from whole blood. One or two drops of fingerstick blood is sufficient for a test, although plasma and serum are also acceptable specimens. Analysis is conducted in batch mode; 1–10 tests of any combination, that is, different tests and different specimens, can be assayed in each run, and results are ready in 8–10 min.

Three steps are required to perform a test on the system. Blood is drawn in a customized capillary tube and inserted into the test pack. Alternatively, the user can add one or two drops of venipuncture sample into the pack's sample well. The test pack is loaded into the analyzer, which can hold any 10 test packs. After the run button is pressed, the analyzer automatically spins down the sample to plasma, mixes it with reagents, measures the absorbance, and calculates and prints the results. The analyzer will flag a warning if the specimen is hemolyzed, icteric, or lipemic, or if insufficient sample is in the test pack.

B. Instrument Performance (Ng *et al.*, 1986)

I found the Vision very easy to use and without technique-dependent steps in the entire procedure. Its ability to automatically separate plasma from whole blood simplifies the testing process and circumvents potential analytical problems from assaying whole blood directly. The self-contained reagent test packs, liquid controls, and calibrators are ready to use. Thus, potential errors from preparing these materials are eliminated. The "walk-away" capability for up to 10 tests at a time and in any combination is also an advantage with this system. The drawback of this system may be the relatively high costs of the instrument and reagents, that is, $14,995.00 for the instrument, $6.25 for a theophylline test, and $4.50 for a thyroxine test.

The calibration is stable for approximately 4–6 weeks with the immunoassays, compared to up to 3 months with other Vision tests.

At present, theophylline and thyroxine are the immunoassays available on the VISION system.

C. Theophylline Assay

1. Principles of the Method

The method is a homogeneous enzyme-inhibitor immunoassay. In this test, the theophylline in the sample competes with an enzyme inhibitor (a theophylline conjugate), which is structurally similar to theophylline, for binding sites on a specific antibody. The amount of free theophylline conjugate present is proportional to the concentration of theophylline in the specimen. Because only the free but not the antibody-bound theophylline conjugate is a potent inhibitor of acetylcholinesterase (EC 3.1.1.7), the enzyme in the assay, the theophylline concentration in the sample is inversely proportional to the activity of the enzyme:

Antibody (theophylline conjugate) +
acetylcholinesterase ⟶ active enzyme

Free theophylline conjugate +
acetylcholinesterase ⟶ inactive enzyme

The activity of acetylcholinesterase is measured by the enzymatic hydrolysis of acetyl-beta-(methylthio)choline iodide (substrate) to the free thio product, beta-(methylthio)choline. Reaction of this thio product with 5,5′-dithiobis (2-nitrobenzoic acid) (DTNB) generates a colored thionitrobenzoate anion, which absorbs at 417 nm.

2. Performance of the Method

Chan *et al.* (1987) reported that within-day precision (coefficient of variation, CV) was 1.8 and 3.1% at theophylline concentrations of 15.2 and 25.2 μg/ml, respectively; between-day CV was 3.5 and 4.8% at 14.9 and 24.4 μg/ml, respectively. Bilirubin (14.3 mg/dl) and triglycerides (740 mg/dl) did not interfere; hemoglobin at 200 mg/dl reduced the theophylline value by 10–15%. Comparison of the Vision method (y) with the Abbott TDx system (x) showed $y = 0.978x - 0.27$ μg/ml; $r = 0.978$; $Sy.x = 1.0$ μg/ml. The Vision method gave comparable theophylline values for serum, plasma, and whole-blood samples. Capillary blood samples collected by fingerstick can be used interchangeably with blood samples collected by venipuncture for monitoring theophylline therapy. The dynamic range of the Vision theophylline method is 0.4–30.0 μg/ml.

D. Thyroxine Assay

1. Principles of the Method

The principles of the thyroxine (T_4) assay are same as those of the theophylline test.

2. Performance of the Method

The manufacturer claimed total CV of 6.9 and 3.2% at 4.5 and 15.2 μg/dl, respectively. The dynamic range is 1.0–24.0 μg/dl. Comparison of the Vision method (y) with the TDx procedure showed $y = 0.97x - 0.14$ μg/dl, $r = 0.97$. The following substances, at the given concentrations, showed less than 10% interference at approximately 7.0 μg/dl thyroxine: bilirubin, 20 mg/dl; hemoglobin, 250 mg/dl; triglycerides, 400 mg/dl.

III. DUPONT ANALYST

A. Instrument Description

The Analyst (DuPont, Wilmington, Delaware) is designed to perform discrete and profile (up to 12 different analytes) testing (Hodgson, 1987). The reagents for each profile or discrete analysis are contained in a disposable plastic rotor. The size of the instrument is 63.5 cm wide, 21.6 cm high, and 33.0 cm deep (19 kg); the pipettor/dilutor is 13.2 cm wide, 25.9 cm high, and 21.8 cm deep (6.7 kg).

To perform an analysis, the operator needs to perform three steps: (1) dilute the patient's serum or plasma sample with the automatic pipettor/dilutor (a 100-fold dilution is required for the theophylline assay), (2) dispense the sample and the control material into two wells located in the center of the rotor, and (3) place the rotor into the instrument and press the start button.

The system then mixes and equilibrates each sample by spinning the rotor at various speeds, reaching 3000 rpm. Centrifugal force pushes the diluted specimens through capillaries into the reaction cells along the rotor's perimeter. These cells contain the reagent tablets. The system's spectrophotometer measures the resulting reactions in the cells at 6-s intervals for 5 min.

B. Instrument Performance

The Analyst is simple to use. However, all specimens must be diluted and dispensed manually with the pipettor/dilutor, which requires some training of any new user. The device is also used to deliver diluents to reconstitute calibrators and controls (Ng *et al.*, 1988).

The Analyst would be ideal for profile testing in the physician office if there were a greater variety of rotors with different test configurations.

Presently there is only one immunoassay (thoephylline test) on the Analyst; it uses a rotor specific for theophylline. The throughput of the system is relatively low (results of one patient and one control in 7–10 min). Comparable to the Vision, the costs for the Analyst system are $14,900 for the analyzer and $6.95 for each theophylline rotor.

C. Theophylline Assay

1. Principles of the Method

The theophylline rotor utilizes the PETINIA (particle-enhanced turbidimetric inhibition immunoassay) technology introduced by DuPont in 1983 for the theophylline method on the *aca* analyzer.

The theophylline rotor contains a latex particle with theophylline linked to the surface. Aggregates of these particles are formed when a theophylline-specific monoclonal antibody is introduced. Theophylline present in a sample competes with the particles for the antibody, thereby decreasing the rate of aggregation. Hence, the rate of aggregation, measured turbidimetrically at 340 nm, is inversely proportional to the concentration of theophylline in the sample.

The theophylline rotor has been designed to assay a patient specimen and a control sample concurrently. The assay range is 2–40 μg/ml. Calibration using three levels of serum-based liquid calibrators is recommended every 2 months.

2. Performance of the Method

Vaughn *et al.* (1989) reported within-day CV of 4.2–4.6%, and between-day CV of 5.4–5.6%. Comparison of patients' results with other methods showed:

Comparative method	Slope	Intercept	*r*	Sy.*x*	*n*
HPLC	1.069	−0.375	0.965	2.65	98
Abbott TDx	1.000	0.396	0.972	2.37	99
Syva EMIT	1.096	−0.708	0.970	2.49	99
DuPont *aca*	1.045	−0.309	0.978	2.11	99

No interference was found with hemoglobin (600 mg/dl), bilirubin (29 mg/dl), or triglycerides (650 mg/dl).

IV. MILES SERALYZER

A. Instrument Description

The Seralyzer System (Miles Inc., Elkhart, Indiana) consists of the Seralyzer blood chemistry analyzer (28 cm wide, 14 cm high, 46 cm deep; 10 kg in weight), plug-in test modules, an electronic pipette system (for the Seralyzer III model), test strips containing dry reagents, and multilevel calibrators (Ng, 1986).

A large selection of tests is available with this system—13 colorimetric methods and five immunoassays. Each test method requires a specific test module, which programs the electronic pipette and the reflectance photometer for the test to be performed. When inserted into the analyzer, the test module sets the analysis time, verifies that the proper test strip (bar code) is used, and provides the proper wavelength of light for the test. Together with the analyzer's microprocessor, each test module processes the reflectance signal from the test strip, calculates the result, and relays it to the instrument's digital display.

To perform a test, the user inserts the desired test module into the Seralyzer and hydrates the integrating sphere (''readhead'' or reflectance chamber) by pipetting 30 μl of water onto a used strip and letting it remain inside the analyzer for 2 min. Thirty microliters of a diluted sample is applied to the desired test strip, which must be placed inside the analyzer within 4 s. The test result is displayed on the analyzer's display panel after an incubation (80–90 s for an immunoassay). There is no printer in the analyzer, but a printer port and an RS232 port are present for hookup to a printer or a computer. All immunoassays of the Seralyzer system require manual dilution of serum prior to analysis. The user is provided with an electronic pipette system for this purpose. The Seralyzer test strips require no refrigeration.

Calibration of immunoassays is recommended every 14 days, whenever a new bottle of strips (25 per bottle) is first opened, and whenever the room temperature is more than 6°C (11°F) above or below the room temperature during the previous calibration for that test. Two levels of calibrators are used.

B. Instrument Performance

The main advantages of the Seralyzer system are its large menu of tests and relatively low cost, that is, $4,495 for the Seralyzer III system, $3.84 for each ARIS reagent strip, $6.95 for a digoxin test, and $495 for a Digoxin Sample Processor (see Section IV.D.1).

The system requires proper pipetting technique and manual dilution of the sample prior to analysis. Calibration is needed more frequently than the Vision or the Analyst.

C. ARIS Tests

1. Principles of the Method

Carbamazepine, phenobarbital, phenytoin, and theophylline are ARIS (apoenzyme reactivation immunoassay system) tests currently available on the Seralyzer. In this system, an antibody to the specific drug is incorporated into the reagent strip. In the absence of the drug, a drug conjugate labeled with flavine adenine dinucleotide (FAD) binds to the antibody and is unavailable for further reaction with apoglucose oxidase in the reagent. In the presence of the drug competing for the antibody binding sites, conjugate that is not bound by antibody is available for reactivation of apoglucose oxidase, the protein component of glucose oxidase (EC 1.1.3.4) remaining after FAD is removed. Active enzyme is detected by a blue color product produced through a coupled reaction with peroxidase. The intensity of the color is proportional to the concentration of the drug in the sample. The Seralyzer measures reflectance at 740 nm.

As pointed out by the manufacturer, ambient moisture can be a source of error. Moisture can initiate the holoenzyme regeneration and cause higher test results (Croci *et al.*, 1988). The reagent strip should be used promptly after removal from the bottle, which contains desiccants and should be capped tightly.

2. Performance of the ARIS Tests

a. Carbamazepine Within-run CV of 2.7–4.4% and between-run CV of 1.9–4.1% have been reported (Sheehan and Caron, 1987; Croci *et al.*, 1988). Parker (1987) found overall CV of 3.3–8.7% in the reference laboratories, and 3.2–9.9% in physician office laboratories. The test is linear between 1.5 and 18.0 μg/ml. Comparison of patient results with other methods showed:

Comparative method	Slope	Intercept	*r*	*Sy.x*	*n*
HPLC	0.993	0.14	0.990	0.54	96
Abbott TDx (Croci *et al.*, 1988)	1.010	−0.02	0.994	0.39	96
Syva EMIT (Sheehan and Caron, 1987)	0.997	−0.06	0.991	—	196

Croci *et al.* (1988) found no interference at the indicated concentrations for total bilirubin (4.5 mg/dl) and uric acid (14.5 mg/dl). Carbamazepine was slightly underestimated (by about 10%) in specimens with high concentrations of cholesterol (490 mg/dl) and triglycerides (380 mg/dl), and in a strongly hemolyzed specimen (hemoglobin, 400 mg/dl).

b. Phenobarbital Croci *et al.* (1987) reported within-run CV of 1.3–5.0% and between-run CV of 2.1–6.1% with the Seralyzer phenobarbital assay. The test is linear between 5 and 60 μg/ml. Comparison of patient results with other methods showed:

Comparative method	Slope	Intercept	*r*	Sy.*x*	*n*
HPLC (Burnett *et al.*, 1987)	1.00	1.65	0.994	1.15	53
Syva EMIT (Croci *et al.*, 1987)	0.998	0.50	0.994	1.70	50
Abbott TDx (Data from the manufacturer)	0.95	0.97	0.99	—	218

Croci *et al.* (1987) reported that bilirubin, uric acid, and triglycerides at levels up to four times those of normal plasma did not affect the test result (underestimation by <10%); a slight hemolysis (hemoglobin up to 25 mg/dl) has no significant effect (underestimation by <8%).

c. Phenytoin (Sommer et al., 1986) Within-run CV of 2.3–5.6% and between-run CV of 2.7–6.5% have been reported (Sommer *et al.*, 1986; Croci *et al.*, 1987). The test is linear between 3 and 30 μg/ml. Comparison of patient results with other methods showed:

Comparative method	Slope	Intercept	*r*	Sy.*x*	*n*
HPLC (Sommer *et al.*, 1986)	1.03	0.33	0.99	1.27	92
Syva EMIT (Croci *et al.*, 1987)	1.040	−0.27	0.992	1.54	50
Abbott TDx (Brettfeld *et al.*, 1989)	1.028	−0.79	0.985	—	30

Sommer *et al.* (1986) found no interference at the indicated concentrations for total bilirubin (10 mg/dl), uric acid (16 mg/dl), cholesterol (500 mg/dl), and triglycerides (700 mg/dl). Hemoglobin did not interfere at 100 mg/dl but decreased the apparent phenytoin value by 2 μg/ml for each 100 mg/dl increase above this value.

The effect of renal failure on test results has not been extensively studied. Oles *et al.* (1986) found that phenytoin values from several patients with end-stage renal failure differed by 25% when compared to results obtained with the Abbott TDx method. Sommer *et al.* (1986) reported that the Seralyzer phenytoin method showed a 20% crossreactivity at a very high concentration (7 μg/ml) of HPPH, a phenytoin metabolite that accumulates in renal failure.

d. Theophylline (Rupchock, 1985) Within-run CV of 3.5–5.9%, and between-run CV of 3.3–7.6% have been reported (Rupchock, 1985; Cheung and Soldin, 1986) with this assay. The test is linear between 3 and 30 μg/ml. Comparison with other methods showed:

Comparative method	Slope	Intercept	*r*	Sy.*x*	*n*
HPLC	1.08	−0.4	0.99	1.11	110
Syva EMIT (Rupchock, 1985)	1.08	0.5	0.98	1.98	45
Abbott TDx (Cheung and Soldin, 1986)	1.08	−0.3	0.98	1.64	79

Rupchock *et al.* (1985) found no interference at the indicated concentrations for total bilirubin (16 mg/dl), cholesterol (500 mg/dl), triglycerides (760 mg/dl), and hemoglobin (200 mg/dl).

This Seralyzer test is a competitive immunoassay with a monoclonal antibody. It showed good specificity except in patients receiving dimenhydrinate or suffering from renal failure. Dimenhydrinate (Dramamine) is the 8-chlorotheophylline salt of the antihistamine diphenyhydramine. A normal metabolite of theophylline, 1,3-dimethyluric acid, accumulates in uremic patients to levels that interfere with the test.

D. The Digoxin Assay

1. Principles of the Method

The Seralyzer digoxin assay is a monoclonal immunometric assay that involves an initial sample extraction step with the sample processor, followed by an analysis with a dry chemistry strip.

In this assay, the sample processor holds an assembly of two vials of reagent—a "signal antibody" (antidigoxin Fab′-beta-galactosidase monoconjugate in excess) and a capture phase (digitoxigenin attached to a cross-linked, beaded polyacrylamide gel). Each assembly of two reagent vials is for measuring one specimen, that is, "unit-dose" packaging. A hollow connector connects the tops of the two vials. Thirty microliters of serum or plasma sample containing digoxin is pipetted into the conjugate reagent, and the binding is allowed to reach equilibrium (automatic rocking for 2 min and standing for 6 min) in the sample processor. The sample processor then rotates the vial assembly to mix the liquid with the capture phase for 4 min. The conjugate that did not bind digoxin is bound by the capture phase. The connector is removed, a filter is inserted in the vial containing the mixture, and a 30-μl sample of the filtrate (containing the patient's digoxin bound to the conjugate) is transferred to a reagent strip on the Seralyzer instrument so that its beta-galactosidase activity can be determined in the degradation of dimethylacridinone galactoside to galactose and dimethylacridinone. The enzyme activity, monitored as the rate of color development in 60 s at 630 nm, is proportional to the concentration of digoxin in the sample. The entire assay can be completed with the result ready in 15 min.

2. Performance of the Method

Within-run CV of 2.3–7.5% and between-run CV of 1.5–8.8% have been reported (Sommer *et al.*, 1988; Butch *et al.*, 1989; Iosefsohn *et al.*, 1989).

Comparison of patients' results with other methods showed:

Comparative method	Slope	Intercept	*r*	Sy.x	*n*
NML RIA	0.96	0.06	0.98	0.15	100
Abbott TDx	1.03	−0.01	0.98	0.16	100
(Sommer *et al.*, 1988)					

The calibration curve is stable for 30 days with this assay. The test is linear between 0.3 and 5.0 ng/ml.

Interference studies have revealed that drug metabolites in patients receiving spironolactone may produce falsely high digoxin results (Iosefsohn *et al.*, 1989). This cross-reactivity has been demonstrated to occur with other digoxin immunoassays (Stone *et al.*, 1988). Unlike many digoxin assays, the Seralyzer method is almost completely free from interference by digoxinlike immunoreactive factors (Matheke and Valdes, 1989).

V. MILES CLINIMATE-TDA

A. Instrument Description

The Clinimate-TDA is a smaller version of the Seralyzer to be used with the therapeutic drug assays available on the Seralyzer. The Clinimate-

TDA is 18.6 cm wide, 9.4 cm high, 18.5 cm deep, and weighs 0.96 kg. It requires reagent strips and sample volume identical to those for the Seralyzer. The cost of the Clinimate-TDA is $1495.

B. Theophylline Assay

The Clinimate-TDA is a newly released instrument; only the theophylline test is presently available. Other drug assays from the Seralyzer system will soon be available on the Clinimate-TDA.

VI. TEST KITS

Test kits involving double-antibody enzyme immunoassays are available from many manufacturers for the measurements of choriogonadotropin (hCG) in serum and urine. One of the two antibodies is immobilized on a bead or a filter membrane. These manual procedures are referred to as "rapid in-office testing methods" since they can be completed usually within 10 min. The user is required to add the specimen and several reagents onto a disposable support matrix (test cylinder, test cell, test pack, etc). The color of the reaction product is read either visually (for qualitative results) or with a reader (for quantitative results).

Test kits involving an immobilized antibody are also used for the detection of:

1. Urinary luteinizing hormone (LH) to predict ovulation
2. Illicit drugs in urine
3. Immunoglobulin E (IgE) in serum or whole blood
4. Various infectious agents, such as group A streptococcal antigen, Herpes simplex virus, and *Chlamydia trachomatis* antigen

The test kits described above are available from various manufacturers, including Abbott Diagnostics, Eastman Kodak, Hybritech, Medix Biotech, Quidel, Roche Diagnostics, and Tambrands.

VII. CONCLUSION

The availability of small, nonisotopic, automated immunoassay systems enables the performance of more complicated tests in the physician's office. The limiting factors in their rapid growth include small test menu and relatively high cost. With some systems, technique dependency and low throughput also limit their acceptance.

I believe the following immunoassays are desirable for use with automated systems in the physician's office: thyroxine, thyroid-stimulating hormone (TSH), choriogonadotropin, luteinizing hormone, progesterone, ferritin, theophylline, digoxin, phenytoin, phenobarbital, carbamazepine, tricyclic antidepressants, apolipoproteins, hepatitis B surface antigen, and various infectious agents. Continued development in medical technology can certainly make these tests available in small, automated systems in the near future.

REFERENCES

Brettfeld, C., Gobrogge, R., Massoud, N., Munzenberger, P., Nigro, M., and Sarnaik, A. (1989). Evaluation of Ames Seralyzer for the therapeutic drug monitoring of phenobarbital and phenytoin. *Ther. Drug Monit.* **11,** 612–615.

Burnett, D., Goudie, J. H., and Tabossi-Reynolds, C. (1987). Seralyzer reagent-strip system evaluated for measurement of phenobarbital in serum [Technical Brief]. *Clin. Chem.* **33,** 191. *Clin. Chem.* **35,** 1109.

Butch, A., Shelton, M., Matheke, M. L., and Valdes, R., Jr. (1989). Evaluation of a dry reagent digoxin immunometric assay performed on a physician's office analyzer [Abstract].

Chan, K. M., Koenig, J., Walton, K. G., Francoeur, T. A., Lau, B. W. C., and Ladenson, J. H. (1987). The theophylline method of the Abbott "Vision" analyzer evaluated. *Clin. Chem.* **33,** 130–132.

Cheung, C. M., and Soldin, S. J. (1986). Clinical evaluation of a dry chemistry strip theophylline assay. *Ther. Drug Monit.* **8,** 205–210.

Croci, D., Nespolo, A., and Tarenghi, G. (1987). Quantitative determination of phenobarbital and phenytoin by dry-phase apoenzyme reactivation immunoassay system (ARIS). *Ther. Drug Monit.* **9,** 197–202.

Croci, D., Nespolo, A., and Tarenghi, G. (1988). A dry-reagent strip for quantifying carbamazepine evaluated. *Clin. Chem.* **34,** 388–392.

Hodgson, J. C. (1987). In-office chemistry system for discrete and profile testing. *American Clinical Laboratory* **6**(1), 12–15.

Iosefsohn, M., Soldin, S. J., and Hicks, J. M. (1989). A dry-strip immunometric assay for digoxin on the Ames Seralyzer [Abstract]. *Clin. Chem.* **35,** 1168.

Matheke, M. L. and Valdes, R., Jr. (1989). A physician's office-based digoxin assay (Seralyzer) evaluated for interference by endogenous digoxin-like immunoreactive factors. *Ann. Clin. Lab. Sci.* **19,** 168–174.

Ng, R. H. (1986). Selecting instrumentation for physician's office testing. *Clin. Lab. Med.* **6,** 305–315.

Ng, R. H., Altaffer M., and Statland, B. E. (1986). Analytical performance of the Abbott Vision system [Technical Brief]. *Clin. Chem.* **32,** 1413.

Ng, R. H., Altaffer, M., and Statland, B. E. (1988). Performance of the Du Pont Analyst physician's office profiler [Technical Brief]. *Clin. Chem.* **34,** 988–989.

Oles, K. S., Parker, D. R., and Penry, J. K. (1986). Clinical evaluation of photometric immunoassays for phenytoin and phenobarbital [Abstract]. *Clin. Chem.* **32,** 1114–1115.

Parker, D. R. (1987). Experience in three physicians' office laboratories with a carbamazepine dry reagent strip system [Abstract]. *Clin. Chem.* **33,** 1019.

Rupchock, P., Sommer, R., Greenquist, A., Tyhach, R., Walter, B., and Zipp, A. (1985). Dry-reagent strips used for determination of theophylline in serum. *Clin. Chem.* **31,** 737–740.

Schultz, S. G., Holen, J. T., Donohue, J. P., and Francoeur, T. A. (1985). Two-dimensional centrifugation for desk-top clinical chemistry. *Clin. Chem.* **31,** 1457–1463.

Sheehan, M., and Caron, G. (1987). Evaluation of a dry reagent strip for carbamazepine [Abstract]. *Clin. Chem.* **33,** 1019.

Sommer, R., Nelson, C., and Greenquist, A. (1986). Dry-reagent strips for measuring phenytoin in serum. *Clin. Chem.* **32,** 1770–1774.

Sommer, R. G., Belchak, M. L., Bloczynski, S. J., Boguslawski, S. J., Clay, D. L., Corey, P. F., Foltz, M. M., Fredrickson, R. A., Halmo, B. L., Johnson, R. D., Marfurt, K. L., Runzheimer, H.-V., and Morris, D. L. (1988). An immunometric digoxin assay for use with dry reagent strips and a reflectance photometer [Abstract]. *Clin. Chem.* **34,** 1252.

Stone, J., Bunting, P., and Soldin, S. J. (1988). Carenoate interference with Abbott TDx Digoxin II FPIA [Abstract]. *Clin. Chem.* **34,** 1252.

Vaughn, R., Lewis, L. M., Biagini, A. V., and Lee, C. K. (1989). Evaluation of a theophylline rotor for the DuPont Analyst [Abstract]. *Clin. Chem.* **35,** 1108.

Index

Printed in Dunstable, United Kingdom

91343655R00214